AF181622

Puerto Rican Women and Children

Issues in Health, Growth, and Development

TOPICS IN SOCIAL PSYCHIATRY

Series Editor: Ellen L. Bassuk, M.D.
The Better Homes Foundation
Newton Centre, Massachussetts
and Harvard Medical School
Boston, Massachussetts

ANATOMY OF PSYCHIATRIC ADMINISTRATION
The Organization in Health and Disease
Milton Greenblatt, M.D., in collaboration with Paul Rodenhauser, M.D.

HOMELESSNESS
A National Perspective
Edited by Marjorie J. Robertson, Ph.D., and Milton Greenblatt, M.D.

PUERTO RICAN WOMEN AND CHILDREN
Issues in Health, Growth, and Development
Edited by Gontran Lamberty, Dr. P.H., and Cynthia Garcia Coll, Ph.D.

RESPONDING TO THE HOMELESS
Policy and Practice
Russell K. Schutt, Ph.D., and Gerald R. Garrett, Ph.D.

A Continuation Order Plan is available for this series. A continuation order will bring delivery of each new volume immediately upon publication. Volumes are billed only upon actual shipment. For further information please contact the publisher.

Puerto Rican Women and Children

Issues in Health, Growth, and Development

Edited by

Gontran Lamberty, Dr. P.H.

Maternal and Child Health Bureau, DHHS
Rockville, Maryland

and

Cynthia Garcia Coll, Ph.D.

Brown University School of Medicine
Providence, Rhode Island, and
Wellesley College
Wellesley, Massachusetts

SPRINGER SCIENCE+BUSINESS MEDIA, LLC

Library of Congress Cataloging in Publication Data

Puerto Rican women and children: issues in health, growth, and development / edited by Gontran Lamberty and Cynthia García Coll.
p. cm.—(Topics in social psychiatry)
Includes bibliographical references and index.
ISBN 978-1-4613-6053-7 ISBN 978-1-4615-2472-4 (eBook)
DOI 10.1007/978-1-4615-2472-4
1. Puerto Rican women—Health and hygiene—Congresses. 2. Puerto Rican children—Health and hygiene—United States—Congresses. I. Lamberty, Gontran. II. García Coll, Cynthia T. III. Series.
[DNLM: 1. Child Welfare. 2. Maternal Welfare. 3. Health Status. 4. Maternal Health Services—Puerto Rico. 5. Maternal Health Services—United States. 6. Child Health Services—Puerto Rico. 7. Child Health Services—United States. WA 310 P977 1994]
RA448.5.P83P84 1994
362.1'089687295073—dc20
DNLM/DLC 93-49633
for Library of Congress CIP

ISBN 978-1-4613-6053-7

©1994 Springer Science+Business Media New York
Softcover reprint of the hardcover 1st edition 1994
Originally published by Plenum Press in 1994

All rights reserved

No part of this book may be reproduced, stored in a retrieval system, or transmitted in any form or by any means, electronic, mechanical, photocopying, microfilming, recording, or otherwise, without written permission from the Publisher

Contributors

LUZ E. ALVARADO, New York State Psychiatric Institute, New York, New York 10032

KATHERINE BAISDEN, Center for Chicano Research, Stanford University, Stanford, California 94305

JEANNE BROOKS-GUNN, Department of Developmental Psychology, Teachers College, Columbia University, New York, New York 10032

SUSAN A. BRUNELLI, College of Physicians and Surgeons, Columbia University and New York State Psychiatric Institute, New York, New York 10032

KEN G. CASTRO, Division of HIV/AIDS, National Center for Infectious Diseases, Centers for Disease Control and Prevention, Atlanta, Georgia 30333

CYNTHIA GARCIA COLL, Department of Pediatrics, Brown University School of Medicine, Women and Infants' Hospital of Rhode Island, Providence, Rhode Island 02905, and The Stone Center, Wellesley College, Wellesley, Massachusetts 02181-8268

CLEMENTE DIAZ, Department of Obstetrics and Gynecology, University of Puerto Rico School of Medicine, San Juan, Puerto Rico 00936-5067

Jack Elinson, Division of Sociomedical Sciences, Columbia University School of Public Health, New York, New York 10032, and Medical and Health Research Association of New York City, Inc., New York, New York 10013

Marta Gwinn, Division of HIV/AIDS, National Center for Infectious Diseases, Centers for Disease Control and Prevention, Atlanta, Georgia 30333

Kenji Hakuta, School of Education, Stanford University, Stanford, California 94305

Barbara Kilbourne, Division of HIV/AIDS, National Center for Infectious Diseases, Centers for Disease Control and Prevention, Atlanta, Georgia 30333

Gontran Lamberty, Maternal and Child Health Bureau, HRSA, Public Health Service, U.S. Department of Health and Human Services, Rockville, Maryland 20857

Sally Ann Lederman, Center for Population and Family Health, School of Public Health, Columbia University, New York, New York 10032

Penny Liberatos, Medical and Health Research Association of New York City, Inc., New York, New York 10013

Cecelia M. McCarton, Department of Pediatrics, Rose F. Kennedy Center for Research in Mental Retardation and Human Development, Albert Einstein College of Medicine, Bronx, New York, 10461

Millie Martin, Department of Obstetrics and Gynecology, University of Puerto Rico School of Medicine, San Juan, Puerto Rico 00936-5067

Reynaldo Martorell, Center for International Health, Emory University School of Public Health, Atlanta, Georgia 30329

Fernando S. Mendoza, Department of Pediatrics, Lucile Salter Packard Children's Hospital at Stanford University, Stanford, California 94305

Margaret J. Oxtoby, Division of HIV/AIDS, National Center for Infectious Diseases, Centers for Disease Control and Prevention, Atlanta, Georgia 30333

Ivan G. Pawson, Koret Center for Human Nutrition, San Francisco General Hospital, San Francisco, California 94110

Virginia A. Rauh, Center for Population and Family Health, Columbia University School of Public Health, New York, New York 10032

Clara E. Rodriguez, Russell Sage Foundation, New York, New York 10021, and Division of Social Sciences, Fordham University, The College at Lincoln Center, New York, New York 10023

Josefina Romaguera, Department of Obstetrics and Gynecology, University of Puerto Rico School of Medicine, San Juan, Puerto Rico 00936-5067

Pedro J. Santiago-Borrero, Department of Pediatrics, University of Puerto Rico School of Medicine, San Juan, Puerto Rico 00936-5067

Diana Sierra, Center for Population and Family Health, School of Public Health, Columbia University, New York, New York 10032

Glenn S. Takata, Division of General Pediatrics, Children's Hospital of Los Angeles, Los Angeles, California 90027

James Tonascia, Department of Biostatistics, Johns Hopkins School of Hygiene and Public Health, Baltimore, Maryland 21205

Marta Valcarcel, Department of Pediatrics, University of Puerto Rico School of Medicine, San Juan, Puerto Rico 00936-5067

Stephanie J. Ventura, Division of Vital Statistics, National Center for Health Statistics, Centers for Disease Control and Prevention, U.S. Public Health Service, Hyattsville, Maryland 20782

Gail Wasserman, College of Physicians and Surgeons, Columbia University, and New York State Psychiatric Institute, New York, New York 10032

Iris Zavala-Martinez, Mental Health Division, San Juan Health Department, San Juan, Puerto Rico 00907

Carmen Zorrilla, Department of Obstetrics and Gynecology, University of Puerto Rico School of Medicine, San Juan, Puerto Rico 00936-5067

Preface

Julio Morales describes the Puerto Rican nation as being comprised of those individuals who identify themselves as Puerto Ricans. This includes almost 6.2 million people who live primarily, but not exclusively, on the island of Puerto Rico, and in the northeastern United States.

One gets to be a Puerto Rican by various means. You are Puerto Rican if you are born in Puerto Rico, although at the same time you are an American because you were born there. You are Puerto Rican if your parents are Puerto Rican, even if you have never visited the island, have never eaten *arroz y habichuelas,* and have never spoken a word in Spanish. You can be a second and third generation Puerto Rican of mixed marriage, be highly acculturated to American culture, but when asked, you say proudly, "I am a Puerto Rican." You can meet some of us whose world is bicultural, a world where English and Spanish are easily interchanged, where traditional Thanksgiving turkey is followed by *lechon asado* at Christmas as the main treat, where *salsa* or *bolero* are enjoyed with the same passion as rock'n roll or the big band sound. It is a world where various cultures have merged and the historical forces of slavery and Spanish and American colonialism have left their indelible marks on the psyche.

For those of us whose primary residence is in one of the contiguous

48 states, what unites us can be many things. It can be the language, the childhood stories and recollections of the way it used to be for us, our parents or grandparents, the anger that we felt upon experiencing racism for the first time on the mainland, or the nostalgia that is generated when we speculate about going back to the island. Whatever it means to be a Puerto Rican still perdures after 500 years of struggle to forge a national identity devoid of colonial vestiges.

This book attempts to put forward our current knowledge and the issues surrounding the health, growth, and development of an important component of the U.S. population—Puerto Rican mothers and children, whose primary (or at least current) residency is on the mainland. Our main purpose is to attract attention to the special needs of this population group. Most of the indicators (socioeconomic, demographic, health, development) of the well-being and future of these Americans are quite negative and, if we do not deal with these issues, a young and potentially productive part of our nation will be lost.

As two Puerto Ricans living on the mainland, we feel a responsibility to bring the issues to the forefront of the political and academic debates. Most of the contributors to the book are established researchers or scholars, some who have dedicated their lives to the welfare of these women and children; others who are interested in research questions that are relevant to Puerto Ricans. Regardless, they all have something to say, something to contribute. The mix of theoretical orientations, methodologies, and disciplines used in their contributions to this volume represents a unique but necessary spectrum in which to discuss the complex issues that today face Puerto Ricans on the mainland and in Puerto Rico.

This book would not have been possible without the support of many individuals and organizations. The work was partially funded by grant MCJ-440569 from the Maternal and Child Health Bureau (Title V, Social Security Act), Health Resources and Services Administration, Department of Health and Human Services. However, the bureau was much more instrumental than just supporting the conference on which this book is based. Vince Hutchins, the bureau's director at the time of the conference, Woodie Kessel, and Jim Papai contributed to the success of the project through constructive criticism, and through their commitment as federal officials to improving the conditions and the life chances of all mothers and children. Jim Papai also contributed to the book through his editing of some of the chapters and through his enviable ability to translate complex ideas into simple declarative statements.

Linda Steinberg, with her hard work and efficiency, kept the revisions of the manuscript going between Rockville, Maryland, and Providence, Rhode Island.

The Department of Pediatrics at Brown University School of Medicine, under the direction of William Oh, cosponsored the conference and contributed resources to the production of the final manuscript. We are especially grateful to Brenda Carr, whose dedication to this project made it all possible. Her steadfast commitment to the task, attention to detail, her persistence with all the contributors, and her continuous smile throughout the long process were especially important. The commitment of Ellen Bassuk, series editor of *Topics in Social Psychiatry*, to social issues made this volume a reality. We are also grateful to Mariclaire Cloutier for her support and patience.

The first editor dedicates this volume to his wife Esther, sons Gontran and Phillip, and to the *Anasquenos* of New London, Connecticut, of whom he was one.

The second editor dedicates this volume to her children, Nataniel, Andres, and Gabriela, who, as second generation Puerto Ricans on the mainland, need to be reminded not only of all the wonderful privileges they have had, but more importantly, where they in part come from.

GONTRAN LAMBERTY
CYNTHIA GARCIA COLL

Contents

Overview

GONTRAN LAMBERTY
AND CYNTHIA GARCIA COLL

INTRODUCTION

In 1990 there were 6.2 million Americans of Puerto Rican ancestry, 44% of whom lived on the U.S. mainland and the remainder in Puerto Rico. Puerto Ricans constituted 21.8% of all Americans claiming a Hispanic origin in 1990; 12.2% if only Puerto Ricans residing on the mainland are considered. About 40% of the 6.2 million Puerto Ricans are less than 20 years of age, an age group which carries rich possibilities for achievement and high odds for failure. Whether the life course of most of these 2.5 million young Americans follows the route of achievement or failure will depend on how much we as a nation are willing to invest in their future.

As Americans, Puerto Ricans have played a unique role in our nation's history. Their island became a possession of the United States in 1898 as part of the spoils of the Spanish-American War. From that

GONTRAN LAMBERTY • Maternal and Child Health Bureau, HRSA, Public Health Service, U.S. Department of Health and Human Services, Rockville, Maryland 20857. CYNTHIA GARCIA COLL • Department of Pediatrics, Brown University School of Medicine, Women and Infants Hospital of Rhode Island, Providence, Rhode Island 02905, and The Stone Center, Wellesley College, Wellesley, Massachusetts 02181-8268.

Puerto Rican Women and Children: Issues in Health, Growth, and Development, edited by Gontran Lamberty and Cynthia Garcia Coll. Plenum Press, New York, 1994.

time on Puerto Ricans, first as colonial subjects, and then as citizens of the United States, have lingered at the periphery of our bountiful national life. This has been the case despite their impressive political loyalty to the United States during the tumultuous years of the Cold War; their collective low participation rates in the urban violence and civil disobedience characterizing the United States in the 1960s and the 1970s; their individual achievements in the sciences, literature, music, theater, and the arts; and an unsurpassed record of taking part in all of the wars and armed conflicts this nation has participated in during the first 93 years of the 20th century. Slightly over a decade after their island became a possession of the United States, Puerto Ricans, as American doughboys, fought in the European trenches of World War I. They did the same in World War II in much greater numbers and with much higher casualties. The first contingent of American troops to reach the Yalu River during the Korean conflict were members of the all-Puerto Rican 65th Infantry Regiment. Puerto Rico had one of the largest per capita participation and casualty rates of any state or territory during the Vietnam War. Some of the first Americans who died in the recent Gulf War and in the Somalian humanitarian rescue mission were Puerto Ricans.

The sacrifices of Puerto Ricans, as Americans, on the battlefields of Europe, Asia, and the Middle East, stand in sharp contrast to the collective rewards they have reaped during their 95 years of being either U.S. colonial subjects or citizens. On the mainland, Puerto Ricans, as a group, have ranked next to last in practically every indicator of socioeconomic status, health, and social well-being. Contrary to the established track records of former European immigrant groups, Puerto Ricans, as a group, have been unable to break away from the poorest, most physically dilapidated, and most crime-ridden areas of our largest urban centers. Despite their heavy concentrations in these less than hospitable places, until recently they have been unable to muster enough political power in their communities and congressional representation in Washington for this to have a significant impact on their daily life. The problems of a lack of political power and congressional representation are greater for Puerto Ricans residing in Puerto Rico, who by law cannot vote in presidential or national congressional elections.

The failure of Puerto Ricans on the mainland to move forward as a group has been attributed by some scientists and scholars to be the result of a number of causes. Some of these include: (1) original migration cohorts being considerably skewed toward those with low educational attainment, with little or no capital to invest on the mainland, and being substantially composed of persons of color; (2) areas where Puerto Ricans have settled have typically been in the process of undergoing drastic dislocations in their industrial economies along with massive unemployment; (3) settlement communities ruled by intractable patterns of job discrimination and residential segregation based on an imputed racial identity; and (4) ongoing population processes within the migrant communities which have selectively pushed out the most promising or the already successful, and replaced them with new, less skilled arrivals from Puerto Rico.

Competing for primacy with the causes listed above has been the old concept of the "culture of poverty," a sort of latent variable that other scientists and scholars feel explains the relatively low rank exhibited by mainland Puerto Ricans in most areas of national life. While these scholars and scientists correctly allude to poverty as a likely causal variable in their considerations, they disregard the fact that a lot of the poverty in this country is ascribed, and that most of that ascribed poverty derives from the way our society is socially stratified and the ways it has chosen to distribute its rewards. Such a system of social stratification, defines a large number of our nation's children from birth as inferior, on the basis of outdated stereotypes about gender, social class, ethnicity, and race. The same system then proceeds to assure that they get to be inferior by denying them the resources and experiences necessary to develop into competent and socially contributing adults.

GOALS AND OBJECTIVES OF THE CONFERENCE

This collection of papers was presented at a Conference held on November 29–30, 1990 at Brown University, Providence, Rhode Island. The Conference's main goal was to focus national attention on the health and development of an often overlooked part of the U.S. population—Puerto Rican mothers and children residing on the mainland—and to discuss, without regard to political proprieties, the likely social origins of their suboptimal experiences in the realms of health and development.

Conceptually, the organizers of the Conference viewed social differentials in health and development in sociological terms. At its most general level, this view posits that most societies are socially differentiated partly on the basis of the division of labor and partly on the basis of other attributes, the nature and significance of which appear to be historically variable and unique. Social differentiation in turn is associated with differential conditions which either restrict or enhance opportunities for individuals to achieve their full potential, including that of health and development.

In terms of specifics, the Conference sought to do the following: (1) collect empirical information on the reproductive health of Puerto Rican women residing on the mainland and on the health, growth, and development of their children; (2) assess how the situation compared for these women and children relative to the United States as a whole and other Hispanic subgroups; (3) identify and catalog for future research, cause-and-effect conjectures based on the information that was evaluated; and (4) identify information gaps and develop recommendations for service, research, and policy.

From the outset, Conference planners saw a need for obtaining information on residents of Puerto Rico comparable to that gathered for Puerto Ricans on the mainland. The scarcity of published works and ongoing research about Puerto Ricans residing on the island precluded that line of development, and to the Conference planners' dismay, what was available for Puerto Ricans residing on the mainland was little better. The planners settled for what material of reasonable quality was available for both locations, which favored the mainland. But a good beginning was made, and it is hoped, as a result of the publication of the Conference proceedings in this volume, considerably more research will follow in the years to come.

There are grounds for optimism. Recently, several federal agencies issued special requests for research applications on the growth and development of minority children. In addition, the newly revised Public Health Service research application form (PHS-398) requires that women and minorities be included in all proposed research unless a compelling rationale is offered for not doing so. Not only will this new requirement foster a comparative as well as a race/ethnic-specific framework in federally supported biomedical, health services, and child development research, but it will also be conducive to making research on racial and ethnic minorities attractive once again to both mainstream and minority researchers.

BACKGROUND TO THE PAPERS

The opening chapter by Rodriguez accomplishes three things: (1) it describes the historical context of Puerto Rican migration to the mainland and the patterns of settlement that evolved; (2) it discusses some of the possible reasons why this migration occurred and continues to this day; and (3) it examines the current demographic and socioeconomic status of Puerto Ricans on the mainland. To Rodriguez, Puerto Ricans have migrated and continue to migrate to the mainland for the same reasons that continue to lead many other Americans to migrate from one state to another: They are in search of a better job, more pay, a brighter future for their children, and the attraction of adventure. She calls for the separate collection, interpretation, and publication of information about Puerto Rican mainland and island residents, as well as for the two communities combined. This makes sense in at least two ways: It would, as Rodriguez has stated, allow us to make comparisons, and these comparisons would "help us to better understand the distinctions and commonalities of both island and mainland communities." Combining the two components would eliminate the long-standing practice of artificially treating Puerto Ricans residing in Puerto Rico as if they were not an integral part of the U.S. population. This practice has been conducive to an "out of sight, out of mind" treatment of Puerto Rico's problems by Congress and federal officials.

Zavala-Martinez's chapter on the dialectics of being a Puerto Rican American takes up where Rodriguez's paper leaves off by discussing some of the psychological consequences of migration. She views the historical course of Puerto Rican migration to the United States as a dynamic process of collective as well as individual adaptation to conflicting cultural and contextual demands. She labels this process *entremundos* or "between worlds," and, as a consequence, posits conflicts of identity and difficulties in adapting to the demands of the two cultures. This conflict of identity and uncertainty as to what is culturally binding is hardly ever resolved, suggests Zavala-Martinez. Because of circular migration and the unresolved political status of the island, marginality is also likely to be a state of mind for both the mainland and the island-born residing in Puerto Rico. Consequences for adult mental and physical health, as well as for the socioemotional development of adolescent children, are implied in Zavala-Martinez's attempts to explicate the concept of *entremundos*.

Chapter 3 by Santiago-Borrero and Valcarcel describes the health care system serving the Commonwealth of Puerto Rico and analyzes selected demographic, morbidity, and mortality data for residents of the island. The morbidity and mortality data examined for the Commonwealth population suggest health levels comparable to most developed countries of the world, but below practically all of the mainland states.

The disparities between the Commonwealth and the mainland are greatest in the areas of obstetrical outcomes and infant survival. The authors are of the view that sizable reductions in current levels of maternal and child morbidity and mortality will not be forthcoming for the island unless health care resources in the public sector are considerably expanded and sizable improvements take place in employment, housing, and overall levels of living.

Chapter 4 on acquired immune deficiency syndrome (AIDS) by Zorrilla et al. describes the situation in Puerto Rico as it applies to mothers and children. In 1991, among U.S. states and territories, Puerto Rico had the second highest number of per capita AIDS cases among women (rate per 100,000). The rate of increase for this devastating disease in Puerto Rico is currently highest for women and children. The sheer volume of cases and the inherent complexities of medically and psychologically treating the affected mothers and children is monumental, and is straining an already maximally burdened public health care system.

Reproductive Health

Chapters 5, 6, and 7 are concerned with the reproductive health of mainland Puerto Rican women. Two have a national perspective; one focuses on a large city—New York. Both chapters use a race/ethnic comparative framework which permits the evaluation of the Puerto Rican experience relative to that of other Hispanic subgroups, non-Hispanic whites, and African-Americans.

Without equivocation, Chapters 5 and 6 by Ventura, and Lederman and Sierra respectively support the conclusion that the reproductive health of Puerto Rican women residing on the mainland is characterized by an extremely high risk of undesirable perinatal and postneonatal outcomes. This high degree of risk is reflected in demographic and socioeconomic characteristics, in the high incidence of teenage pregnancy, in prior reproductive and obstetrical histories, and in pregnancy-related behaviors such as unprotected sex, late or no prenatal care, and substance abuse. With few exceptions, all of these risk-enhancing characteristics and patterns of undesirable pregnancy-related behaviors occur at a higher incidence among Puerto Ricans than among other Hispanic subgroups; the levels are lower than among African-American women, however. Of interest is the much better experience recorded for Puerto Rican women residing on the mainland who were born in Puerto

Rico. These differences favoring women born outside the mainland appear in other Hispanic subgroups as well.

The inherently high risk for Puerto Rican women in reproductive health translates into high levels of undesirable outcomes. For example, the proportion of infants weighing less than 2500 grams at birth among Puerto Rican women residing on the mainland is currently about one-third higher than among other Hispanic and non-Hispanic Caucasian women, but lower than the rate among African-American women. Not surprisingly, race/ethnic differentials of similar magnitude and direction are evident with respect to neonatal and postneonatal mortality also.

Chapter 7 by Kilbourne et al. on human immunodeficiency virus (HIV) infection and AIDS among Hispanic women residing on the mainland (Puerto Ricans included) describes a situation similar to that reported by Zorrilla et al. for Puerto Rico. These two chapters more than any others in this volume underscore the interconnection between the mainland and the island and in most cases support the treatment of the two populations as one. It also suggests that bidirectional streams of influence are operating between the two communities, most likely through revolving door migration.

Growth and Development

According to Martorell et al., in Chapter 8, Puerto Rican children residing on the mainland are similar in height to the general U.S. population before adolescence, begin to fall behind during the early teenage years, and, by 18 years of age, their median height falls at the 25th percentile of the U.S. reference growth curves. This pattern of growth is similar for males and females except that for females growth deceleration appears earlier. A similar pattern of growth has been described for Mexican-American and Cuban-American children based on comparable data from the Hispanic Health and Nutrition Examination Survey (HHANES).

The data on sexual maturation indicate some minor differences when mainland Puerto Rican children are compared to Mexican-American and Dutch children. It appears that Puerto Rican children mature slightly earlier than Mexican-American children and slightly later than the Dutch children used in the analyses as the second reference group. Normative data on sexual maturation are not available for the United States as a whole. The significance of the differences just described for health or for other domains is not apparent. No evidence appears in the HHANES data indicative of extremes in acceleration or retardation in sexual development for mainland Puerto Rican children. In Puerto Rico, precocious menarche has been a much debated issue in years past.

Examination of the body mass index (BMI) medians, triceps, and subscapular skinfolds thickness for Puerto Rican children and adults residing on the mainland indicates a greater incidence of overweight and obesity at almost all ages. There is also a tendency, particularly in adult males, for fat to be deposited in the trunk. Similar patterns have been reported for Mexican-American and Cuban-American children.

Chapter 9 by Wasserman et al. on the cultural context of adolescent childrearing is one of three chapters in this volume based on findings from hypothesis-testing research. The paper is noteworthy in other respects. The subjects are adolescent mothers who are of Puerto Rican, Dominican, or African-American descent, and of low economic and educational attainment. Adolescent mothers constitute about one-fourth of all women given birth among Puerto Ricans residing on the mainland and, because of age and life circumstances, are able to provide a less than optimal child-rearing environment. Most importantly, the study sought to unravel the effects of age and ethnicity on parenting attitudes and practices and the effects of these attitudes and practices on developmental outcomes, taking into consideration, indirectly, the possible effects of acculturation.

McCarton et al. (Chapter 10) report on the effects of a health and home-based and center-based early intervention service directed at low-birth-weight infants of various race/ethnic and socioeconomic backgrounds. Findings indicate an increase in the cognitive functioning of Hispanic and African-American study subjects. The effects on cognitive functioning were most pronounced in those areas where, traditionally, low-birth-weight infants have lagged. These effects patterns are present among Puerto Rican children participating in the New York City study site. Whether the cognitive results continue into school is currently being evaluated by another study following study subjects until the early school years. McCarton et al.'s findings also indicate that Puerto Rican infants as a group have higher rates of serious morbidity, accounted for mainly by higher respiratory tract infections and by asthma attacks requiring hospitalization and lengthy periods of convalescence at home. The latter findings validate similar findings reported by other investigators, including those reported by Mendoza and Takata (Chapter 12) in this volume.

As in the case of Chapter 13 by Elinson and Liberatos, the McCarton et al investigation failed to stratify initially on race and ethnicity and consequently missed the opportunity to conduct more robust race- and ethnic-specific analyses.

Hakuta's Chapter 13 on language shift among mainland Puerto Rican and Mexican-American children teases out nuances of the process and relates somewhat to acculturation as a variable to be considered in understanding disease patterns and health services use by ethnic minorities.

Health and the Use of Health Services

Information on the health of Puerto Rican children residing on the mainland included in this volume comes from two main sources—the National Health Interview Survey (NHIS) and the HHANES. The NHIS relies strictly on questionnaires to gather the information and does not include an actual medical examination, which is the case with the HHANES.

Based on NHIS data, Mendoza and Takata report that parents of Puerto Rican children residing on the mainland reported 50 to 100% greater prevalence of acute conditions, limitations due to chronic medical conditions, and restrictive activity than non-Hispanic Caucasian, Mexican-American, Cuban-American, and African-American children. The NHIS data also show that Puerto Rican children residing on the mainland have the highest health care utilization rates of any of the groups studied and that this utilization is overwhelmingly public clinic based. The picture that evolves from the HHANES data is slightly more favorable. In general, mainland Puerto Rican children exhibit higher prevalence rates of chronic conditions than Mexican-American and Cuban-American children. Among chronic conditions, asthma and anemia were the most significant problems. High prevalence rates were also reported for neurodevelopmental conditions. The incidence rates for speech, psychological, and behavioral problems, as reported by mothers for Puerto Rican children, were considerably higher than for Mexican-American and Cuban-American children. Puerto Rican mothers reported a higher rate of treatment for medical and for neurodevelopmental conditions.

Elinson and Liberatos's study contains features worthy of emulation. The researchers took advantage of a naturally occurring experiment to evaluate the effectiveness of a comprehensive health care delivery model. Although not specifically designed to address racial/ethnic differences, the study was able to look at differences multivariately and to roughly assess the impact of the delivery model on health status and use of services. More could have been done if the race and ethnicity variables had been initially incorporated into the structure of the study design.

SUMMARY

The overall picture that emerges from the chapter reviewed above is not a particularly enviable one. The worst maternal and child health experience of any of the mainland Hispanic subgroups examined in this volume is that documented for Puerto Ricans, the second worst in the United States, when the experience is assessed under a much broader race/ethnic framework. This was expected, although not to the degree documented by the papers contained in this volume. What was not expected was the almost total absence of research efforts and systematic data collection on Puerto Ricans that goes beyond documenting that socioeconomic and health problems exist. If something of an enduring nature will be contributed by this volume it may well be the documentation, by omission, that key information needed to develop and mount intervention programs for mainland or Island Puerto Ricans is not available.

No official support or endorsement of the views in this book by DHHS or the Public Health Service is intended or should be inferred.

1

A Summary of Puerto Rican Migration to the United States

CLARA E. RODRIGUEZ

THE HISTORICAL CONTEXT

The most important element in understanding Puerto Rican migration is perhaps the least visible one: the historical context. In the nineteenth century, Puerto Rico had been receiving people, rather than exporting them. Yet by the middle of the twentieth century, Puerto Rico began to experience a concentrated exodus of people (see Figure 1). Although this migration has fluctuated, the flow has continued. In net terms, it has been so significant that it has been referred to as the "Puerto Rican diaspora."[1] The net result of this unprecedented migration is that by 1980 over 40% of Puerto Ricans lived outside Puerto Rico, primarily on

CLARA E. RODRIGUEZ • Russell Sage Foundation, New York, New York 10021, and Division of Social Sciences, Fordham University, The College at Lincoln Center, New York, New York 10023. Sections of this chapter have been excerpted from the author's book *Puerto Ricans: Born in the U.S.A.* London: Unwin Hyman, Inc., 1989; by permission of Westview Press, Boulder, Colorado, 1991.

Puerto Rican Women and Children: Issues in Health, Growth, and Development, edited by Gontran Lamberty and Cynthia Garcia Coll. Plenum Press, New York, 1994.

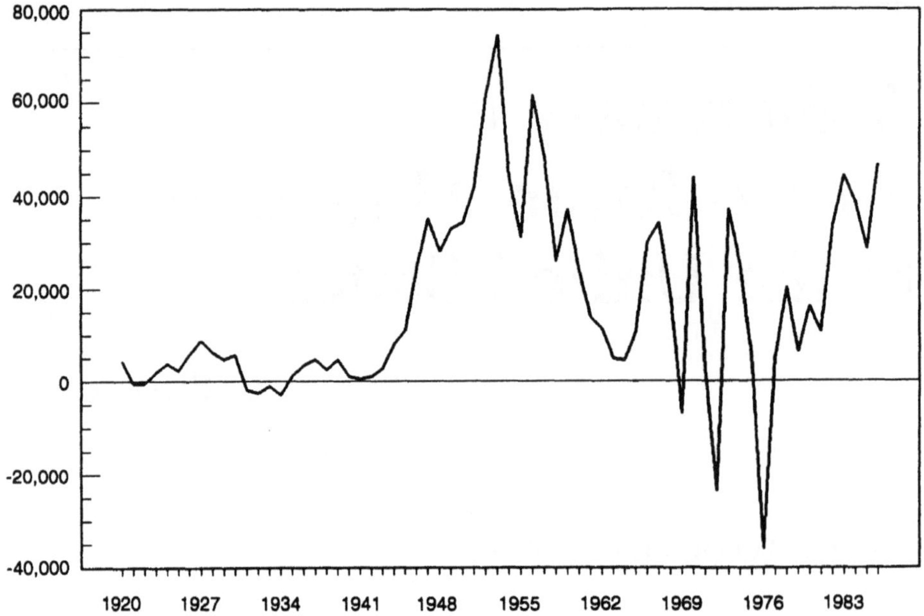

Figure 1. Net migration of Puerto Ricans, 1920–1986.

the U.S. mainland.[2] Aldorondo (1990) projects that by the year 2000, 38.8% of Puerto Rico's population will have migrated to the mainland.[3]

Causes of Twentieth-Century Out-Migration

Why have so many Puerto Ricans left the island during the twentieth century? Early theorists like Chenault and Handlin argued that overpopulation in Puerto Rico was the major factor inducing migration.[4,5] Others have argued that this overpopulation had come about as a result of health and medical improvements made under U.S. mainland policies. Senior and Watkins,[6] Mills et al.,[7] and Perloff[8] have posited that job opportunities elsewhere were the major factor motivating migration.[6–8]

More recently, researchers have tended to see migration in more macro terms, i.e., as the response of surplus labor to the economic transformations occurring in Puerto Rico. Influenced by the larger context of economic and political dependence on the mainland, these transformations are seen to have yielded increasingly larger numbers of displaced and surplus workers who were forced to migrate elsewhere for jobs.[2,9–13]

Microlevel analyses have focused on economic push and pull factors.[9,14–19] For example, when the mainland national income goes up and unemployment goes down, Puerto Rican migration increases. Relative wages and unemployment rates in Puerto Rico and the mainland have also been found to affect migration to the mainland and back to Puerto Rico.[15,20] In essence, Puerto Ricans migrate when job opportunities look better on the mainland and/or when they look worse in Puerto Rico. It has also been found that Puerto Ricans do not migrate to secure greater welfare benefits.[20]

Other scholars have emphasized the role of mainland companies in recruiting Puerto Rican labor to work on the mainland.[2,12,21–23] A 1944 issue of *Business Week* confirms this recruitment.[24] In an article entitled "Labor Recruited" it noted that three large mainland firms were recruiting skilled Puerto Rican workers for jobs on the mainland in cooperation with the War Manpower Commission. It also noted that the Commission expected that more workers would be recruited by other firms.

According to Morales, Puerto Rican labor was attractive to employers on the mainland because Puerto Ricans were citizens and because of their agricultural background.[12] He notes that Puerto Ricans were "greatly valued" by their employers and they were seen to be "excellent workers." The low wage rates paid to these workers also produced "substantial profits" for these employers and enhanced the attractiveness of Puerto Rican laborers.

Other scholars have cited the role of the government of Puerto Rico in encouraging migration.[6,13,21,23] Although the official position of the government during Operation Bootstrap was that it did not encourage or discourage migration, some authors dispute this. Padilla[13] maintains that the Puerto Rican government requested that the Federal Aviation Administration (FAA) set low rates for air transportation between Puerto Rico and the mainland, while Lapp argues that the government's Migration Division Office in New York facilitated migration.[23]

Undoubtedly, migration has resulted from a combination of these factors. There are additional factors that have received less attention. Sanchez-Korrol points out that the mainland's 1921 legislation restricting immigration and the conferring of citizenship status on Puerto Ricans in 1917, induced Puerto Ricans to migrate.[19] After the Second World War, there may also have been era-specific factors that contributed to the migration, such as greater participation in the armed forces; pent-up travel demand; surplus aircraft and pilots making for cheaper and more accessible air travel; and greater opportunities on the mainland. What is perhaps the most important factor in propelling the Puerto Rican migration, however, is what is perhaps least visible to the migrants. This is the political and economic relationships between Puerto Rico and the mainland.

The Political and Economic Relationship

The political relationship between Puerto Rico and the mainland resulted not just in political dependence, but also in economic dependence. Changes in the Puerto Rican economy after the mainland invasion were dramatic. The economy went from a diversified subsistence economy around the turn of the century with four basic crops produced for export (tobacco, cattle, coffee, and sugar) to a sugar-crop economy with 60% of the sugar industry controlled by absentee owners from the mainland.[25,26] The decline of the sugar cane-based industry (combined with no reinvestment and continued population growth) in the twenties resulted in high unemployment, poverty, and desperate conditions in Puerto Rico. These factors propelled the first waves of Puerto Ricans to the mainland in search of a better life. The thirties saw more migration as workers sought to deal with the then stagnant economic situation on the island.

In the forties, the Second World War boosted the flagging economy somewhat. The Puerto Rican government initiated a series of reforms and entered into what has been variously called its "state capitalist development phase," or its "socialist" venture.* A series of government-owned enterprises were established and run by the Puerto Rican Development Corporation. These included glass, pulp and paper, shoe leather, and clay products corporations as well as a hotel and a textile mill that were financed but not run by the government. Influenced by the New Deal philosophy, this program stressed both "social justice and economic growth" goals. In these regards, the program was "ahead of its time."[27] Had this program succeeded, greater economic independence would have been achieved. These efforts were frustrated, how-

*For analyses of the New Deal period in Puerto Rico see Stahl,[29] Gonzalez, A.,[26] Reynolds,[9] Hanson,[30] Goodsell,[3] Lewis, G.,[32] Carr,[28] Dietz,[27] and Wells.[33]

ever, by a combination of technical problems, ideological opposition from conservatives in the U.S. Congress, the local press, business interests both in Puerto Rico and on the mainland, and government bureaucrats.[27,28]

Between 1947 and 1951 there was a changeover from government development of industry to promotion of private investment. The new approach, which was firmly established by 1951, was called "Operation Bootstrap." A forerunner of the economic development strategies subsequently developed throughout the world, the idea was to industrialize Puerto Rico by luring foreign companies, mainly from the U.S. mainland, to Puerto Rico with the promise of low wage and tax incentives. The tourism industry was also developed at this time. Puerto Rico began its thrust toward industrialization and its clear incorporation into an emerging global economy.

Much in Puerto Rico improved during this period, e.g., education, housing, drinking water, electrification and sewage systems, road and transportation facilities. To the residents of Puerto Rico there was a clear and present sense of development and progress and, for some, the perception of a more equitable distribution of income.

The industries that were attracted to the island turned out to be increasingly capital intensive, however, to have little commitment to the development of the island, and to be integrated into sourcing and distribution networks on the mainland or other countries, not in Puerto Rico. As a result, these industries had little indirect employment effects and did not provide sufficient jobs. With increased population growth and displacement from traditional labor pursuits, the result was a growing surplus population that could not be accommodated in Puerto Rico's new industrial order. Much of the surplus labor migrated to the mainland.[2,11,12]

Thus, Operation Bootstrap in Puerto Rico foreshadowed what was to happen in numerous former colonies and developing countries, namely the development of off-shore operations by foreign capital or multinational corporations which siphon off profits so that there is little or no economic benefit to the island. Today, the distinctions between colonies and client states have become less clear-cut. In today's world economy we may no longer need a colonial framework to find conjunctions of political and economic dependence that induce migration. Economic and political dependence are no longer so clearly distinguishable when it comes to the flow of labor, capital, or goods.

The political and economic ties between Puerto Rico and the mainland also helped to fan the migration in a number of other ways. For example, without the ties, tax breaks would not have been granted to mainland firms doing business in Puerto Rico; duty-free exports and imports would not have been allowed between Puerto Rico and the mainland; capital could not have flowed without controls; and American factories and American management would not have come to Puerto Rico in such large numbers during the fifties and sixties. In addition, without this context, increases in national income or employment on the mainland would not have provoked emigration as quickly from Puerto Rico; there would not have been open borders, a military experience for Puerto Rican men and women, citizenship status, accessible and frequent air travel, and early communications and education systems that were tied to the U.S. mainland. In the end, this context made Puerto Ricans "colonial immigrants," i.e., similar to Algerians, Tunisians, Moroccans, and West or East Indians who have immigrated to English, French, and Dutch "fatherlands" over the past two decades.

Thus, within this larger structure, we see that economic push and pull factors were involved in the decision to migrate, and they still are. The most recent analysis of migrants leaving Puerto Rico found that the majority (69%) were not employed, and this was especially the case for women.[29] As the Junta de Planificacion points out, however, employment was not the decisive factor for all those leaving because 52% of those with 16+ years of education had jobs before they left.[34]

But pull factors have also always been important. Puerto Ricans were (and are) pulled by the promise (or hope) of a better life, a life like the one they perceived Americans to have—a life to which they, as American citizens, were also entitled. They were also undoubtedly pulled by connections to family that were already living on the mainland. These connections expanded into networks that became self-reinforcing pulls; these pulls grew as the migration continued. Finally Puerto Ricans were pulled by an adventurous perspective—one that proposed they try their luck in a new land, that they strive for something better.

PATTERNS OF SETTLEMENT

There have been Puerto Ricans, and even Puerto Rican organizations, in New York since the nineteenth century.[19,35] However, it was only after 1900 that significant numbers of Puerto Ricans came to the city, while the bulk of the migration occurred in the fifties and sixties (see Figure 1). The migration of Puerto Ricans after the U.S. takeover in 1898 has been classified into three major periods.[36] During the first period, 1900–1945, the pioneers arrived. The majority of these "pioneros" settled in New York City, in the Atlantic Avenue area of Brooklyn, El Barrio in East Harlem, and other sections of Manhattan such as the Lower East Side, the Upper West Side, Chelsea, and the Lincoln Center area, while some began to populate sections of the South Bronx. During this period, industrial and agricultural labor under contract also arrived and "provided the base from which sprang many of the Puerto Rican communities" outside of New York City.[21]

The second phase of the migration, 1946–1964, is known as "the great migration" because the largest numbers of Puerto Ricans arrived. During this period the already established Puerto Rican communities of East Harlem, the South Bronx, and the Lower East Side increased their numbers as well as their borders. Settlements in new areas of New York, New Jersey, Connecticut, Chicago, and other areas of the country appeared and grew, but the bulk of the Puerto Rican population continued to reside in New York.

The last period, from 1965 to the present, is termed "the revolving door migration," and involves a fluctuating pattern of net migration as well as greater dispersion to other parts of the mainland. As Figure 1 illustrates, the last few years have shown net outflows from Puerto Rico that begin to rival those experienced in the early fifties. By 1980, the majority of Puerto Ricans on the mainland were living outside of New York State.[37]

Contract laborers have been another stream in the Puerto Rican migration. They have generally received less attention in the literature because many returned to Puerto Rico after their contracts were completed, while others moved quickly out of agricultural contract labor and settled in more urban settings. Initially recruited by companies and then by family members and word-of-mouth, these migrants formed the nucleus of Puerto Rican communities that would subsequently develop in less urban areas or in areas outside of the New York metropolitan area. The communities in Hawaii, Arizona, and other southwestern states, San Francisco, Gary, Indiana, and Lorain, Cleveland, and Youngstown, Ohio began in this way.[6] Contract labor migration began soon after 1898 an continued throughout the twentieth century. Indeed, the very first wave of migration after the 1898 takeover of Puerto Rico by the United States was a contract labor group that went to Hawaii.

The class composition of the Puerto Rican communities has changed over time, but the communities have always retained a distinctive diversity. The late nineteenth century Puerto Rican community on the mainland was made up of generally well-to-do merchants, political activists closely allied with the Cuban Revolutionary movement, and skilled workers, many of whom were "tabaqueros" (skilled tobacco workers).[19,35] By the first quarter of the twentieth century the Puerto Rican community is described by a number of scholars as consisting of people who were employed in predominantly working-class occupations.[4,5,38] It was in the post-World War II period that migration from Puerto Rico to the mainland accelerated, causing the communities to grow rapidly. The composition of these communities continued to reflect diversity but with a strong working-class base.

PUERTO RICANS' SOCIOECONOMIC STATUS: A PERSISTENT DISADVANTAGE

For quite some time now, Puerto Ricans on the mainland have been in a most difficult and highly vulnerable economic situation. Soon after the "great migration" of Puerto Ricans to the mainland in the fifties, government and scholarly reports began to highlight the economic adversities Puerto Ricans were experiencing on the mainland. Despite these early warnings, little was done and the situation of Puerto Ricans received little attention by policy-makers.

More recently, however, there has been an emerging interest in the "persisting disadvantage" of Puerto Ricans. Much of the current interest in Puerto Ricans derives from the results of new studies that have found them to be uniquely disadvantaged relative to other groups in mainland society. That is to say, while other minorities experienced a period of socioeconomic advancement during the 1960s, followed by a phase of limited gains during the 1970s, the Puerto Rican experience is one of continuously growing disadvantage since 1960. During the 1980s, government data and research reports provided growing evidence of the uniquely disadvantaged position of Puerto Ricans within postwar U.S. society.[39,40]

The deteriorating relative position of Puerto Ricans is reflected in a variety of indicators. In 1960, Puerto Rican median family income was lower than that of African-Americans, other Hispanics, and Native Americans. Puerto Ricans were the only Hispanic group not to have narrowed the family income gap relative to Caucasians during the seventies.[39] By 1980 the difference had widened. In 1987, median family income for Puerto Ricans was less than half that of Caucasians.[40]

Moreover, during the late eighties, the incidence of poverty among Puerto Ricans continued to be higher than for any other group, remaining similar to the poverty rate of a decade earlier.[40] Data on labor force participation present the same story of relative disadvantage. Puerto Ricans (in 1980) exhibited participation rates lower than that of other groups, and those employed worked fewer hours on the average.[41] Analysis of trends by gender indicates that participation rates for Puerto Rican males steadily declined between 1960 and 1980, while that of women improved modestly during the same period.[39] The disadvantaged situation of Puerto Ricans, relative to other groups, has been so severe that it has led some to speculate about whether Puerto Ricans are becoming a Hispanic underclass.[42]

Figures 2 through 9, based on data published by the U.S. Bureau of

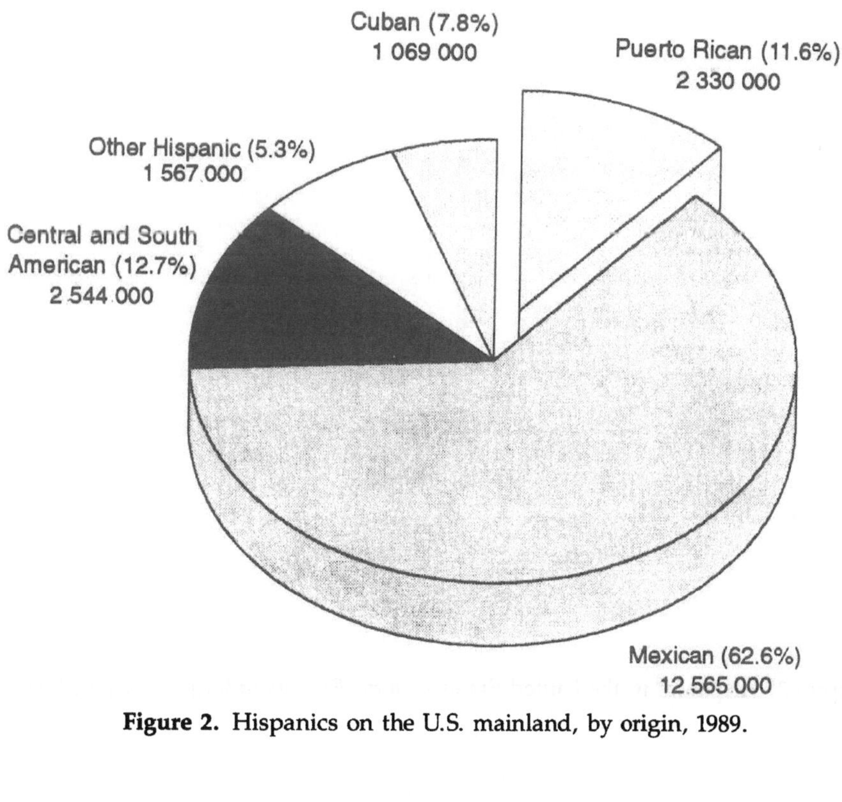

Figure 2. Hispanics on the U.S. mainland, by origin, 1989.

the Census, present selected aspects of the current situation of Puerto Ricans relative to non-Hispanics and other Hispanic groups on the U.S. mainland. Figure 2 shows the number and percentage distribution by origin of Hispanics on the mainland. Figure 3 presents similar information with Puerto Ricans living in Puerto Rico added to the mainland total. As may be seen in Figures 2 and 3, the Puerto Rican share of the total mainland Hispanic population rises from 11.6 to 24.7% if those living in Puerto Rico are included. Given that government programs and other funding activities often extend to Puerto Rico, it would seem important to include Puerto Ricans in Puerto Rico as part of the total U.S. Hispanic population.

Figure 4 presents the poverty rate (% of families below the poverty level) for the various Hispanic groups residing on the mainland. The poverty rate is a widely used indicator of socioeconomic disadvantage, and Puerto Ricans have the highest rate. Figure 5 shows the median household income for Hispanics, which is another indicator of relative disadvantage. On this indicator, Puerto Ricans score the lowest. Associated with poverty, as cause or consequence, is a low participation rate in

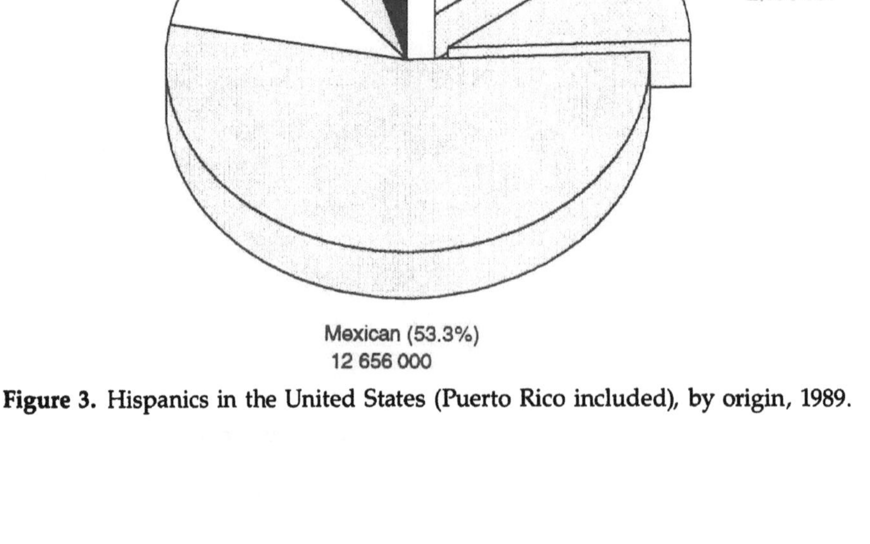

Figure 3. Hispanics in the United States (Puerto Rico included), by origin, 1989.

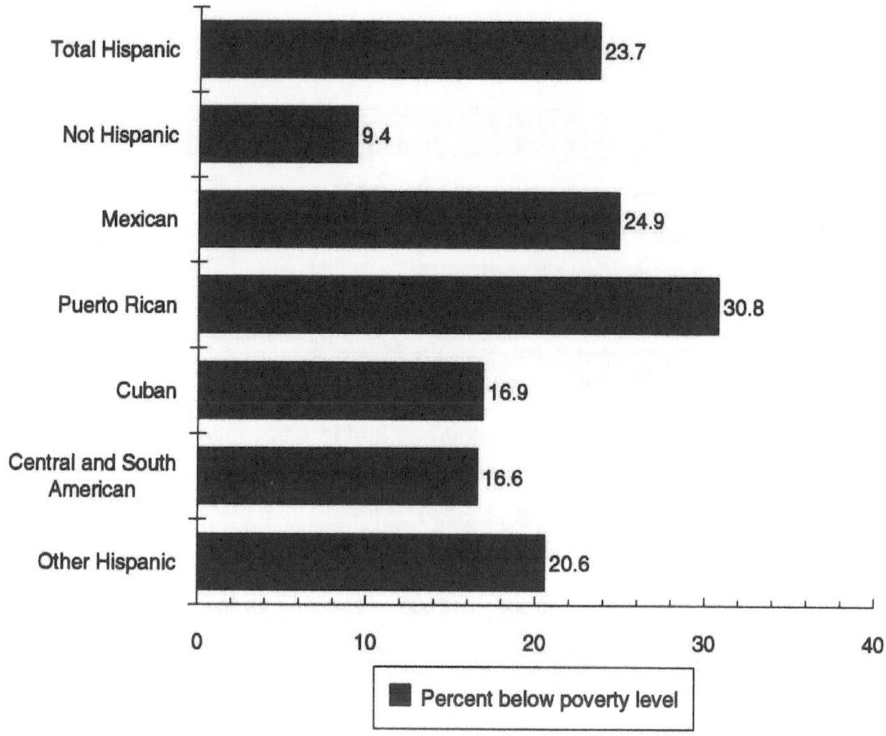

Figure 4. Percent of all Hispanic families residing on the U.S. mainland who are below poverty level, by origin, 1989.

the labor force. Figure 6 indicates that Puerto Rican women have the lowest labor force participation rate of all Hispanic groups. Figure 7 shows another distinguishing characteristic of Puerto Ricans residing on the mainland: a high percentage of female-headed households and a low percentage of male-headed households.

Educational attainment is also an indicator of a group's relative socioeconomic advantage/disadvantage. Figure 8 shows the percentage of the mainland population that has completed 4 years of high school or more according to Hispanic/non-Hispanic origin and two broad age groups. In both age groups, Puerto Ricans rank below the total for non-Hispanics; considerably below the total for Hispanics in the 35 years and over age group, but substantially above in the 25 through 34 years of age. While, irrespective of origin, younger adults have more schooling than older adults, the age disparity is wider in Puerto Ricans than in

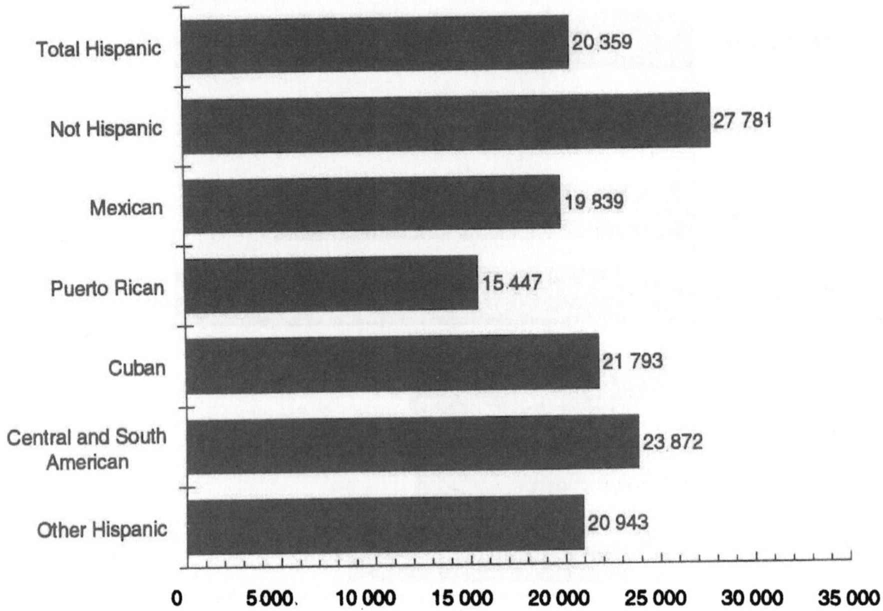

Figure 5. Median household income of Hispanic families residing on the U.S. mainland, by origin, 1989.

other Hispanic groups, suggesting recent gains for Puerto Ricans (see Figure 9). This, in all probability, reflects recent gains achieved by mainland-born Puerto Ricans as well as gains achieved by the Puerto Rico-born migrating to the mainland.

CONCLUSION

It is clear from the scholarly information reviewed that the causes for the migration of Puerto Ricans to the mainland are many, complexly interwoven, and difficult to extricate from the mass of data. Economic and social changes in both the U.S. mainland and Puerto Rico appear to have created a series of pull and push factors that seem to explain the peaks and valleys observed in year to year net migration figures. The most propelling force for the original and the continuing migration, however, is likely to be the unique political relationship existing between Puerto Rico and the mainland. This relationship, relatively

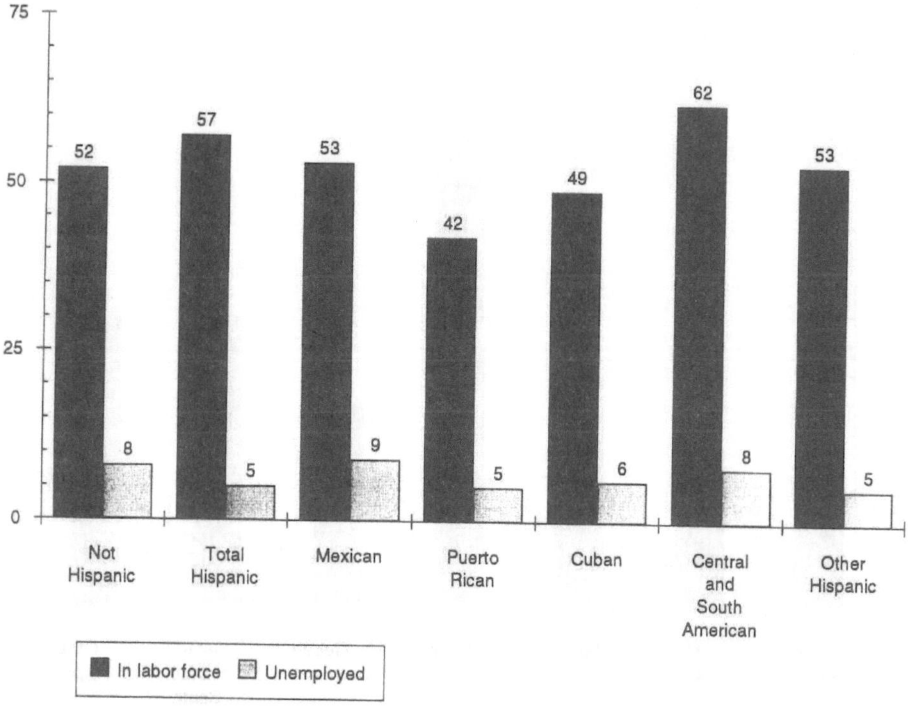

Figure 6. Percent of all Hispanic women 16 years and over residing on the U.S. mainland who are in the civilian labor force and unemployed, by origin, 1989.

speaking, makes movement from the island to the mainland effortless because it is a right of citizenship. The right is not any different from the right that residents of the 50 U.S. states have to cross state boundaries either temporarily or permanently. That is not to say that without the unique political relationship, migration would not occur. It is conjectured that it would not be as great, and as in the case of Cubans, politics would play a larger role. In addition, the socioeconomic characteristics of those migrating would be more likely to be skewed toward the upper rather than the lower socioeconomic levels.

This chapter has also reviewed the socioeconomic disadvantage of Puerto Ricans on the mainland over time, as well as in comparison to other Hispanic and non-Hispanic groups at a particular point. The persistence of the disadvantage over the years and the size of the current disadvantage relative to other Hispanic and non-Hispanic

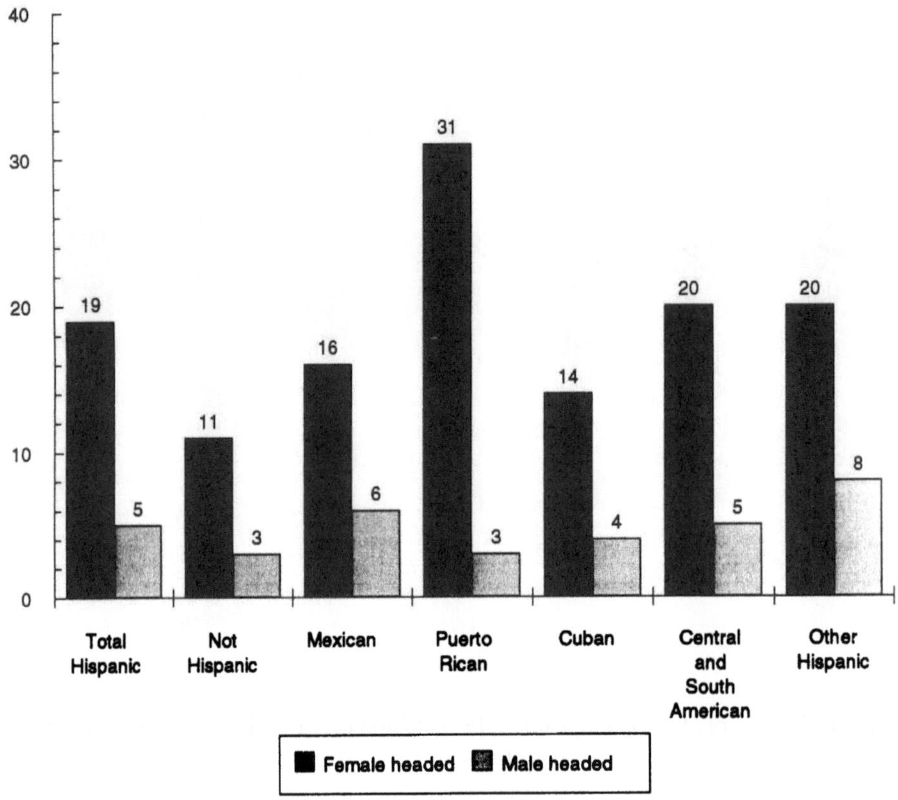

Figure 7. Percent of all Hispanic family households on the U.S. mainland headed by a male or a female, by origin, 1989.

groups begs for explanations supported by facts. Unfortunately, only conjectures are possible. One such conjecture is the pattern of settlement which has led to the concentration of Puerto Ricans in the most decaying urban regions of the U.S. mainland. These regions also happen to be experiencing drastic dislocations in their industrial economies and to be suffering from extremely high levels of unemployment. This, coupled with intractable patterns of job discrimination and residential segregation based on social class and/or imputed racial identity, is creating a situation of persistent poverty for many Puerto Ricans that would be hard for any group to escape.

Indications are that the Puerto Rican population on the mainland may have increased between 18 and 29% since 1980, making Puerto

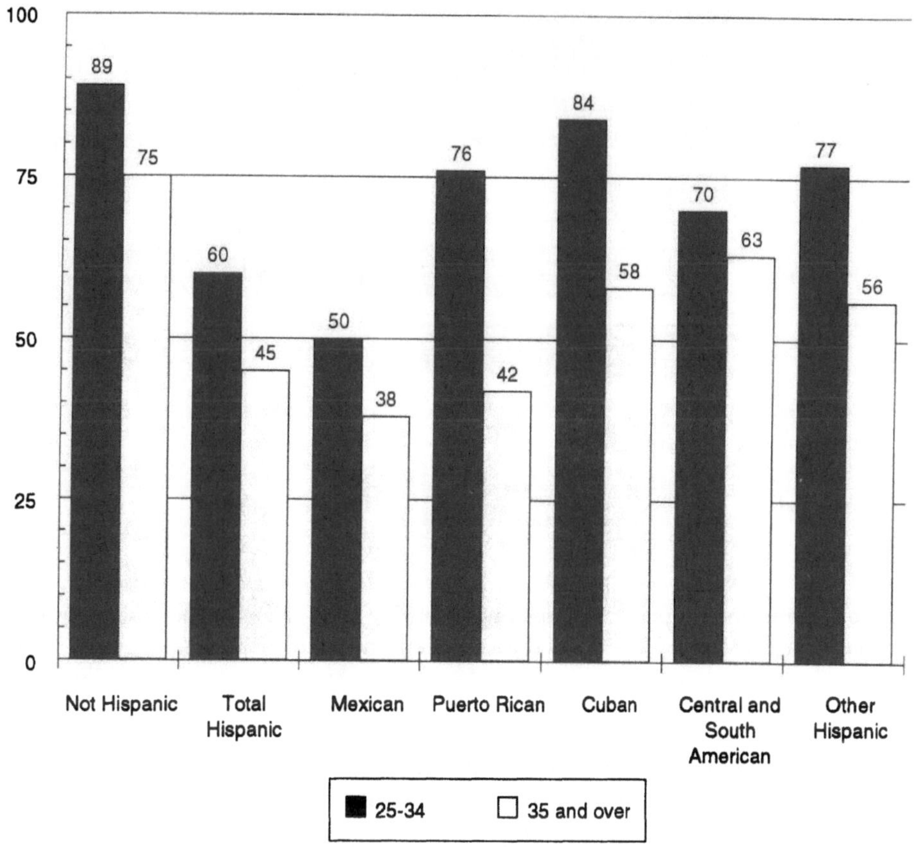

Figure 8. Percent of all Hispanic persons residing on the U.S. mainland who have completed four years of high school or more, by origin, 1989.

Ricans one of the fastest growing ethnic groups on the mainland. Close to 40% of all Puerto Ricans currently residing on the mainland are below 20 years of age, with about one-fourth of that 40% being 5 years of age or under. Typically, these are the age groups with the greatest health, education, and social needs, which, in conjunction with the extremely high rates of poverty and female-headed households, translate into a high demand for publicly supported services. Such high demands can only be met to a very limited degree as Puerto Ricans are concentrated in localities with inadequate public services and with economies likely to remain drastically impaired for years to come. A series of well-financed initiatives to improve the situation described is

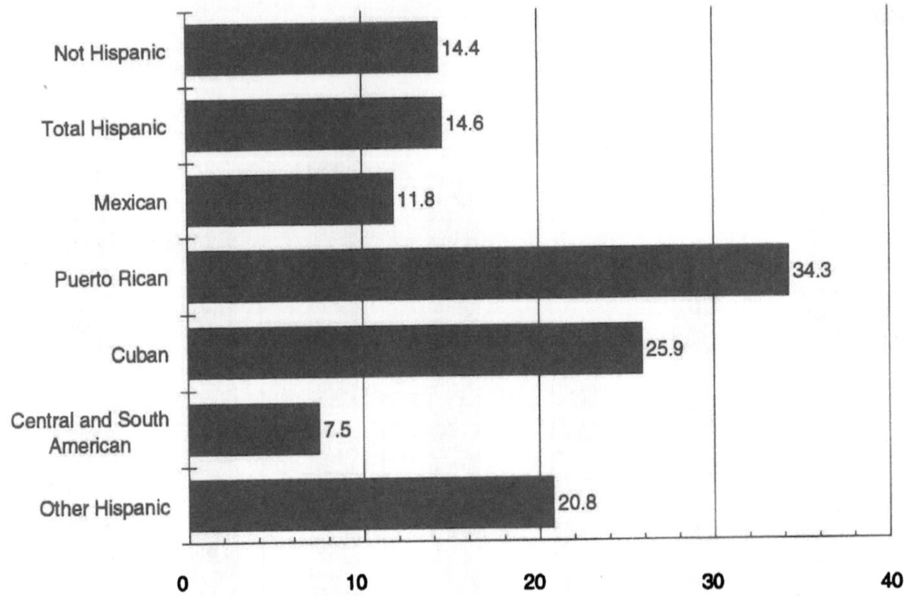

Figure 9. Difference in percent completing 4 years of high school or more between U.S. mainland Hispanics aged 25–34 and those 35 years and over (Hispanics, by origin, 1989).

justified. This would require a high level of cooperation between the states where Puerto Ricans are concentrated, the Commonwealth of Puerto Rico, and agencies of the federal government. A joint commission similar to the one operating along the U.S.–Mexico border should be considered.

REFERENCES

1. Lopez A, Petras J: *Puerto Rico and Puerto Ricans*. Cambridge, MA, Schenkman, 1974
2. Uriarte-Gaston M: *Organizing for Survival: The Emergence of a Puerto Rican Community*, Doctoral dissertation, Boston University, Boston, MA, 1987
3. Aldorondo, E: *Perfil de la Comunidad Puertorriquena en los Estados Unidos*. Departamento de Asuntos de la Comunidad Puertorriquena en los Estados Unidos, 1990
4. Chenault L: *The Puerto Rican Migrant in New York City*. New York, Columbia University Press, 1938, 1970
5. Handlin O: *The Newcomers: Negroes and Puerto Ricans in a Changing Metropolis*. Cambridge, MA, Harvard University Press, 1959
6. Senior C, Watkins DO: Toward a balance sheet of Puerto Rican migration, in *Status of Puerto Rico: Selected Background Studies* (prepared for the U.S.–Puerto Rico Commission on the Status of Puerto Rico). Washington, DC: Government Printing Office, 1966
7. Mills CW, Senior C, Goldsen R: *The Puerto Rican Journey: New York's Newest Migrants*. New York, Harper Bros, 1950

8. Perloff H: *Puerto Rico's Economic Future*. Chicago, University of Chicago Press, 1950
9. Reynolds, LG, Peter G: *Wages, Productivity and Industrialization in Puerto Rico*. Chicago, Richard D. Irving, 1965
10. Maldonado-Denis M: *Puerto Rico: A Socio-Historic Interpretation*. New York, Random House, 1972
11. Bonilla F, Campos R: A wealth of poor: Puerto Ricans in the new economic order. *Daedulus* 110:133–176, 1981
12. Morales J: *Puerto Rican Poverty and Migration: We Just Had to Try Elsewhere*. New York, Praeger, 1986
13. Padilla F: *Puerto Rican Chicago*. Notre Dame, IN, University of Notre Dame Press, 1987
14. Fleisher BH: *Some Economic Aspects of Puerto Rican Migration to the United States*. Doctoral dissertation, Stanford University, Stanford, CA, 1961
15. Fleisher BH: Some economic aspects of Puerto Rican migration to the United States. *Rev. Econ. & Statistics* 45:245–253, 1963
16. Glazer N, Moynihan DP: *Beyond the Melting Pot*, 2nd ed. Cambridge, MA, MIT Press, 1970
17. Pantoja A: *Puerto Rican Migration*. Preliminary Report to the U.S. Commission on Civil Rights of Puerto Ricans, New York, January 31, 1972
18. Rodriguez C: *The Ethnic Queue: The Case of Puerto Ricans in the U.S.* San Francisco, CA, R & E Research Associates, 1974
19. Sanchez-Korrol V: *From Colonial to Community: The History of Puerto Ricans in New York City, 1917–1948*. Westport, CT, Greenwood Press, 1983
20. Maldonado R: Why Puerto Ricans migrated to the United States in 1947–73. *Monthly Labor Rev.*, September 1976, pp. 17–18.
21. Maldonado E: Contract labor and the origins of Puerto Rican communities in the United States. *Internat. Migrat. Rev.* 13:103–121, 1979
22. Piore M: *Birds of Passage: Migrant Labor and Industrial Societies*. New York, Cambridge University Press, 1979
23. Lapp M: *The Migration Division of Puerto Rico and Puerto Ricans in New York City, 1948–1969*. New York Historical Society, New York, 1986
24. Labor recruited. *Business Week* April 29, 1944, p 114.
25. Steward J: *The People of Puerto Rico*. Chicago, University of Illinois Press, 1965
26. Gonzalez AJ: La Economia y el Status Politico. *Revista de Ciencias Sociales* 10:5–50, March, 1966
27. Dietz JL: *Economic History of Puerto Rico: Institutional Change and Capitalist Development*. Princeton, NJ, Princeton University Press, 1986
28. Carr R: *Puerto Rico: A Colonial Experiment*. New York, New York University Press, 1984
29. Stahl JE: *Economic development through reform in Puerto Rico*, doctoral dissertation. Iowa State University, Ames, IA, 1965
30. Hanson EP: *Puerto Rico: Land of Wonders*. New York, Alfred A. Knopf, 1960
31. Goodsell C: *Administration of a Revolution*. Cambridge, MA, Harvard University Press, 1965
32. Lewis GK: *Puerto Rico: Freedom and Power in the Caribbean*. New York, Monthly Review Press, 1963
33. Wells H: *The Modernization of Puerto Rico: A Political Study of Changing Values and Institutions*. Cambridge, MA, Harvard University Press, 1969
34. Junta de Planificacion de Puerto Rico: *Caracteristicas de la Poblacion Migrante de Puerto Rico*. Santurce, P.R., 1986
35. Iglesias CA: *Memorias de Bernardo Vego: Una Contribucion a la Historia de la Comunidad Puertorriquena en Nueva York*. Rio Piedras, P.R., Ediciones Huracan, 1977, 1980
36. Stevens-Arroyo A, Diaz-Stevens, M: Puerto Ricans in the United States: A struggle for identity, in Dworkin AG, Dworkin, RJ, (eds): *The Minority Report: An Introduction to*

Racial, Ethnic and Gender Relations, 2nd ed. New York, CBS College Publishing, Holt, Rinehart & Winston, 1982
37. US Bureau of the Census: *Persons of Spanish Origin By State: 1980*, Supplementary Report PC80–S1–7, August. Washington, DC: Government Printing Office, 1982
38. Gosnell Aran P: *The Puerto Ricans in New York City*, doctoral dissertation. New York University, New York, 1945
39. Bean F, Tienda M: *Hispanic Population in the U.S.* Russell Sage Foundation, New York, 1988
40. Center on Budget and Policy Priorities: *Shortchanged: Recent Developments in Hispanic Poverty, Income and Employment*, Washington D.C., 1988
41. Borjas G: Jobs and employment for Hispanics, in San Juan Cafferty P, McCready WC (eds): *Hispanics in the United States*. New Brunswick, NJ: Transaction Books, 1985
42. Tienda M: Puerto Ricans and the underclass debate. *Annals* 501:105–119, January, 1989

2

Entremundos: The Psychological Dialectics of Puerto Rican Migration and Its Implications for Health

IRIS ZAVALA-MARTINEZ

Since World War II, "one of the greatest population exoduses registered in contemporary history began."[1] Massive migrations to the United States in the early 1950s and during the 1960s have resulted in a Puerto Rican diaspora and "this massive transfer, dispersal, and circulation of population constitutes a dismemberment of the Puerto Rican nation that has yet to run its course . . ."[1] According to the 1990 Census, there are 2.7 million first, second, and third generation Puerto Ricans now living in the United States, constituting a diverse and vital Puerto Rican community.[2]

IRIS ZAVALA-MARTINEZ • Mental Health Division, San Juan Health Department, San Juan, Puerto Rico 00907.

Puerto Rican Women and Children: Issues in Health, Growth, and Development, edited by Gontran Lamberty and Cynthia Garcia Coll. Plenum Press, New York, 1994.

This chapter discusses the psychological dialectics associated with the migration of Puerto Ricans to the United States and how this relates to and impacts on health and the use of health services by mothers, children, and adolescents. This chapter's principal thesis argues that the complex experience of migration generates this psychological dialectic for Puerto Ricans which in turn becomes the dynamic context for their adaptive struggles as well as for the process of ongoing socialization and regeneration. This context has propelled interacting psychosocial dimensions which seem to define and identify aspects of the Puerto Rican experience of migration. This situation is one in which a growing number of Puerto Ricans are born and socialized into an experience that can be best described as being between two worlds, or *entremundos*, with all the ambiguities and complexities that such a reality creates. Puerto Ricans as a people are caught up between two worlds: between the United States and the island of Puerto Rico; between speaking Spanish or English, both, or neither well; between being born in the United States or on the island; between feeling nationalistic on the one hand yet feeling apologetic or feeling victimized by historical circumstances they could not control. Puerto Ricans experience not only being between two worlds, but also having to forge multiple identities within these contexts or often feeling marginal or alienated from any one or all of these situations. This process occurs while simultaneously adapting to the taxing demands of a constantly changing, highly urbanized technological society. According to a Puerto Rican who migrated to the U.S. mainland, "uno no sabe si va o viene" (one does not know if one is coming or going), or as another described it, "You know, I sit here in New York and I'm homesick for Salinas, I go home to Salinas, and I'm homesick for New York. I don't know what the hell I am."[3] Although it may appear that this experiential definitional problem would apply only to Puerto Ricans born and/or raised in the United States, the impact of circular migration and the reality of Puerto Rico's sociopolitical status renders related but not identical effects for the residents of the island. For Puerto Ricans, *entremundos* is part of an ongoing polemic on national identity that has permeated Puerto Rico's colonial history and most likely will continue to be a salient experiential issue in the future.

Moreover, the psychological *entremundos* experience is part of a complex dynamic process which is also influenced by other variables such as gender, social class, race, personal values, political forces, and generational status. To handle these multiple forces, Puerto Ricans have resorted to coping strategies and survival skills that are acquired as part of their socialization or are generated in response to the demands and limitations of their life situations.[4–9] Similarly, their community life and transactions have been affected as well. The challenge of being the "new kid on the block" was conducive to recreating the island barrios in New York City from the 1930s through the 1950s. This led to the challenges of the surging new generations of Puerto Ricans of the 1960s and 1970s who were caught up in the throes of trying to adapt to their poverty-stricken and often discriminatory urban contexts while seeking a collective political and cultural voice and identity. During the 1980s, additional challenges ensued when having to negotiate with the different needs of first, second, and third generation Puerto Ricans and those of other Latino immigrants fleeing from wars and economic injustice in Central and South America. Now the 1990s, the threshold of the twenty-first century, may witness a renewed struggle toward an integrated definition of the Puerto Rican experience.

In summary, the psychological experience of *entremundos* has forged subjective life and behavioral actions that from a dialectical perspective has generated conflictual identity stress and confusion. For Puerto Ricans *entremundos* may be part of the historical struggle toward defining the national family, one that is not a single-parent nation, or a step or reconstituted family nation, or a foster one, but a dispersed family that has maintained, persevered, and affirmed its commonalities and collective sense of identity.

MIGRATION AND PSYCHOSOCIAL HEALTH

Such a complex migration and experiential context inevitably affects the health and psychosocial development of those who experience it. The psychological literature on Puerto Rican immigrants highlights the stress of adaptation, discrimination, and prejudice, the feelings of loss and confusion, the survival struggles resulting from recurrent poverty, and cultural and family conflicts.[9–15] The general literature on migration and mental health has in fact addressed many of these same issues for other migrants and has noted the impact and interaction between social conditions and immigrant mental health.[16,17] Migration provokes family disruptions, role confusions, fragmented social support networks, generational conflicts and language variations, often within a context permeated by poverty, discrimination, racism, and the absence of growth promoting experiences for the young. More needs to be learned, however, about numerous Puerto Rican families who did and do, in fact, surmount severe difficulties and are able to transform their situation through the help of religion, personal strengths, social support, family networks, economic stability, and other health promoting factors. Unfortunately, the literature has generally paid limited attention to this crucial aspect of Puerto Rican migration to the United States. The importance, however, of the support provided by the extended Puerto Rican family has been noted in the published literature as exemplified in Rogler[18] and Bravo et al.[19]

The literature indicates that for Puerto Ricans in the United States, stress-induced "ataques," suicidal fits, psychosomatic symptoms, and anxiety were the most prevalent socioemotional and behavioral manifestations along with alcohol and drug abuse.[11,20–22] But the corrosive impact of unemployment, poor parenting skills, and family instability most probably underlie many of these manifestations. In fact, what is most often being attended to by many health care practitioners are by and large the cumulative effects of social and economic inequality.[21] It may be that the chronic psychosocial stress of poverty, and the recurrent multiple transitions and dislocations among Puerto Ricans underlie most of these negative psychosocial health effects.

A variation of these stresses and of the *entremundos* experience, for example, is that experienced by young Puerto Ricans who return to the island with their parents who are full of nostalgic longing. Now the young are the ones who experience culture shock, and experience what their parents already had experienced as culture shock upon emigrating to the United States. Return migration and its psychological impact has received recent attention as it brings the psychological dialectics of migration full circle. Returning Puerto Ricans, whether first, second, or third generation, undergo a process of readaptation to a Puerto Rico of the 1990s and not the Puerto Rico of 15, 20, or 30 years ago. This process can be highly distressing and confusing for adults because they have to reconnect with a social history that they did not experience and with the emotional and cultural dimensions of that history. In a sense, they have an experiential lacuna and no memory of a collectively shared past.

For the returning adolescents who have lived their early years in the United States, the disconnection is similar and perhaps more salient given the underlying developmental processes they are experiencing. Adolescents often experience great stress upon returning or coming for the first time to the island as they experience the *entremundos* reality with more intensity, and often harbor confused feelings about what is happening and why they may be frustrated and angry. The following case illustrates some of these points.

> José was a 16-year-old youth who returned with his parents to a rural island town from the urban, working class section of Chicago after living there all his life. He spoke a battered Spanish and was excruciatingly self-conscious of this. His parents nagged him to speak more Spanish but in Chicago they had encouraged him to speak English. José, previously Joey, was experiencing a form of culture shock and what is defined here as an *entremundos* experience. José did not know the island's history, did not understand "folkish" ways, and felt angry, confused, shortchanged, and frustrated. He had become sullen and withdrawn.

In essence, José was caught between two worlds and suffered the subjective distress borne out of the migratory experiences of his family, which reflect a microcosm of the collective social history of the Puerto Rican family.

The degree of stress related to this readaptation and relocation process has to be investigated more closely. What are the coping strategies used and to what degree are these similar to those extant in the United States? Are they effective? Further, bilingual youth and adults often express that they feel discriminated against by island born and raised Puerto Ricans or feel ostracized for speaking English rather than Spanish. On the other hand, those in Puerto Rico sometimes complain that "Nuyoricans" think themselves superior, take their jobs, and are not "real" Puerto Ricans. This situation creates a tension between victimization borne out of the irony and contradictions of historical and socioeconomic processes, which are directly related to Puerto Rico's colonial status and its migration history.

It is crucial that the *entremundos* dynamics be critically analyzed and understood, so that appropriate action plans are made to ensure the well-being of returning youth and their families. Such a process will help to develop an integrated definition of what is a Puerto Rican, and a critical understanding of the complex psychological dialectics of migration. It is imperative to ensure that health care practitioners, educators, and Puerto Ricans on the island and in the United States do not fall prey to the dynamics of victimization and to obscuring the true source of the problem.

SUMMARY AND DISCUSSION

In this chapter, the psychological dialectic for Puerto Ricans has been described as a dynamic process that grows out of the migration experience and results in a subjective experience labeled *entremundos* or "between two worlds." As a consequence of being *entremundos*, conflicts of identity and difficulties in adapting to the demands of the two cultures can evolve. This conflict of identity and uncertainty may permeate areas of the overall Puerto Rican experience related to circular migration and the unresolved political status of the island. Feelings of marginality or alienation may also be experienced for both U.S. and island born or raised Puerto Ricans. Consequences for adult mental and physical health, as well as for the socioemotional development of adolescents and children, have been postulated to derive from the *entremundos* experience.

What are the implications of the *entremundos* concept for the health care of Puerto Rican mothers, children, and adolescents in the United States?

First, this concept emphasizes that a complex dynamic process is operating which affects the health and development of Puerto Ricans. This process derives from the interaction of multiple factors operating within the boundaries of the immigration experience. It is within this dynamic process that Puerto Rican mothers, children, and adolescents need to be understood. Practitioners in health care centers experience the various manifestations of this process and, for the most part, fail to recognize them as such. It is necessary but not sufficient to be culturally sensitive. Practitioners must be responsive to the diverse ways in which people embody and manifest their culture and life histories. This requires the adoption of an open method of inquiry. It is necessary for the health care practitioner to be sensitive to the ways in which, for example, a particular economic situation impinges on a person's health, or how stresses deriving from changing sex-role expectations may be influencing recurrent complaints of headaches. It is also important to ascertain how unprocessed, underlying feelings of dislocation and nostalgia, for example, may be propelling insomnia; how the marital discord a family is operating under may affect the management of asthma in a child; or how perceived attitudes and institutional barriers force mothers to shop around for health care practitioners with whom they can feel comfortable.[23,24] These skills might not generally be considered a part of the necessary repertoire of practitioners in health care centers. Given the fact that Puerto Ricans frequently use emergency rooms and primary care facilities, however, it is often the primary care physician, the nurse, and the social worker in such settings who will become the conduit for channeling health and illness concerns that may have a social dynamic origin rather than a biomedical one.[25]

Second, we must initiate a collaborative history-taking process which is engaging, dynamic, and geared to educate both the patient and the health practitioner. Such an interview can elicit vital information that helps us to understand health problems within their social contexts. As such, the recommended approach supports a biopsychosocial model of health which is consistent with the open and dynamic method of inquiry proposed. Canino, Vela, and Passalaqua,[26] described a systematic method of inquiry which draws forth information on key areas of an individual's sociocultural experience in order to avoid stereotypic generalizations and to identify salient social, economic, and cultural factors that may impact on somatic and mental health while placing the person in a dynamic context. Although these authors focus their inquiry around the themes of migration, spiritualism, racism, and child-rearing practices in evaluating persons for mental health treatment, an abbreviated version of their recommended process could be highly useful in primary care settings. It is imperative that practitioners not take for granted what they have read or heard about Puerto Ricans, but inquire into their actual experiences and social histories. The practitioner should explore diverse scenarios and examine the symptoms within their sociocultural contexts. Factors such as the language of preference, time in the United States, support systems available, and economic resources need to be considered, as well as how the family defines health and what function health plays in the matrix of their lives. In summary, it would behoove health practitioners to develop a more personal interviewing style that promotes trust and *confianza* while eliciting valuable and needed health information.

Third, health care practitioners must be aware of specific patterns of health care use and preferences of Puerto Ricans. The literature on health utilization by Puerto Ricans[21,24] suggests that besides frequent use of emergency room and primary care facilities, the following should be taken into consideration:

1. They tend to make limited use of preventive services (prenatal or otherwise) when, in fact, true health prevention and promotion from a social change perspective would be crucial here.

2. They are likely to have high expectations of being informed of

any medical problem in ways that they can understand and relate to, that is, using terms and concepts that are unambiguous, not emotionally charged, and consistent with their world views (e.g., using the word *nervios* versus saying mental illness, *enfermedad mental*, or *locura*).

3. Care needs to be exercised in the use of translators: other family members may withhold data if they judge it to be loaded; English-dominant children may temporarily exert a role that does not correspond to them or may become parentified; and other Latinos' vernacular may contain words and phrases not used by Puerto Ricans.

4. It is useful to consider that most Puerto Ricans tend to feel more comfortable with practitioners who are warm, show concern, maintain a certain measured informality, yet who demonstrate respect with a personally attentive style.

This work would not be complete, however, if we did not provide a vision of progressive health care for the Puerto Rican community that encourages patient responsibility, empowerment, community development, self-support, and integral socially conscious health practices. Health care providers need to actively engage their patients in their own health care as a way of fostering participation and validating respect for a person's healing potential.[9,15,27] Encouraging dependency through the expert medical model of allopathic medicine may not be conducive to optimal health because a person's own resources are not maximized or developed. If providers engage patients in a participatory health care process, we could gradually develop a more health conscious community as a preventive strategy. Prevention could be related intimately to community education and development, and to the equitable distribution of knowledge, resources, and skills.[15] Given the distressing health and socioeconomic statistics of Puerto Ricans, participatory and democratizing models of health care should be advocated to reflect the vision outlined in this chapter. Seeking and maintaining health would become a proactive praxis and patients could then become true participants in the crucial process of appropriating their own history and constructing their own healthy future.

REFERENCES

1. Vasquez Calzada JL: Demographic aspects of migration, in Center for Puerto Rican Studies (ed.): *Labor Migration Under Capitalism: The Puerto Rican Experience*. New York, Monthly Review Press, 1981, p. 224
2. Rodriguez C: *Puerto Ricans: Born in the USA*. Boston, Unwin Hyman, 1989

3. Hamill P: Coming of age in Nueva York, in Cordasco, F, Bucchioni, E (eds.): *The Puerto Rican Experience*. Totowa, NJ, Littlefield, Adams and Co, 1973, pp 198–212
4. Canino, IA, Canino G: Impact of stress on the Puerto Rican family: Treatment considerations. *Amer. J. Orthopsychiatry* 50:535–541, July 1980
5. Mizio E: Impact of external systems on the Puerto Rican family. *Soc. Casework* 55: 76–89, 1974
6. Rodriguez C, Sanchez Korrol V, Alers JU (eds.): *The Puerto Rican Struggle: Essays on Survival in the United States*. New York, Puerto Rican Migration Research Consortium, 1980
7. Sluzki CE: Migration and family conflict. *Fam. Process* 18:379–390, 1979
8. Zavala-Martinez I: En La Lucha: Economic and socioemotional struggles of Puerto Rican Women in the United States, in Letkowitz R, Withorn A, eds., *For Crying Out Loud: Women and Poverty in the United States*. New York, Pilgrim Press, 1986a, pp. 111–124
9. Zavala-Martinez I: En La Lucha: The economic and socioemotional struggles of Puerto Rican women. *Women & Therapy* 6:3–24, 1988
10. Alers JU: *Puerto Rican and Health: Finding from New York City*. Monograph 1. New York, Hispanic New York Center, 1978
11. Fitszpatrick JP, Gould RE: Mental illness among Puerto Ricans in New York: Cultural condition or intellectual misunderstanding? *Amer. J. Orthopsychiatry* 40:238–239, 1970
12. Inclan J: Psychological symptomatology in second generation Puerto Rican women of three socioeconomic groups. *J. Commun. Psychol.* 11:334–345, 1983
13. Rendon M: Transcultural aspects of Puerto Rican mental illness in New York. *Internat. J. Soc. Psychiatry* 20:18–24, 1974
14. Zavala Martinez I: *Mental Health and Puerto Ricans in the United States: A Critical Literature Review and Comprehensive Bibliography* (Unpublished manuscript, Dept. of Psychology, University of Massachusetts). Amherst, MA, 1981
15. Zavala-Martinez I: Praxis in psychology: Integrating clinical and Community orientation with Latinos. *Commun. Psycholog.* 19:11, 1986b
16. Grinberg L, Grinberg R: *Psicoanalisis de la Migración y del exilio* (Psychoanalysis of Migration and Exile). Madrid, Alianza Editorial, 1984
17. Kantor M: Internal migration and mental illness in: Plog SC, Edgerton RB, eds. *Changing Perspectives in Mental Illness*, New York, Holt, Rinehart, and Winston, 1969, pp. 364–394
18. Rogler L: Help patterns, the family, and mental health: Puerto Ricans in the United States. *Internat. Migrat. Rev.* 12:248–259, 1979
19. Bravo M, Canino G, Rubio-Stipec M, Serrano-Garcia I: Importancia de la familia como recurso de apoyo social en Puerto Rico [The importance of the family as a social support resource in Puerto Rico]. *Puerto Rico Health Sci. J.* 10:149–156, 1991
20. Abad V, Boyce E: Issues in the psychiatric evaluation of Puerto Ricans: A sociocultural perspective. *J. Operat. Psychiatry*, 10:23–39, 1979
21. Harwood A: Mainland Puerto Ricans. In: Harwood A, ed. *Ethnicity and Medical Care*. Cambridge, MA, Harvard University Press, 1981, pp. 397–481.
22. Trautman EC: The suicidal fit: A psychology study on Puerto Rican immigrants. *Arch. Gen. Psychiatry* 5:76–83, 1961
23. Guarnaccia P: Puerto Ricans, asthma, and the health care system. Unpublished studies paper, Dept. of Anthropology and Community Medicine, University of Connecticut, 1979
24. Irigoyen M, Zambrana R: The utilization of pediatric health services by Hispanic mothers. In Zambrana R (ed.), *Work, Family, and Health: Latina Women in Transition*. Monograph No. 7, New York Center, 1982, pp. 63–74.
25. Mishler E: Viewpoint: Critical perspectives on the biomedical model. In: Mischler EG,

Amarasingham LR, Hauser S, Liem R, Osherson S, Waxler N, eds.), *Social Contexts of Health, Illness, and Patient Care*. New York, Cambridge University Press, 1981, pp. 1–23
26. Canino I, Vela M, Passalaqua E: Clinico-cultural factors relevant to Puerto Ricans. *World J. Psychosynth.* 10:19–22, 1978
27. Zavala-Martinez I: Toward an emancipatory clinical practice in human services. In: Gil D, Gil E, (eds.) *Toward Social and Economic Justice*. Cambridge, MA, Schenkman, 1985, pp. 55–62

3

Maternal and Child Health and Health Care in Puerto Rico

PEDRO J. SANTIAGO-BORRERO
AND MARTA VALCARCEL

INTRODUCTION

An understanding of the health and developmental problems faced by Puerto Ricans residing on the U.S. mainland requires knowledge about the health of Puerto Ricans living on the island, as well about the systems of private and public health care serving them. Not only do these two groups share a common set of cultural values, attitudes, and perceptions affecting health and health service use, but there is also a sizable back and forth movement of individuals and families between the island and the mainland. The movement is suspected of being selectively skewed toward low socioeconomic status, low levels of education, a high prevalence of complex personal and family problems, and dependency on the public sector for health care services. Health

PEDRO J. SANTIAGO-BORRERO and MARTA VALCARCEL • Department of Pediatrics, University of Puerto Rico School of Medicine, San Juan, Puerto Rico 00936-5067.

Puerto Rican Women and Children: Issues in Health, Growth, and Development, edited by Gontran Lamberty and Cynthia Garcia Coll. Plenum Press, New York, 1994.

professionals have conjectured that this shared, floating, high-risk population contributes significantly to the poor health outcomes documented for Puerto Ricans residing on the mainland as well as in Puerto Rico.

HEALTH INDICATORS IN PUERTO RICO

The Commonwealth of Puerto Rico has a population of approximately 3.5 million of which over 37% are children and adolescents.[1,2] The island's crude birth rate in 1989 was 19.1 per 1000 inhabitants, a rate essentially unchanged since 1984 (see Table 1). The crude mortality rate of the island in 1989 was 7.3 per 1000 inhabitants, compared to 5.4 for the mainland.[3] In 1989, life expectancy for males residing in Puerto Rico was 70.1 years; 78.6 for females. This compares well with the life expectancies documented for mainland males and females. Marriage and divorce rates are considerably higher in Puerto Rico than on the mainland at a rate of 12.5% per 1000 for marriages and 5.5% per 1000 for divorce, and so is the crude fertility rate (the number of live births per 1000 women is 80, in females ages 15 through 44).

The ten leading causes of death for the Commonwealth in 1989 were practically the same reported for the mainland[1–3] (see Table 2). Exceptions were (1) homicide and suicide are leading causes for the mainland but not for Puerto Rico; and (2) hypertensive diseases and the human immunodeficiency virus (HIV) were leading causes of death in Puerto

Table 1 Key Demographic Indicators: Puerto Rico, 1950–1989

Indicator	1989	1980	1970	1960	1950
Population*	3 493 975	3 203 956	2 716 000	2 360 000	2 218 000
Crude birth rate**	19.1	22.8	24.8	32.2	38.5
Crude fertility rate***	80	96.8	—	—	—
Crude mortality rate**	7.4	6.4	6.7	6.7	9.9
Life expectancy—males	74.14	69.88	68.96	67.14	59.45
Life expectancy—females	78.57	76.87	75.18	71.88	62.43
Marriage rate**	9.3	8.7	10.9	8.7	9.3
Divorce rate**	5.5	6.9	3.6	2.3	1.6

Source: Commonwealth of Puerto Rico Department of Health.
* as of July 1, 1990
** rates per 1,000 population
***rates per 100,000 women in ages 15 through 44

Table 2 Ten Leading Causes of Death: Puerto Rico and the United States, 1989

Rank	Causes of death	Rate per 100 000	% of all deaths
	Puerto Rico		
1.	Diseases of the heart	178.7	24.4
2.	Malignant neoplasms	114.2	15.3
3.	Diabetes mellitus	46.1	6.2
4.	Pneumonia and influenza	36.4	4.9
5.	Accidents	35.3	4.8
6.	Cerebrovascular diseases	33.4	4.5
7.	Human immunodeficiency virus	27.2	3.7
8.	Chronic obstructive pulmonary diseases	26.7	3.6
9.	Hypertensive diseases	26.3	3.5
10.	Chronic liver disease and cirrhosis	21.3	2.9
	United States		
1.	Diseases of the heart	155.9	34.1
2.	Malignant neoplasms	133.0	23.1
3.	Cerebrovascular diseases	28.0	6.8
4.	Accidents	33.8	4.4
5.	Chronic obstructive pulmonary diseases	19.4	3.9
6.	Pneumonia and influenza	13.7	3.6
7.	Diabetes mellitus	11.5	2.2
8.	Suicides	11.3	1.4
9.	Chronic liver disease and cirrhosis	8.9	1.2
10.	Homicides	8.4	1.1

Sources: Commonwealth of Puerto Rico Department of Health and National Center for Health Statistics.

Rico but not on the mainland. Acquired Immune Deficiency Syndrome (AIDS) is quickly emerging as a leading cause of death in Puerto Rico. When all causes of deaths were considered, it was the eighth leading killer of both men and women in the age group 20 through 49 in 1988, and the seventh in 1989.

In summary, the Commonwealth of Puerto Rico compares fairly well with most of the developed countries of the world in terms of overall mortality, life expectancy, and pattern of leading causes of death. This is so despite the fact that only one-third of its population has private health insurance. Private health insurance in many instances does not cover chronic, nor many serious illnesses, thus requiring that in Puerto Rico insured persons turn to the public sector for the needed care.

THE PUBLIC HEALTH CARE SYSTEM

A regionalized public health care system exists in Puerto Rico, administered by the Commonwealth Department of Public Health.[4] A few of the larger municipalities have their own public health care facilities. These are in one way or another linked to the Commonwealth regionalized system of health care. The private sector is strong only in the largest cities, such as San Juan, Ponce, and Mayaguez. Even in these cities, however, the private facilities provide services to less than 50% of the population.

The public health care system of Puerto Rico consists of the traditional four levels of care: primary, secondary, tertiary, and supra-tertiary. This particular organizational mode has been proven to be an efficient one for Puerto Rico and has been used as a model by other developing countries.[4]

Within the public health care system primary care is offered in Diagnostic and Treatment Centers as well as in Family Health Centers located in small towns on the island and in some sectors of the larger cities. Preventive, ambulatory, and emergency care are also provided in these primary health care units. Secondary health care is offered in Area Hospitals, each of which serves five to six small towns. Tertiary care is rendered in six regional hospitals and medical centers scattered throughout the island. Regional hospitals and medical centers have at least the major medical and surgical specialties represented, including obstetrics and gynecology and pediatrics. These hospitals and centers also have neonatal intensive care units, differing in the complexity of the care they can handle.

Highly specialized maternal and child health services are provided at the University of Puerto Rico Medical School Hospital and at the University Pediatric Hospital. Both are located at the Puerto Rico Medical Center in Rio Piedras, a municipality which is part of San Juan Metropolitan Area. The Neonatal Intensive Care Unit of the University Pediatric Hospital provides specialized services to severely ill neonates referred from all over the island, including private hospitals.

MATERNAL AND INFANT HEALTH

Official statistics from the Commonwealth Department of Health indicate that in 1988 there were 64 081 live births recorded in Puerto

Rico; and there were 66 489 in 1989 (see Table 3). Of these births about 9.0% weighed less than 2500 grams at birth, a figure that has remained virtually unchanged since 1980[1,2] (see Table 4). The very low-birth-weight rate (under 1500 grams) was substantial (1.2%) in 1989. The corresponding low-birth-weight rate for the mainland in 1989 was 6.8% and the very low-birth-rate was 1.2%.[3] The persistence in Puerto Rico of a low-birth-weight rate close to 9% suggests a lack of progress in controlling the major risk factors affecting birth outcomes, such as adolescent and unwed pregnancies, inadequate prenatal care, substance abuse during pregnancy, small interval between births, and premature labor.[5]

In 1989, the infant mortality rate for the island was 14.3 per 1000 live births, a figure 13.5% higher than the rate of 12.6 recorded in 1988, but lower than the rates recorded between 1980 and 1985 (Table 5). The corresponding 1989 figure for the U.S. mainland was 9.8. Based on the slow, but overall declining trend of the period 1970–1980, there are reasons to expect that the infant mortality rate will be reduced to approximately 8.2 per 1000 live births by the year 1998.

Table 6 shows the 10 leading causes of infant mortality in Puerto Rico and on the mainland for 1989. In general, the two jurisdictions exhibit similar patterns of leading causes, with congenital malformations and conditions related to short gestation and low birth weight ranking highest in both distributions. Rates for infectious causes (i.e., influenza and pneumonia) are higher in Puerto Rico than on the

Table 3 Live Births According to Selected Characteristics and Type of Medical Facility: Puerto Rico, 1989

Characteristic	All facilities	Public	Private
Number of live births	66 489	41 332	25 157
Percent of all live births	100	62.2	37.8
Percent of live births weighing 2500 grams or less	9	10.6	6.4
Percent of live births weighing 1500 grams or less	1.2	1.6	0.5
Infant deaths per 1000 live births	14.3	18.1	7.3
Percent of adolescent births (under 20 years)	18.1	26	5
Percent of initiating care late (no care + 3rd trimester)	5.3	6.8	2.9
Percent of mothers with less than 12 years of school	33.8	49.5	8.2
Percent of live births to unwed mothers	35.2	48.5	13.4

Source: Commonwealth of Puerto Rico Department of Health.

Table 4 Percent of All Live Births Weighing 2500 Grams or Less at Birth: Puerto Rico and the United States, 1980–1989

		United States	
Year	Puerto Rico	All races	White
1980	9.0	6.84	5.72
1981	8.8	6.81	5.69
1982	8.7	6.75	5.64
1983	9.0	6.82	5.69
1984	9.1	6.72	5.61
1985	8.9	6.75	5.65
1986	8.9	6.81	5.66
1987	8.8	6.90	5.70
1988	8.8	6.93	5.67
1989	9.0	7.05	5.72

Source: Commonwealth of Puerto Rico Department of Health and National Center for Health Statistics.

mainland, and represent an area where significant reductions could be achieved.

Despite some improvement in the last decade, the maternal death rate in Puerto Rico remains very high, 19.5 per 100,000 live births in 1989. This rate is 2.5 times that of 7.9 recorded for the mainland in the same year, and considerably above the mainland national goal of less than 5 chosen for the 5-year period ending in 1990.[5]

Evidence suggests that the quality of obstetrical and infant care in the public health care sector of Puerto Rico needs attention.[6,7] Vazquez Calzada and Rivera-Acevedo have indicated that great geographical disparities exist in the quality of prenatal care received by pregnant women throughout the island.[6] The highest rates of low birth weight and infant mortality were recorded for municipalities far removed from the capital city, San Juan, particularly those located in the northern, southern, and western regions of the island. Vazquez-Calzada and Rivera-Acevedo's findings are supported by a 1988 evaluation of the island's system of regionalized perinatal care. Becerra et al.[7] examined the weight-specific neonatal death rates for Puerto Rico and found them to be higher than any on the mainland. These investigators also found that nearly one-half of the infants weighing less than 1500 grams at birth had been delivered at hospitals without neonatal intensive care units.

Table 5 Deaths Under 1 Year of Age per 1,000 Live Births: Puerto Rico and the United States, 1950–1989

		United States	
Year	Puerto Rico	All races	White
1989	14.3	9.8	8.2
1988	12.6	10.0	8.5
1987	14.2	10.1	8.6
1986	13.7	10.4	8.9
1985	14.9	10.6	9.3
1984	15.7	10.8	9.4
1983	17.3	11.2	9.7
1982	17.2	11.5	10.1
1981	18.6	11.9	10.5
1980	18.9	12.6	11.0
1979	19.9	13.1	11.4
1978	18.5	13.8	12.0
1977	20.1	14.1	12.3
1976	20.2	15.2	13.3
1975	20.9	16.1	14.2
1974	23.0	16.7	14.8
1973	24.2	17.7	15.8
1972	27.1	18.5	16.4
1971	27.5	19.1	17.1
1970	28.6	20.0	17.8
1969	29.7	20.9	18.4
1968	29.2	21.8	19.2
1967	32.7	22.4	19.7
1966	37.6	23.7	20.6
1965	43.0	24.7	21.5
1964	51.7	24.8	21.6
1963	44.8	25.2	22.2
1962	28.6	25.3	22.3
1961	42.3	25.3	22.4
1960	43.7	26.0	22.9
1959	48.1	26.4	23.2
1958	53.7	27.1	23.8
1957	50.3	26.3	23.3
1956	55.3	26.0	23.2
1955	55.1	26.4	23.6
1954	57.8	26.6	23.9
1953	63.3	27.8	25.0
1952	66.6	28.4	25.5
1951	67.1	28.4	25.8
1950	68.3	29.2	26.8

Source: Commonwealth of Puerto Rico Department of Health and the National Center for Health Statistics.

Table 6 Leading Causes of Infant Mortality: Puerto Rico and the United States, 1989

Rank	Rate per 100,000 live births	Percent of all deaths
Puerto Rico		
All Causes	1427.5	100.0
1. Disorders related to short gestation and unspecified low birth weight	323.9	22.7
2. Congenital malformations	263.9	18.5
3. Respiratory disease syndrome	245.9	17.2
4. Pneumonia and influenza	67.5	4.7
5. Infections specific to the perinatal period	42.0	2.9
6. Sudden infant death syndrome	27.0	1.9
7. Accidents	25.5	1.8
8. Intrauterine hypoxias and birth asphyxia	21.0	1.5
9. Meningitis	21.0	1.5
10. Newborn affected by complications of the placenta, cord, and membranes	13.5	0.9
United States		
All Causes	981.3	100.0
1. Congenital malformations	200.9	20.5
2. Sudden infant death syndrome	139.4	14.2
3. Disorders related to short gestation and unspecified low birth weight	97.3	9.9
4. Respiratory disease syndrome	89.9	9.2
5. Newborn affected by maternal complications of pregnancy	38.0	2.5
6. Accidents and adverse effects	24.6	2.5
7. Newborn affected by complications of placenta cord and membranes	24.4	2.5
8. Infections specific to the perinatal period	22.1	2.2
9. Intrauterine hypoxia and birth asphyxia	17.9	1.8
10. Pneumonia and influenza	15.7	1.6

Source: Commonwealth of Puerto Rico Department of Health and National Center for Health Statistics.

They concluded that problems existed in access and quality of the neonatal health care being offered in Puerto Rico and recommended that primary preventive efforts focus on strategies to lower the proportion of low and very low-birth-weight infants. They also recommended that secondary prevention efforts concentrate on early detection of high risk cases and referral to the appropriate health care level. These investigators stressed that tertiary care should aim to decrease the neonatal mortality rate.[7]

The nature and quality of maternal and infant care in the public system has been significantly affected by the sheer size of its load (annually, 62.2% of all women giving birth in the Commonwealth of Puerto Rico do so in public hospitals), and the demographic and socioeconomic composition of the population it serves[2] (see Table 3). Users of·this system have a substantially greater inherent risk for morbidity in reproductive outcomes than those receiving care from the private sector. For example, in 1989, 49.5% of all the women giving birth in public hospitals had less than 12 years of education compared to 8.2% for the private sector. A greater proportion of public than private users were adolescents who had received inadequate care (48.5% versus 13.4%) and delivered low-birth-weight infants (10.6 versus 6.4%). The infant mortality rates for users of the public health system in 1989 was 2.5 times greater than that of users of the private health care system (18.1 versus 7.3), reflecting not only the much lower low-birth-weight rate but also in all probability much lower weight-specific death rates. As a matter of fact, the rate of 7.3 infant deaths per 1000 live births recorded for users of the private health care system of Puerto Rico in 1989 was 11% lower than the rate of 8.2 recorded for Caucasians on the mainland in the same year.

Family planning has been used as an important tool to reduce maternal and infant mortality in Puerto Rico. Vazquez Calzada and Morales del Valle, conducted a large-scale study on the use of contraceptive methods.[8] They found that 69% of all women between the ages 15 to 49 had used contraceptives. The five more commonly used methods were: female sterilization (57.1%); contraceptive pills (18.6%); condoms (6.0%); intrauterine devices (4.9%); and male sterilization (4.1%). Among women married for over 20 years, more than 80% had been sterilized.

CHILDREN'S HEALTH

The leading causes of morbidity and mortality for children in Puerto Rico are those typical of developed countries (see Table 7). These conditions include: congenital malformations, accidents, including poisoning; neoplastic diseases; heart and pulmonary diseases; homicides, genetic diseases; and infections, such as pneumonias, acute gastroenteritis, Dengue, and AIDS.

Congenital malformations, especially of the neural tube variety,

Table 7 Five Leading Causes of Childhood Mortality by Age: Puerto Rico, 1989

Rank	Cause	Number of deaths	Percent of all deaths	Rate per 100,000
	1–4 Years of Age			
	All causes	112	100.0	45.4
1.	Accidents	14	12.5%	5.7
2.	Congenital malformations	13	11.6	5.3
3.	Malignant neoplasms	13	11.6	5.3
4.	Pneumonia and influenza	11	9.8	4.5
5.	Homicides	7	6.2	2.8
	Other causes	54	45.5	21.9
	5–9 Years of Age			
	All causes	61	100.0	18.7
1.	Accidents	15	24.6	4.6
2.	Malignant neoplasms	8	13.1	2.5
3.	Congenital malformations	4	6.6	1.2
4.	Heart diseases	3	4.9	0.9
5.	Pneumonia and influenza	2	3.3	0.6
	Other causes	29	47.5	8.9
	10–14 Years of Age			
	All causes	98	100.0	28.5
1.	Accidents	30	30.6	8.7
2.	Malignant neoplasms	15	15.3	4.4
3.	Heart diseases	7	7.1	2.0
4.	Homicides	3	3.1	0.9
5.	Congenital malformations	3	3.1	0.9
	Other causes	40	40.8	11.6
	15–19 Years of Age			
	All causes	238	100.0	70.8
1.	Accidents	90	37.8	26.8
2.	Homicides	53	22.3	15.8
3.	Malignant neoplasms	11	4.6	3.3
4.	Suicides	8	3.4	2.4
5.	Heart diseases	7	2.9	2.1
	Other causes	69	29.0	20.5

Source: Commonwealth of Puerto Rico Department of Health.

seem to be more common in Puerto Rico than in most other Western countries. Data from a study conducted by the Center for Environmental Health of the U.S. Mainland Public Health Service covering the years 1970 through 1984 indicated an average incidence of neural tube defects (NTD) for Puerto Rico of 17.3 per 10 000 live births.[5] Fernandez et al.[9] found an average incidence rate of NTD of 15.7 per 10 000 births (live births and fetal death combined). This prevalence rate, higher than mainland rates, has remained constant, compared to the declining trends evident for most areas of the mainland and elsewhere. The estimated number of children born with NTD in Puerto Rico since 1975 is 603. Between 1980 and 1983, the Vital Statistics Unit of the Commonwealth Department of Health reported an average of 26 deaths per year from NTD.[5] Due to the economic burden that treatment of NTD entails, the majority of these patients are being treated in public health care facilities, mostly at the University of Puerto Rico Pediatric Hospital. At present, there is a clear need for a centralized registry for congenital malformations and for the provision of counseling services to couples who have had children with severe birth defects.

Puerto Rico, being an island, has a high rate of intermarriage. This has led to a high incidence of genetic diseases. A modest Hereditary Disease Program was started in 1980 which was later expanded by means of P.R. Law 84 in 1987.[10,11] The program is now providing screening, diagnostic, and treatment services for some of the most important genetic and metabolic diseases in children. At present, about 95% of all neonates are being screened for phenylketonuria, hypothyroidism, and hemoglobinopathies. The overall incidence of these conditions is as follows: phenylketonuria, 1 per 18 300 newborns; hypothyroidism, 1 per 3920 newborns; and symptomatic hemoglobinopathies, 1 per 3600 newborns. Approximately 15 cases of symptomatic hemoglobinopathies are being diagnosed annually. The overall incidence of abnormal hemoglobins detected is 3.3%.[11]

Hemophilia is a common disease in some towns in the interior of the island. There are about 150 children with hemophilia and related bleeding disorders registered in the Puerto Rico Pediatric Hemophilia Program. That number accounts for about 50% of the total number of hemophilic patients on the island.[12]

Cancer in children in Puerto Rico is one of the 10 leading causes of death for children up to 20 years of age[1,2] (Table 7). A Pediatric Oncology Program, based at the University Pediatric Hospital, provides services to patients referred from all municipalities of the island. This oncology program is affiliated with several national cooperative groups. It contributes patients to many cancer treatment studies, and collaborates and actively participates in the search for new cancer therapies.[13]

In Puerto Rico, accidents and poisonings are a relatively frequent cause of morbidity and mortality in children above one year of age.[14] Injuries are the leading cause of death in childhood and the most frequent cause of injuries is automobile accidents. Drowning is also a fairly common cause of death at all ages.

Lead poisoning occurs sporadically in Puerto Rico, but data on lead poisoning are scarce. A survey conducted in selected neighborhoods of the City of San Juan and Ponce in 1973 indicated that 11 out of 334 children tested (3%) had excessive lead absorption levels.[15] Another survey was conducted in the town of Cataño in 1986 in which 650 children 1 to 5 years of age were tested at random. In this survey, all children had blood lead levels below 25 μg/dl,[16] but 30% had levels above 10 μg/dl, including 9.6% who were between 15 μg/dl and 24 μg/dl.

Homicides and suicides have become one of the 10 leading causes of death among children under 20 years of age,[1,2] but scientific data are scarce.

Child abuse is an important pediatric health and social problem in Puerto Rico. Some 12 289 abused children were identified in 1988–1989. During the same year there were 20 950 active cases registered in the Department of Social Services files. The high rate of child abuse and domestic violence in Puerto Rico is part of the significant social violence and juvenile delinquency problem currently existing on the island.[17,18]

Mortality due to infections has decreased significantly in Puerto Rico in the last few decades. Infections still remain one of the 10 leading causes of death, however, and one of the leading causes of morbidity.[1,2,5]

Dengue has occurred in Puerto Rico for many years. The disease has become hyperendemic since 1964 with multiple dengue virus serotypes being transmitted simultaneously.[19] This change in the epidemiology of dengue has led to the emergence of the severe dengue hemorrhagic fever and fatal dengue shock syndrome (DHF/DSS). In 1986, a significant number of DHF/DSS cases were recorded for the first time in Puerto Rico's history: 29 per 1000 confirmed cases of dengue. There were three confirmed fatalities, but many others were probably undiagnosed.[19]

As documented in the chapter by Zorrilla et al. in this volume, the island's health care system has been taxed severely by the recent epidemic of HIV infection in Puerto Rico, especially in the lower socioeconomic groups. An ongoing neonatal HIV seroprevalence study in the San Juan Region has shown that one in 67 pregnant women in the public health care system is HIV seropositive.[20] In the private sector the prevalence is one in 1250. The neonatal HIV prevalence survey is being expanded to monitor HIV infection in the entire island. In 1989 AIDS emerged as the seventh leading cause of death among individuals 20 to 49 years of age.[2]

It is estimated that 10 to 12.5% of all persons living in Puerto Rico suffer from a form of mental illness. Rates are especially high among children and adolescents coming from families of low socioeconomic status. In a carefully designed study covering the years 1987 through 1990, Canino et al. demonstrated a high prevalence rate and a wide range of mental illnesses in Puerto Rico.[21]

SUMMARY

Despite significant improvement during the last three decades, some of the health levels of Puerto Rico, such as infant mortality, lag considerably behind practically all of the states on the mainland. The greatest disparities are in evidence for women of reproductive age and in infants, children, and adolescents. Information about Puerto Ricans who live on the mainland are not available in the same detail as for residents of the Commonwealth, thus it is difficult to ascertain whether significant disparities are present and, if they are, in what health areas and favoring which of the two population components. In the area of reproductive health, the available data suggest comparable levels between the Puerto Ricans living on the mainland and the two-thirds of Puerto Ricans living in Puerto Rico who utilize the island's public health care system. For Puerto Ricans living in Puerto Rico, who are users of the private health care system of the Commonwealth, the available data indicate levels of reproductive health comparable to or better than those evident for non-Hispanic Caucasians on the mainland.

Improving the public health care system will not be enough to bring about positive changes in the two-thirds of all Commonwealth residents who rely solely on the public health care system. A wide range of efforts are also needed in a variety of areas: an improvement in the employment rate, better housing, better nutrition, and significant changes in negative life-styles such as early childbearing, unsafe sex practices, and use of licit and illicit drugs.

As stated by Rigau-Perez in 1986, the problem of infant and neonatal mortality in Puerto Rico is clearly defined; and effective methods for dealing with it are known. Puerto Rico also has the physical facilities, personnel, and the organizational infrastructure needed to provide the health care needed to reduce infant mortality, but these systems need reinforcement and refinement to reach all segments of the population to the degree warranted.[5]

REFERENCES

1. *Informe Anual de Estadísticas Vitales 1988, Estado Libre Asociado de Puerto Rico*. Departamento de Salud, Administración de Facilidades y Servicios de Salud, Oficina de Estadísticas de Salud [*Vital Statistics Annual Report 1988, Commonwealth of Puerto Rico*. Department of Health, Office of Health Statistics], San Juan, Puerto Rico, April; 1991
2. *Informe Anual de Estadísticas Vitales 1989, Estado Libre Asociado de Puerto Rico*. Departamento de Salud, Administración de Facilidades y Servicios de Salud, Oficina de Estadísticas de Salud [*Vital Statistics Annual Report 1989, Commonwealth of Puerto Rico*. Department of Health, Office of Health Statistics], San Juan, Puerto Rico, November; 1991
3. Wegman ME: Annual summary of vital statistics, 1988. *Pediatrics* 84:943–956, 1989
4. Arbona G, Ramirez de Aarellano AB: *Regionalization of Health Services: The Puerto Rican Experience*. New York, Oxford University Press, 1978
5. Rigau-Pérez JG: La salud durante el embarazo y el primer año de vida en Puerto Rico: Progreso hacia los objetivos nacionales de salud para 1990 [Health during pregnancy and in the first year of life in Puerto Rico: Progress toward 1990 health objectives] (VIII). *Bol. Asoc. Med. P. Rico* 78:244–252, 1986
6. Vázquez Calzada JL, Rivera-Acevedo S: Prenatal care, infant birth weight and infant mortality in Puerto Rico. *P. Rico Health Sc. J.* 8:283–288, 1989
7. Becerra JE, Pérez de Saliceti N, Smith JC: Evaluation of a regionalized perinatal care system through linked infant birth and death certificates: Puerto Rico 1980–84. *P. Rico Health Sc. J.* 8:305–311, 1989
8. Vázquez Calzada JL, Morales del Valle Z: Female sterilization in Puerto Rico, and its demographic effectiveness. *P. Rico Health Sc. J.* 1:68–79, 1982
9. Fernandez FR, Colón R, Fernandez SA, Fernandez RM: Neural tube defects: A study in Puerto Rico. *Bol. Asoc. Med. P. Rico* 82:57–61, 1990
10. Santiago-Borrero PJ: The Puerto Rican sickle cell disease clinic and its transition into a genetic disease program. *Bol. Asoc. Med. P. Rico* 75:583–540, 1983
11. Santiago-Borrero PJ, Valcarcel M, Caceres M, Montalvo F: Geographical distribution of abnormal hemoglobins in Puerto Rico. *Bol. Asoc. Med. P. Rico* 75:447–451, 1983
12. Santiago-Borrero PJ, Casanova R: Response of patients with hemophilia and Von Willebrand's Disease to DDAVP. *Bol. Asoc. Med. P. Rico* 82:207–210, 1990
13. Clavell LA, Gelber RD, Harvey JC, Hithcock-Bryan J, Cassady JR, Tarbell NJ, et al: Four agent induction and intensive asparaginase therapy for treatment of acute lymphoblatic leukemia. *N. Eng. J. Med.* 315:657–663, 1986

14. Rigau-Pérez JG: Prevención de accidentes y control de lesiones en Puerto Rico: Progreso hacia los objetivos nacionales de salud para 1990 [Accident prevention and control of injuries in Puerto Rico: Progress toward 1990 national health objectives] (IX). *Bol. Asoc. Med. P. Rico* 78:55–60, 1986
15. Rigau-Pérez JG: El control de los agentes tóxicos ambientales en Puerto Rico: Progreso hacia los objetivos nacionales de salud para 1990 [The control of environmental toxic agents in Puerto Rico: Progress toward 1990 national health objectives] (XV). *Bol. Asoc. Med. P. Rico* 79:251–258, 1987
16. Santiago-Borrero PJ, Rivera-Caragol E: Undue exposure to Lead among preschool children in San Juan. *P. Rico Health Sc. J.* 6:172 (abstract), 1987
17. Rigau-Pérez JG: Control de estres y el comportamiento violento en Puerto Rico: progreso hacia los objetivos nacionales de salud para 1990 (VIII). *Bol. Asoc. Med. P. Rico* 78:391–398, 1986
18. Olmo MC: *Abuso y negligencia infantil en Puerto Rico: Consideraciones socioeconomicas* Infant abuse and neglect in Puerto Rico: Socioeconomic considerations]. Doctoral thesis, Centro Caribeño de Estudios Post-graduados, San Juan, Puerto Rico, 1977
19. Gubler DJ: Dengue in Puerto Rico. *Bol. Asoc. Med. P. Rico* 79:343–346, 1987
20. Santiago-Borrero PJ, Rullan J, Garcia M, Gwinn M: HIV seroprevalence in newborns from San Juan and nearby town. *P. Rico Health Sc. J.* 9:272 (abstract), 1990
21. Canino GJ, Bird HR, Shrout PE, Rubio-Stipec M, Bravo M, Martinez R, Sesman M, Guevara LM: The prevalence of specific psychiatric disorders in Puerto Rico. *Arch. Gen. Psychiatry* 44:727–735, 1987

4

Acquired Immune Deficiency Syndrome (AIDS) in Women and Children in Puerto Rico

CARMEN ZORRILLA, CLEMENTE DIAZ, JOSEFINA ROMAGUERA, AND MILLIE MARTIN

Puerto Rico was impacted early in the acquired immunodeficiency syndrome (AIDS) epidemic. The first case reported to the Centers for Disease Control (CDC) Surveillance Unit in the island (Latin American Center for Sexually Transmitted Diseases) was documented early in 1981. As opposed to the pattern seen on the U.S. mainland the epidemic in Puerto Rico primarily involved young male injection drug users (IDU). Sixty percent of all cumulative AIDS cases in adult/adolescent men in Puerto Rico have drug use as a risk behavior contrasted with 25% on the mainland.[1,2] An additional 10% report injection drug use plus homosexual/bisexual behavior as the main risk categories. On the

CARMEN ZORRILLA, CLEMENTE DIAZ, JOSEFINA ROMAGUERA, and MILLIE MARTIN • Department of Obstetrics and Gynecology, University of Puerto Rico School of Medicine, San Juan, Puerto Rico 00936-5067.

Puerto Rican Women and Children: Issues in Health, Growth, and Development, edited by Gontran Lamberty and Cynthia Garcia Coll. Plenum Press, New York, 1994.

mainland this group constitutes 5%. By contrast only 22% of all AIDS cases in men in Puerto Rico have been reported as related to homosexual/bisexual behavior, whereas on the mainland it accounts for 53%. The proportion of AIDS cases in males associated with homosexual/bisexual behavior in Puerto Rico has been stable through the years; nevertheless it is a significant cohort of infected men. Most human immunovirus (HIV) transmission to women comes from drug use or sex with an IDU. Bisexual behavior in the young Puerto Rican population may play a significant role in 10 to 20% of women.[3]

The differences in epidemic profile with most cases related to IDU had a marked influence in subsequent transmission patterns in Puerto Rico. As shown in Figure 1 the cumulative number of AIDS cases in Puerto Rico is steadily increasing. A total of 8561 cases have been reported as of October 1, 1992.[2] The rate of increase is highest for women and children. Figure 2 describes AIDS cases in females and risk factors on the mainland and Puerto Rico.

Heterosexual transmission is the major route for transmitting HIV among women in Puerto Rico. In 1991 it accounted for 58% of all AIDS cases in women on the island. By contrast, 37% of females on the

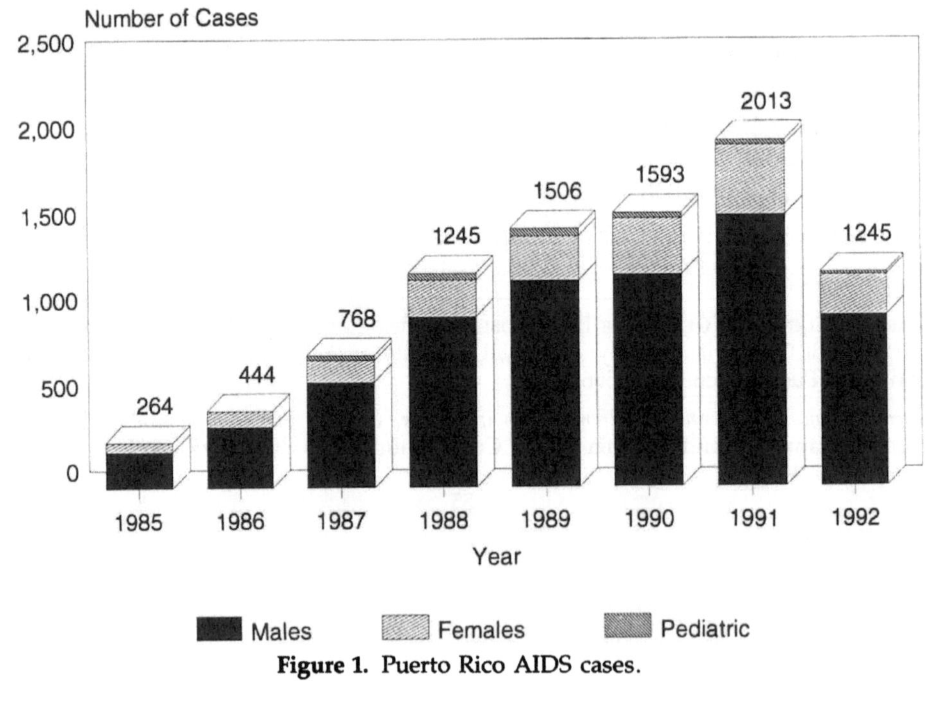

Figure 1. Puerto Rico AIDS cases.

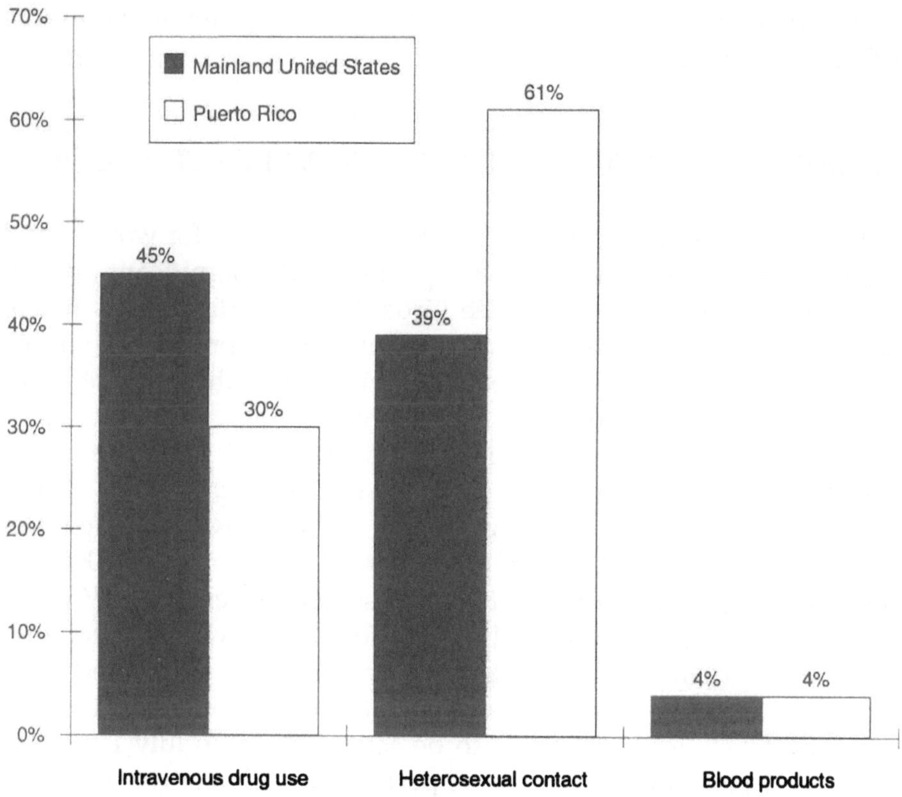

Figure 2. Adult/adolescent AIDS cases (1992) risk factors (Females).

mainland were infected by sexual contact in 1991. The heterosexual transmission of AIDS has been studied by several investigators[4,5] who have found that the transmission of HIV is more efficient from male to female than from female to male.[6] The preferential transmission, from male to female, has been reported to occur with other sexually transmitted infections such as Chlamydia Trachomatis and Neisseria Gonorrhea.[7]

In 1991, Puerto Rico ranked second when compared to other states in AIDS cases in women per capita (rate 25.1 per 100 000 population). Puerto Rico also ranked second in overall AIDS cases (50.9 per 100 000) and third in pediatric AIDS cases (rate 30.4 per 100 000). These grim statistics reflect the overrepresentation of Puerto Ricans in the worldwide HIV pandemic. If Puerto Rico were an independent nation, it would rank fourth in the world in AIDS cases per capita. These facts underscore the major public health challenge this epidemic represents for Puerto Rican society.

PRENATAL AND NEONATAL SEROPREVALENCE STUDIES

Given the high proportion of AIDS cases reported for women and children in Puerto Rico, we would expect to find a significant portion of the population infected with the virus, but in earlier stages where disease is not always apparent. We completed a seroprevalence survey that demonstrates how widespread this virus is in the population of pregnant women in our hospital catchment area.

In 1986 the University of Puerto Rico School of Medicine established a prenatal HIV screening program in the Metropolitan Health Region in Puerto Rico. This region, which includes five municipalities adjacent to the capital city of San Juan, has a population of 400 000 and approximately 5000 deliveries per year. A screening test for HIV infection (Elisa test, Genetic Systems Inc.) is offered to all women attending public prenatal clinics. This screening is voluntary, is offered after counseling, and requires written consent. Of all patients attending these prenatal clinics, 97% agree to be screened. From July 1, 1990 to June 26, 1991 a total of 4700 tests were performed. All positive screening tests are then confirmed by means of a Western Blot (Du Pont). The seroprevalence rate in our region for the period 1987–1988 was 1.4%. This rate was similar to the neonatal seroprevalence rates of Hispanics in New York State for the same period, 1.31% for Hispanic pregnant women[8] (0.13% for Caucasian women, 1.82% for African-Americans).

In contrast to most prenatal seroprevalence studies, the seropositivity rate in our population has been decreasing since 1990. For the period July 1991 to June 1992 a rate of 0.9% was reported. Other seroprevalence surveys show a stable trend.[9] Many factors might explain our decreasing trend: attrition, migration, lack of screening, or decrease in fertility. All of these factors might be contributing except lack of screening because of the universal nature of the HIV counseling and testing available in our hospital. The number of samples obtained through the years parallels the number of deliveries. In our opinion a decrease in the fertility rate is the most important factor and it is probably due to the family planning services offered to HIV-infected women who are participants of this comprehensive program. Out of 100 consecutive patients enrolled for our perinatal transmission study, only two subsequent pregnancies were noted in the first two years of the study.

In sum, the rate of seropositivity during pregnancy for the Puerto Rico Metropolitan Health Region is high. One of every 100 infants born in this region is at risk for acquiring HIV. One of every 100 pregnant women in the region is infected with this virus. Comprehensive intervention that includes family planning options can reduce the number of infants born to HIV-infected women if it is their choice.

How representative are these findings as contrasted with those obtained in the rest of the island? By comparing our data with that of other investigators we can validate our findings. Since 1990 the Centers for Disease Control in Atlanta has sponsored a program for anonymous neonatal HIV testing in Puerto Rico. Initial reports for public hospitals in San Juan showed a 1.45% seroprevalence, which is in agreement with the seroprevalence in our public prenatal screening program. Public hospitals in adjacent towns (Bayamon and Caguas) reported 0.97% prevalence, and private hospitals in San Juan and Bayamon had a 0.08% prevalence rate.[10]

These seroprevalence rates primarily reflect the extent of the epidemic in women of reproductive age. These figures will likely translate into a high seroprevalence rate in children in the future. The prenatal and neonatal seroprevalence studies show that the probability of caring for an HIV-infected mother ranges from one in 67 to one in 1250 deliveries. This reenforces the need for adhering to the currently recommended universal precautions for prevention of transmission. In addition, understanding the natural evolution of HIV infection will be an essential component for providing appropriate care of an increasingly large segment of the population of women and children in Puerto Rico.

WOMEN FOLLOW-UP

Since 1986, a follow-up clinic of HIV-infected women was established at the OB-GYN Department of the University of Puerto Rico School of Medicine. Up to April 1993, more than 400 women have been evaluated. An understanding of the needs of this population will help us anticipate how to care for the future cohort of AIDS cases in women in Puerto Rico.

All seropositive pregnant women from our catchment area are followed by us at a centralized facility. We compared 188 seropositive pregnant women with 101 seronegative controls selected from the same population.

The mean age of the seropositive patients was 25.6 years compared to 25.4 years among the uninfected women. In both groups the age range was from 15 to 42 years, and sociodemographic background was similar. A higher proportion of seropositive women are either single or engaged in consensual unions when compared to the control group. The proportion of patients who were legally married was lower for the seropositive then for the controls. Thus, mandatory HIV testing when obtaining a marriage license would not identify a great number of the infected females. Nevertheless, we have observed that the majority of the seropositive women are engaged in stable long-term (>3 years) consensual relationships (see Table 1).

Risk Assessment in Women

Most of the HIV infected women in our cohort acquired the infection through heterosexual contact (64.6%). The large majority of those women were aware of their partners' risk behavior, but were unable to learn and practice safer sex. Studies in other populations of IDU men showed that among participants with both "steady"and "casual" partners, using condoms all the time was more common with casual (72%) than with steady (30%) partners.[11] Alternative preventive strategies are needed for these women. They have suggested to us that condom use messages should target sexual behavior within primary relationships where partners do not know their HIV status, are discordant for HIV infection, or one or more partners are continuing activities that pose a risk for HIV infection.

A substantial number reported no risk factors upon interview

Table 1 Marital Status

	HIV Positive N = 188	HIV Negative N = 101	Z-Test
Single	23%	6%	*
Married	28%	70%	*
Consensual	35%	17%	*
Separated/Divorced	12%	5%	NS
Widowed	2%	—	NS

* = Less than .5%.

(17.27%). Since these women were unaware of their partner's risk behavior it may well be that this group of women are partners of bisexual men. A recent survey[3] of young men in San Juan showed that 20% of those self-described as heterosexuals had experienced sex with men in the previous three months. Almost the same proportion of self-described homosexual men acknowledged sex with women in the past three months. This group of women would not be identified by campaigns based on the acknowledgment of risk behavior. In this context, these women were at a disadvantage since they were unaware of their own risk. Counseling and screening for HIV infection during pregnancy should be an important component of the care offered to women in high prevalence areas. We recommend that such an option should be available to all women of childbearing age and particularly those attending prenatal clinics.

Life-Styles and Substance Use/Abuse

We have also documented certain life-styles that are more prevalent in women with HIV infection than in the women in our comparison group. These include cigarette smoking and the use of nonintravenous substances such as marijuana, cocaine, and crack (see Table 2). A higher proportion of HIV seropositive women gave histories of cigarette smoking and experimenting with other substances, in particular marijuana, cocaine, and crack. Half of the women who reported using IV drugs engaged in needle sharing. In our opinion cultural patterns of needle-sharing behavior in drug users may partially explain the striking dissemination of HIV in Hispanic and African-American drug users.

Table 2 Life-Styles

	HIV Positive N = 188	HIV Negative N = 101	Chi square
Cigarette smoking (ever)	58%	36%	*
Cigarette smoking (actual)	44%	28%	*
Marijuana (ever)	48%	8%	*
Cocaine (ever)	44%	5%	*
Crack (ever)	39%	1%	*
Intravenous drug user (ever)	18%	2%	*
Sex partner intravenous drug user (ever)	55%	6%	*

* = Less than .5%.

The association between seropositivity and cigarette smoking and/ or other non-IV substance use is a reflection of unhealthy life-styles rather than a biologic cofactor for HIV transmission. A recent study[12] found a higher proportion of smokers among HIV seroconverters but they could not prove a biologic association. They suggested that cigarette smoking may be a surrogate marker for continued high-risk sexual behavior.

Many women continued to smoke cigarettes during pregnancy suggesting that educational campaigns directed against cigarette smoking are not being effective in this group. If these interventions are not working, then interventions in the socially forbidden areas of sexuality may prove also to be ineffective. New approaches are needed and cultural considerations (e.g., male–female relationship) should be incorporated into educational interventions. Efforts need to be directed into empowering women to negotiate sex and use condoms. Research also has to be directed toward developing male-independent female protective methods such as intravaginal virucidal agents and barriers.

In terms of sexual practices, we found a statistically significant increased prevalence of receptive anal intercourse in the group infected with HIV. Two-fifths (40%) of the seropositives and one-third (28%) of the seronegatives reported such a practice, illustrating that heterosexual couples also engage in this HIV risk-behavior, but less frequently.

Receptive anal intercourse was the only sexual practice for which there was a significant statistical difference among the two groups. No differences were found for oral sex (29% vs. 25%), oral sex with male ejaculation (17% vs. 13%), or coitus during menses (20% for both groups).

Although this population of low socioeconomic pregnant women from the adjacent municipalities of San Juan is not a representative sample of the Puerto Rican population, the information presented here is the first data that correlates life-styles, sexual practices, and sociodemographic information with HIV serostatus.

In our population, the proportion of women with identifiable risk factors is four times greater than the proportion found to be HIV infected. Prevention programs directed toward those women at risk could make a significant impact. Acquired immunodeficiency syndrome and HIV prevention are topics that should be included in all pregnancy educational programs in high prevalence regions. A total revision of our current health care delivery practices may be necessary in order to prevent, in a culturally sensitive manner, the heterosexual transmission of AIDS. In order to effectively decrease female participation in high-risk sexual practices both empowerment of women and incorporation of both partners in sexual decision making is imperative.

Gynecological Manifestations

Human immunovirus infected women have been reported to have increased risk for development of cervical cancer and present with advanced stages of cancer at a younger age.[13–14] In this section, we report data from gynecologic evaluations of nonpregnant women followed at a follow-up clinic as described on page 59. Only nonpregnant women are included because pregnancy alters the manifestations of cervical disease. We compared the cervical cytology results (PAP smear) from four different groups: (1) HIV-infected women (N = 46) with associated symptoms (adenopathies, fevers, recurrent vaginitis, diarrhea); (2) HIV-infected women (N = 47) without symptoms; (3) a sample of 119 patients from the general gynecology clinics in our hospital; and (4) a sample of 150 PAP smears reported from a private pathology laboratory located in San Juan.

As seen by other investigators, women with HIV infection are more likely to develop or express coinfection with Human Papilloma Virus (HPV) (16%) than our general gynecologic population (1.7%) or private patients (.7%). In addition, symptomatic HIV-infected women are more likely than asymptomatic HIV-infected women to express HPV (22% vs. 4%). One explanation for this increased expression may be immunosuppression, which may be more evident in the symptomatic women than in the asymptomatic. Cervical cancer and HPV have also been reported in chronically immunosuppressed patients such as renal transplant recipients.[18]

Similarly, the relative frequencies of cervical dysplasia is higher among HIV-infected groups (45% for those with symptoms and 17% for those without symptoms as compared to 1.7% for the general gynecologic population and 2% for private patient). The relationship between HIV infection, HPV coinfection, and the development of cervical dysplasia or cancer is of importance for those caring for HIV-infected women. Since gynecologic malignancies may be an expression of immunosuppression that may precede or accompany HIV symptomatology, these manifestations may be considered a gender specific expression of HIV disease.

Other genital tract manifestations of HIV disease include increased incidence and severity of pelvic infections[19] specifically those associated with sexual transmission. Again, the increased severity of the pelvic infections in these women may be secondary to their immunosuppression.

AIDS IN CHILDREN IN PUERTO RICO

There are two major centers that provide care for children with HIV infection in Puerto Rico: the San Juan City Hospital and the University Pediatric Hospital. Over 500 children with symptomatic HIV diseases have been seen within these two institutions since 1983. The greater San Juan Metropolitan Region is served by the San Juan City Hospital, while the University Pediatric Hospital serves the medical care needs of children from the five adjacent municipalities.

The University Pediatric Hospital (UPH) is also the major tertiary center for the care of children with HIV infection, outside of the San Juan Metropolitan Area. This 90-bed children's hospital is the main teaching and research center for the University of Puerto Rico School of Medicine. Children with HIV infection are referred from primary care centers or any of five secondary level Regional Hospitals. Referral to UPH is made for immunologic evaluation, treatment of acute infections, and longitudinal follow-up. Care for children with HIV infection is provided by a multidisciplinary team in which pediatricians, nurses, and social workers are the central hub. Ambulatory services are offered in a specialized designated unit with access to subspecialty consultation and follow-up; as well as special services like nutritional and respiratory therapy support.

Population Profile

In December 1984 the first child with AIDS was admitted to the UPH. To date, 250 symptomatic children have been followed. As of July 1st, 1992, 64% of the children were alive (see Figure 3). This overall mortality has remained rather stable during the last four years. The marked increase in the number of children seen in our institution with HIV disease is also shown in Figure 4.

The age breakdown of children with symptoms related to their HIV infection is seen in Figure 5. The median age was 59.2 months with a range of 0 to 169 months. The mean age was 62 months. This contrasts

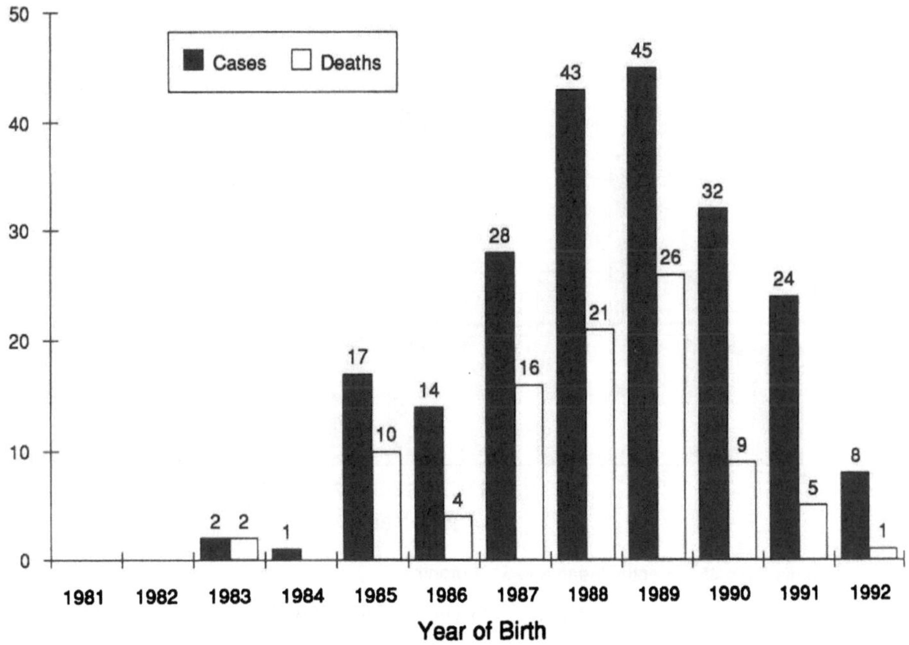

Figure 3. Reported pediatric cases of AIDS in the University Pediatric Hospital, San Juan, Puerto Rico as of October 6, 1992.

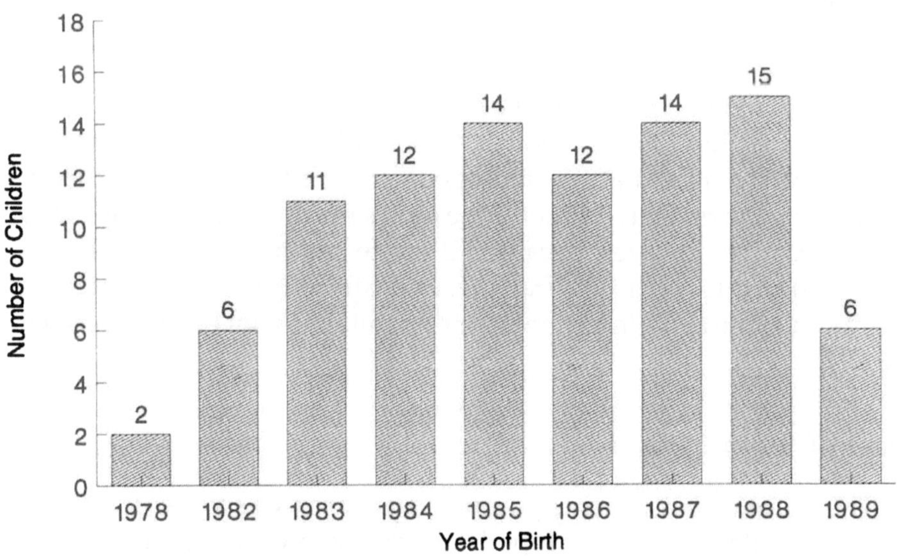

Figure 4. Pediatric HIV disease, University Pediatric Hospital, San Juan, Puerto Rico.

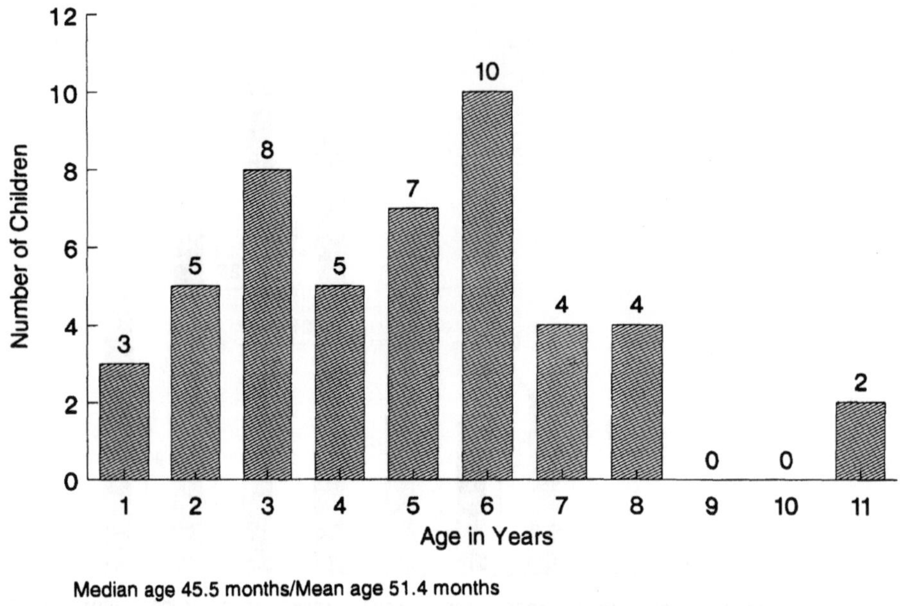

Figure 5. Pediatric HIV disease, University Hospital, San Juan, Puerto Rico.

with our initial experience during 1984–1985 with a younger group of children, mostly below 24 months of age. In our opinion, in agreement with others, this underscores the need for redefining perinatal acquired pediatric HIV disease. This is similar to what has occurred for other chronic diseases of children.

The mode of transmission of HIV infection amongst these 250 children is as follows: In 98% of the cases, transmission of HIV occurred perinatally from an infected mother to her child. Seventy-four percent of the mothers were sexual partners of HIV-infected men, most of whom were IV drug users. Only 26% of these mothers admitted to intravenous drug usage. Two children became HIV infected as a result of sexual abuse from an infected adult. Transfusion-acquired (2% of current cases in our population) HIV infection in our hospital has not been seen since 1986.

Onset of Symptoms

The age range at which symptoms appeared was wide: 1 week of age, in an infant who developed laboratory proven gram negative bacterial sepsis, to 8 years, in a perinatally acquired HIV-infected asymptomatic girl. At that age she developed a decrease in CD4 lymphocyte cell count and progressive neurologic deficits associated with the onset of opportunistic infections.

The median age at which HIV-related symptoms appeared was 8.4 months, while the median age at diagnosis was 22 months. Because of earlier identification and referral, children have been diagnosed at a younger age during the last three years.

The early appearance of symptoms related to HIV infection did correlate with a poor prognostic outcome. Children with onset of HIV-related symptoms prior to the age of 6 months had a mortality rate of 92%, which contrasts markedly with the overall mortality amongst children of 36%. In particular, the appearance of pneumonia caused by Pneumocystis carinii (PCP) during this age period carried a much higher mortality (90% vs. 64%) than when the first episode was diagnosed beyond a year of age.

Signs and Symptoms

Based on our review of clinical data for 1990, a broad range of signs and symptoms related to perinatal HIV acquired infection in children were evident in our population.[9] Nonspecific but frequent findings in children at the time of diagnosis included generalized adenopathy and slow and delayed growth. Infections accounted for the largest share of morbidity in these children. As shown in Table 3, 37 cases of specific opportunistic infections, as listed in the CDC surveillance definition for AIDS, were diagnosed.

Recurrent severe bacterial infections were documented in 40 children. Other specified secondary infectious diseases, such as recurrent

Table 3 Documented Opportunistic Infections in Order of Greater to Lower Frequency, University Pediatric Hospital, San Juan, Puerto Rico

Pneumocystis carinii pneumonia
Systemic or mucocutaneous candidiasis
Disseminated CMV
Persistent cryptosporidiosis
Disseminated herpes simplex
Disseminated *M.* tuberculosis
Cerebral toxoplasmosis
Disseminated histoplasmosis

oropharyngeal thrush or herpes, were present in 47 of our cases. Encephalopathic HIV disease as evidenced by progressive loss of neurologic function, or developmental milestones, was seen in 28 of our patients.

Opportunistic malignancies secondary to HIV infection in our cohort have been seen in eight cases: Burkitt's lymphoma (4), undifferentiated lymphoma (2), acute lymphocytic leukemia (1), and Hodgkin's disease (1).

Mortality

The overall mortality rate has remained stable during the last three years. However, we found different mortality rates in subgroups of children. The different classes in the current classification system for pediatric HIV infection of the CDC[14] had differing probabilities of survival. As would be expected, the highest mortality was associated with the presence of opportunistic infections. Progressive neurologic involvement was also associated with high mortality.

SUMMARY AND RECOMMENDATIONS

Puerto Rico has experienced a disproportionate share of the world's HIV pandemic. The expanding epidemic will have important implications on the delivery of health services on our island.

Based on our experience of being one of the first programs to universally offer HIV counseling and testing during pregnancy we strongly recommend such practice. Major benefits are already evident based on our early initiation of antiretroviral therapy for women and children with evidence of immune impairment even in the absence of symptoms. We also offer pregnant women identified as HIV infected reproductive decision-making options such as pregnancy continuation or interruption, and family planning (short-term or permanent). Another benefit of prenatal HIV testing is the option to intervene during pregnancy with antiretrovirals or vaccines to decrease the perinatal transmission of this virus.

Current CDC guidelines for the care of infants born to HIV-infected women include initiation of preventative strategies to decrease the early mortality caused by Pneumocystis carinii pneumonia (PCP). Effective medication is available to decrease this significant risk and should be initiated at one month of age. The early identification of these infants may be lifesaving.

The clinical management of HIV infected women requires periodic gynecologic evaluations to detect potentially treatable conditions such as pelvic inflammatory disease (PID), recurrent candida vaginitis, or cervical intraepithelial neoplasia.

Research efforts should be directed toward the development of preventive devices for women such as intravaginal virucides or antivirals. Sexual risk reduction messages should address primary as well as casual relationships in a culturally appropriate manner.

Women and children sustain a share of the burden of AIDS in our society. In October 1990 a publication of the World Health Organization (WHO)[20] stated:

> [S]ocial, economic and cultural conditions are fueling the epidemic, contributing particularly to women's risk of acquiring and transmitting HIV infection. Therefore, the ultimate solutions to the AIDS pandemic will not be found without acknowledging and addressing these conditions. One of the most critical of these is the status of women. Such things as inferior social and legal rights, little or no voice in sexual matters, and the added burden of serving as caregivers and managers of their families' daily needs even when they themselves are ill add up to what has been referred to as a social vulnerability to infection among women.

This has already had important social and economic implications for many Puerto Rican women and children. The data presented in this chapter alert us to some of these negative consequences. Yet, the full impact of this crisis and cost to society has still to be felt.

REFERENCES

1. Department of Health and Human Services Public Health Service, Centers for Disease Control (CDC): *HIV/AIDS Surveillance*, Year-end edition, 1992
2. Central Office for AIDS Affairs, Puerto Rico Health Department: *AIDS Surveillance Report*, Puerto Rico, 1992
3. Crandon J: A study concerning HIV related knowledge, attitudes and behaviors in a sample of Puerto Rican men and its relevance to AIDS education, prevention and outreach in San Juan, P.R., in 7th International Conference on AIDS, Abstract No. PoD 5830. Amsterdam, The Netherlands, 1992
4. Rehmet S, Staszweski S, Wangeheim S, Bergmann L, Helm EB, Doerr HW, Stille W: HIV transmission rates and co-factors in heterosexual couples. 6th International Conference on AIDS, Frankfurt FGR Abstract Th.C.582. San Francisco, CA, 1990

5. Falciano M, Ferri F, Macedonio A: Heterosexual transmission of HIV; A 4-year-old follow up. 7th International Conference on AIDS, Abstract M.C., 3070. Florence, Italy, 1991
6. Handsfield HH: Gonorrhea and uncomplicated gonococcal infection, in: Holmekk KK, Maidh PA, Sparling PF, Wiesner PJ (eds): *Sexually Transmitted Diseases*. New York: McGraw-Hill, 1984, pp 205–220
7. Noviek LF, Berns D, Stricof R, Sterns R, Pass K, Wethers J: HIV seroprevalence in newborns in New York State. *JAMA* 261:1745–50, 1989
8. U.S. Department of Health and Human Services, Public Health Service, Centers for Disease Control. *National HIV Surveillance Summary Results through 1990*, Vol. 2, 1990
9. Santiago-Borrero PJ, Rullan J, Garcia M, Gorrin M: HIV seroprevalence in newborns from San Juan and nearby towns. 12th Annual Research Forum, Abstract A-42. University of Puerto Rico Medical Sciences Campus, 1990
10. Noviek LF, Berns D, Stricof R, Sterns R, Pass K, Wethers J: HIV seroprevalence in newborns in New York State. *JAMA* 261:1745–1750, 1989
11. Condom use among male infecting drug users—New York City, 1987–1990. *Morbidity and Mortality Weekly Report* 41:617–620, 1992
12. David N, Burns, Kramer A, Yellin F: Cigarette smoking: A modifier of HIV Type I infection. *J. AIDS* 4:76–83, 1991
13. Rellihan M, Dooley D, Burke T et al: Rapidly progressive squamous cervical cancer in a patient with HIV infection. *Gynecology Oncology* 36:435–438, 1990
14. Schwartz L, Carcangiu M, Bradham L et al: Rapidly progressive squamous cell carcinoma of the cervix with HIV infection: Clinical opinion. *Gynecology Oncology* 41:255–258, 1991
15. Feingold, Vermund S, Burk R, Kelly K: Cervical cytologic abnormalities and Papilloma virus in women infected with HIV. *J. of AIDS* 3:896–903, 1990
16. Maiman M, Tarrcone N, Viera J, Suarez J, Serur E, Boyce J: Colposcopic evaluation of human immunodeficiency virus seropositive women. *Obstet. & Gynecol.* 78:84–88, 1991
17. Zorrilla C, Romaguera J, Corrada R, Diaz C, Diaz R, Zweig M: Increased incidence of cervical intraepithelial neoplasia (CIN) and human Papilloma virus (HPV) in cervical smears of HIV seropositive women in Puerto Rico. 7th International Conference on AIDS, Abstract M.C. 3170. Florence, Italy, 1991
18. Halpert R, Fruchter R, Sedlis A, Butt K, Boyce J, Sillman F: Human Papilloma virus and lower genital neoplasia in renal transplant patients. *Obstet. & Gynecol.* 68:251–258, 1986
19. Hoegsberg B, Abulafia O, Sedlis A, Feldman J, Des Jalais D, Landesman S, Minkoff H: Sexually transmitted diseases and HIV infection among women with pelvic inflammatory disease. *Amer. J. Obstet. Gynecol.* 163:1135–1139, 1990
20. Women and AIDS: The growing crisis. *HIV/AIDS Prevention Newsletter* 2:1–2, 1991

5

Demographic and Health Characteristics of Puerto Rican Mothers and Their Babies, 1990

STEPHANIE J. VENTURA

INTRODUCTION

This chapter presents and analyzes data on births amongst Puerto Rican women residing on the U.S. mainland as they compare to four other Hispanic subgroups and with Caucasian and African-American non-Hispanic women. The data were derived from the official birth certificates submitted by states to the National Center for Health Statistics (NCHS) during the calendar year 1990. Forty-eight states and the District of Columbia contributed to the pooled data on Hispanics, which represented about 99% of the estimated 600 000 total Hispanic births on the mainland in 1990. Of these, nearly 59 000 births were to Puerto Rican mothers.[1]

STEPHANIE J. VENTURA • Division of Vital Statistics, National Center for Health Statistics, Centers for Disease Control and Prevention, U.S. Public Health Service, Hyattsville, Maryland 20782.

Puerto Rican Women and Children: Issues in Health, Growth, and Development, edited by Gontran Lamberty and Cynthia Garcia Coll. Plenum Press, New York, 1994.

Since practically all births are registered, birth certificate data have the unique advantage of offering universal coverage. Moreover, information contained on the birth certificate is very complete for nearly every participating state. Although the information on the birth certificate allows for births to be classified by the national origin of the mother, the father, or both, NCHS has opted to tabulate births according to the Hispanic origin of the mother. The data analyzed for this chapter makes it clear how important it is to differentiate among the various Hispanic subgroups. Data from the U.S. Bureau of the Census on age distribution, income level, family composition, occupation, etc., attest to the importance of making these categorical distinctions.[2]

AGE AND BIRTH ORDER

An important component of the fertility of a given population is the incidence of childbearing by adolescents. Women who begin childbearing at relatively young ages tend to have more low-birth-weight infants and shorter intervals between pregnancies. This places these infants at a higher risk for mortality during their first year of life and for suboptimal growth and development in childhood. Early childbearing also leads to higher overall fertility which impacts on the extent of resources, monetary or otherwise, that will be available per child in a household. This also influences survival during the first year of life and, among those who survive the first year, how healthy a child may turn out to be as a teenager or as a young adult.

In 1990, teenage births accounted for 22% of all births to Puerto Rican mothers, higher than for any other Hispanic group, and nearly as high as the level for African-American non-Hispanic mothers which was 23% (Figure 1). Teenage mothers accounted for 17% of all Mexican births, but only 8% of Cuban-American and 10% of Caucasian non-Hispanic births. Among Puerto Rican teenage mothers, 42% were 17 years or younger, an age group considered to be at high risk for poor maternal and infant outcomes (i.e., early onset of labor, low birth weight, etc.). This is nearly as high as the level for African-American non-Hispanic teenagers, 44%, but considerably above the level for Caucasian non-Hispanic teenagers, 31%. Age-specific birth rates, which measure the level of childbearing for a given age group, were two to three times as high for Mexican-American and Puerto Rican

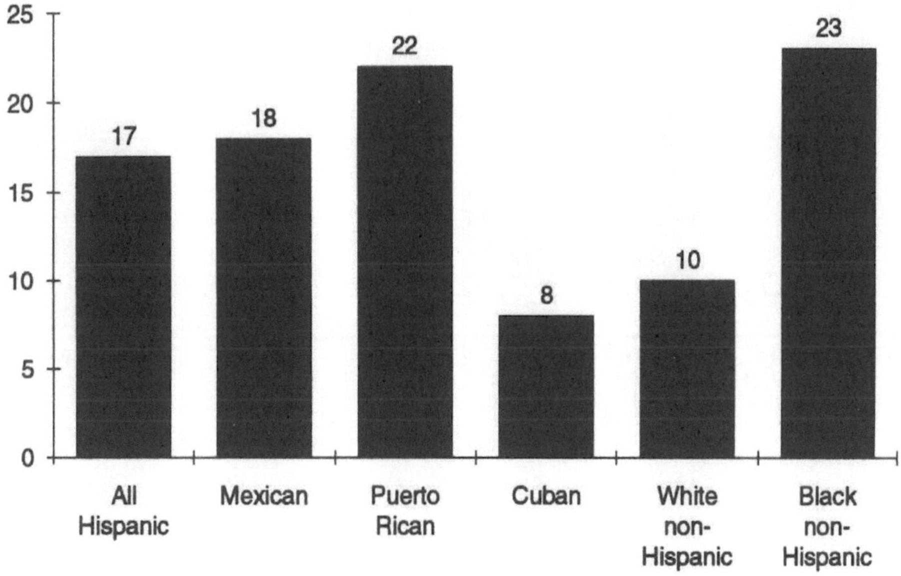

Figure 1. Percent of births to teenage mothers, 1990.

teens (102–108 per 1000) as for Cuban-American and Caucasian non-Hispanic teens (30–43 per 1000).

What may be responsible for the high level of teenage childbearing exhibited by Hispanics of Puerto Rican and Mexican origin? Data from the most recent cycle of the National Survey of Family Growth (NSFG) conducted by NCHS suggest that about half of all Hispanic and non-Hispanic teens are sexually active.[3] Unfortunately, the NSFG sample was not large enough to permit analysis for individual Hispanic subgroups. Information on pregnancy resolution among pregnant teenagers in New York City suggests that abortion is less often used by pregnant Hispanic teens, including Puerto Ricans.[4] A study of abortion from the Alan Guttmacher Institute's 1987 survey also indicated that Hispanic teens who obtain an abortion are less likely to have ever used contraception.[5] This suggests a need for more outreach, education, and family planning services among sexually active Hispanic teens.

Parity, the number of previous live births, is also high for Puerto Rican mothers. About one in eight, or 13%, of all Puerto Rican women giving birth in 1990 was having her fourth or higher order child (Figure 2). This is a somewhat smaller proportion than that observed among

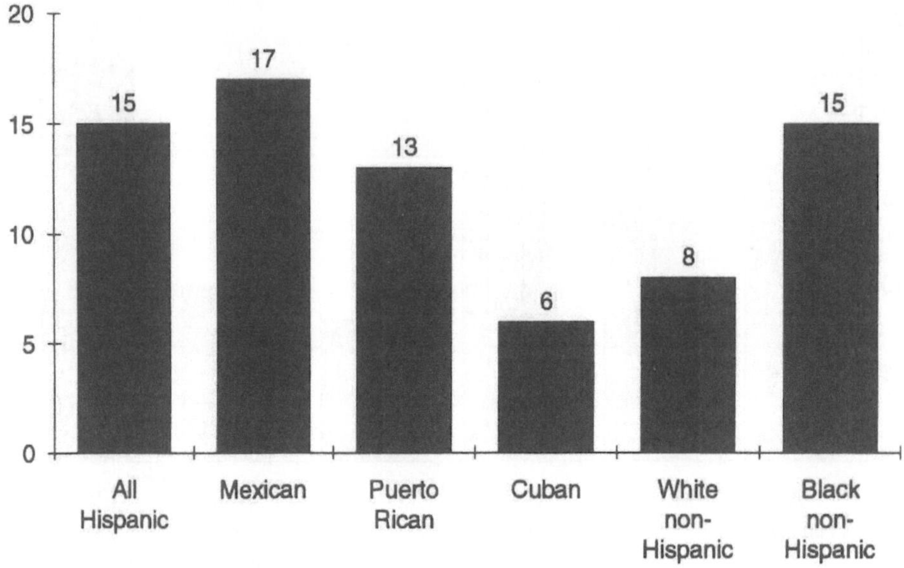

Figure 2. Percent of births 4th and high order, 1990.

Mexican-American women, 17%, but considerably higher than for Cuban-American or Caucasian non-Hispanic women, 6 to 8%. A pattern of early repeat childbearing is also suggested for Puerto Rican mothers when parity is examined independently for teens. Nearly 30% of the births amongst Puerto Rican teenage mothers in 1990 were of second or higher order, compared with 19% of births to Cuban-American and Caucasian non-Hispanic teenage mothers. The levels of repeat teenage childbearing are also high for Mexican-American (26%) and African-American non-Hispanic teenagers (32%).

Not being legally married is an additional risk factor for childbirth. In addition to being younger, unmarried mothers generally are less educated, have lower incomes, and possibly less emotional and other support that would accompany childbearing in a two-parent family.

Childbearing by unmarried mothers has been increasing for Hispanic and non-Hispanic women alike. In 1990, 56% of Puerto Rican mothers were unmarried, a higher level of nonmarital childbearing than for other Hispanic women or Caucasian non-Hispanic women, which ranged from 17 to 41%, but lower than observed for African-American non-Hispanic women (67 percent) (Figure 3, part a). As may be seen in Figure 3, part b, teen mothers of all ethnic and racial origins have a much greater incidence of nonmarital childbearing than

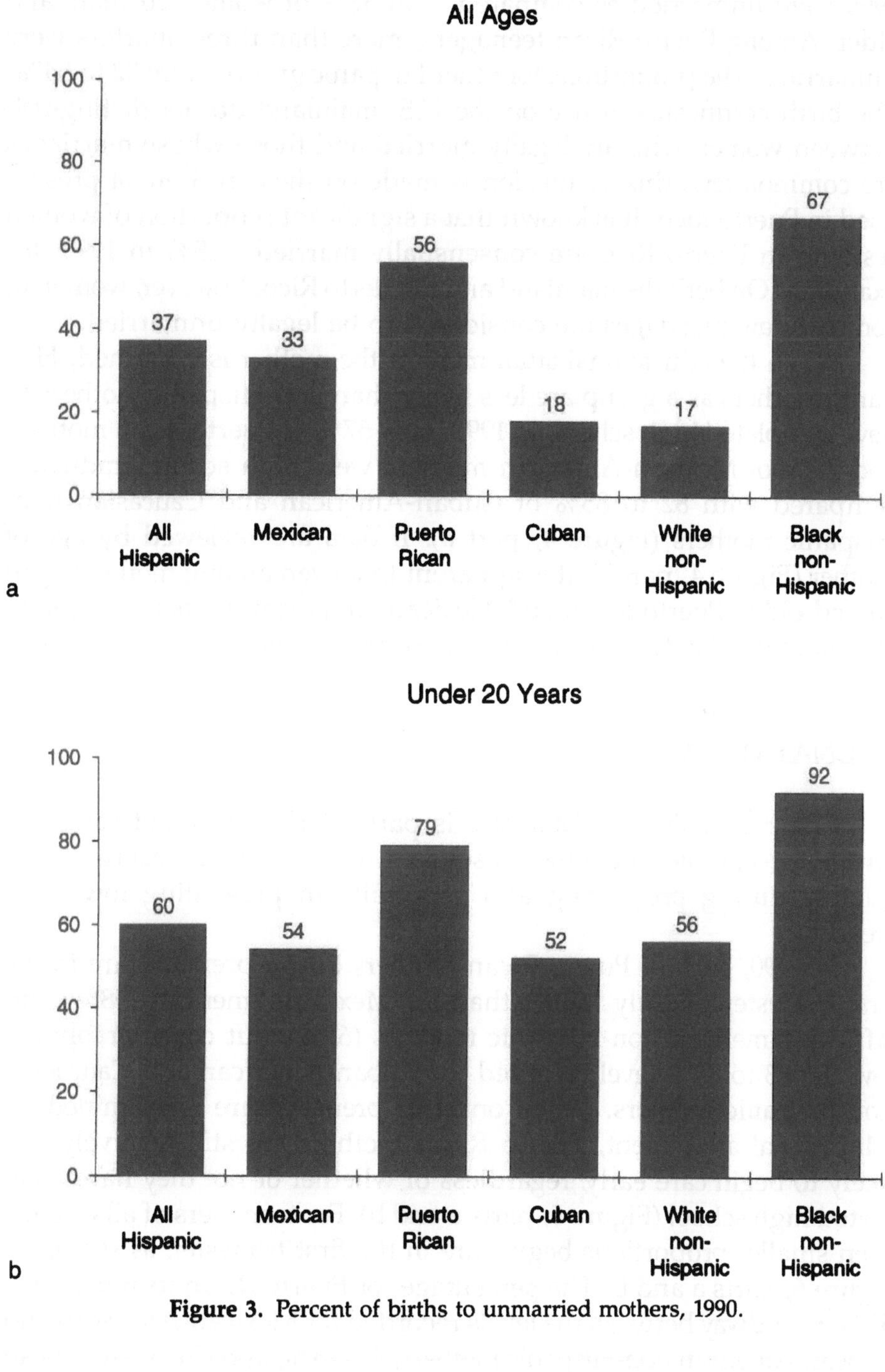

Figure 3. Percent of births to unmarried mothers, 1990.

older women. For example, 60% of all Hispanic teenager mothers in 1990 were unmarried as compared with 32% of women 20 years and older. Among Puerto Rican teenagers, more than three-quarters were unmarried. The proportions for other Hispanic groups were 52 to 54%. The birth certificates in use on the U.S. mainland do not distinguish between women who are legally married and those whose marriages are common law; this distinction is made on the certificate at present used in Puerto Rico. It is known that a significant proportion of women residing in Puerto Rico are consensually married—28% in 1990, for example.[6] On both the mainland and in Puerto Rico, however, women in common law marriages are considered to be legally unmarried.

When the educational attainment of the mother is examined, Hispanic mothers as a group are less likely than non-Hispanic mothers to have completed high school. In 1990, only 57% of Puerto Rican mothers and 39% of Mexican-American mothers were high school graduates, compared with 82 to 85% of Cuban-American and Caucasian non-Hispanic mothers (Figure 4, part a). If data are reviewed by age of mother (Figure 4, part b), it is apparent that even among mothers aged 20 and older, Puerto Rican and Mexican-American mothers were substantially less likely to have completed high school.

PRENATAL CARE

Comprehensive prenatal care is particularly important for those without economic and other resources to care for themselves adequately during pregnancy, and especially in preventing low birth weight.

In 1990, 64% of Puerto Rican mothers began prenatal care in the first trimester, slightly higher than for Mexican-American (58%) and African-American non-Hispanic mothers (61%), but considerably below the 83 to 85% level recorded for Cuban-American and Caucasian non-Hispanic mothers. When onset of prenatal care is examined by educational attainment, Puerto Rican mothers are still relatively unlikely to begin care early, regardless of whether or not they have completed high school (Figure 5, parts a and b). For teenagers of all origins, even smaller proportions begin care in the first trimester, as shown in Figure 6, parts a and b. The percentage for Puerto Rican teen mothers, 53%, is midway between the levels recorded for Mexican-American and African-American non-Hispanic mothers, 47–48%, and Cuban-American and Caucasian non-Hispanic mothers, 62%. Teenagers are particularly

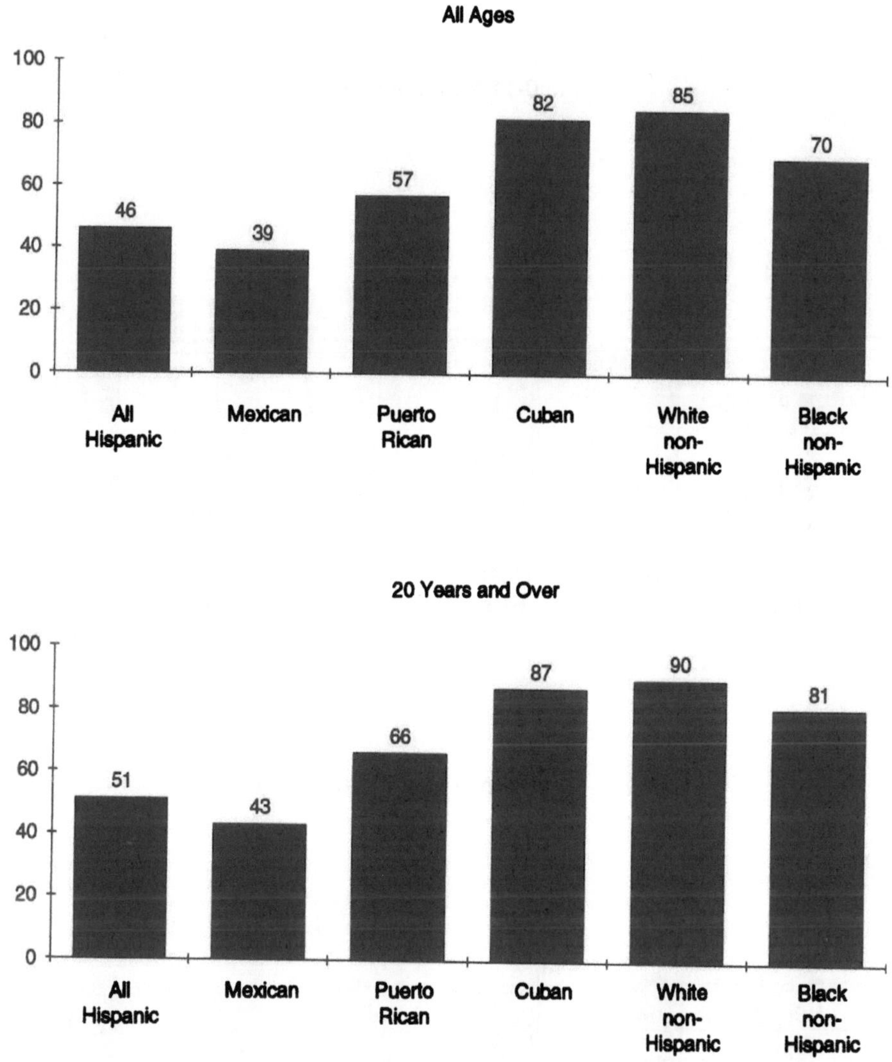

Figure 4. Percent of births to mothers with 12 or more years of education, 1990.

vulnerable to health problems and complications during pregnancy and could benefit from guidance on nutrition and other health and life-style matters during pregnancy.

As would be expected, based on the first trimester data just presented, Puerto Rican, Mexican-American, and African-American non-Hispanic mothers are much more likely than Cuban-American or Caucasian non-Hispanic mothers to delay their first prenatal care visit until the third trimester or to have no care at all (Figure 7, part a).

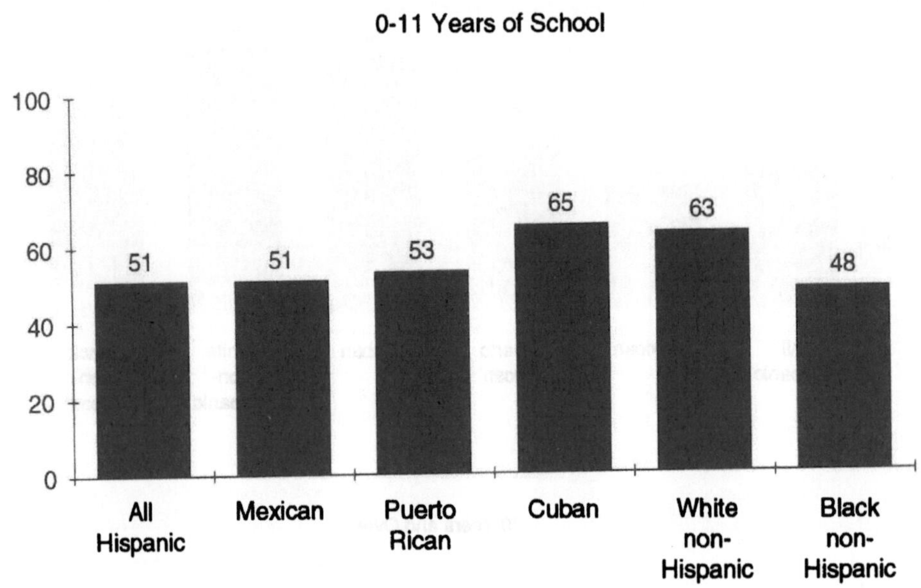

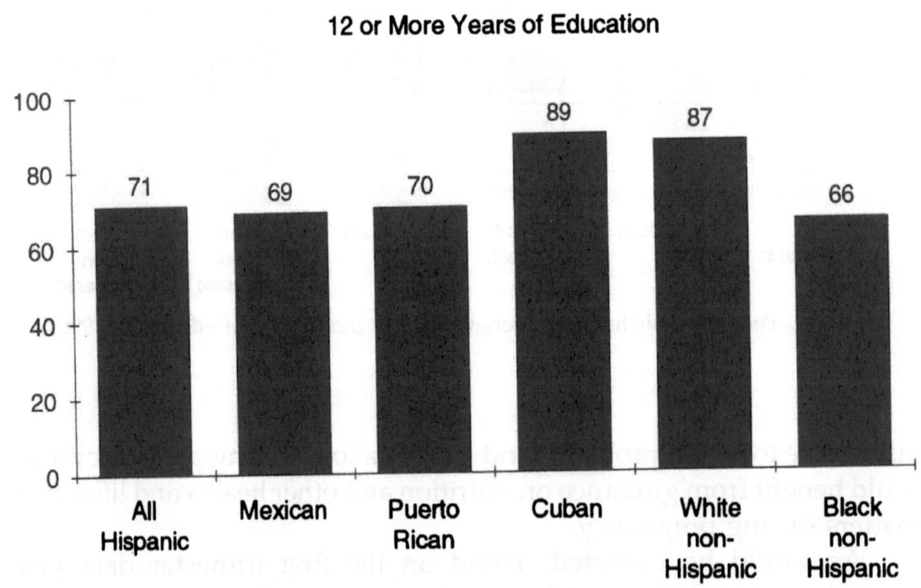

Figure 5. Percent of mothers beginning prenatal care in first trimester by education, 1990.

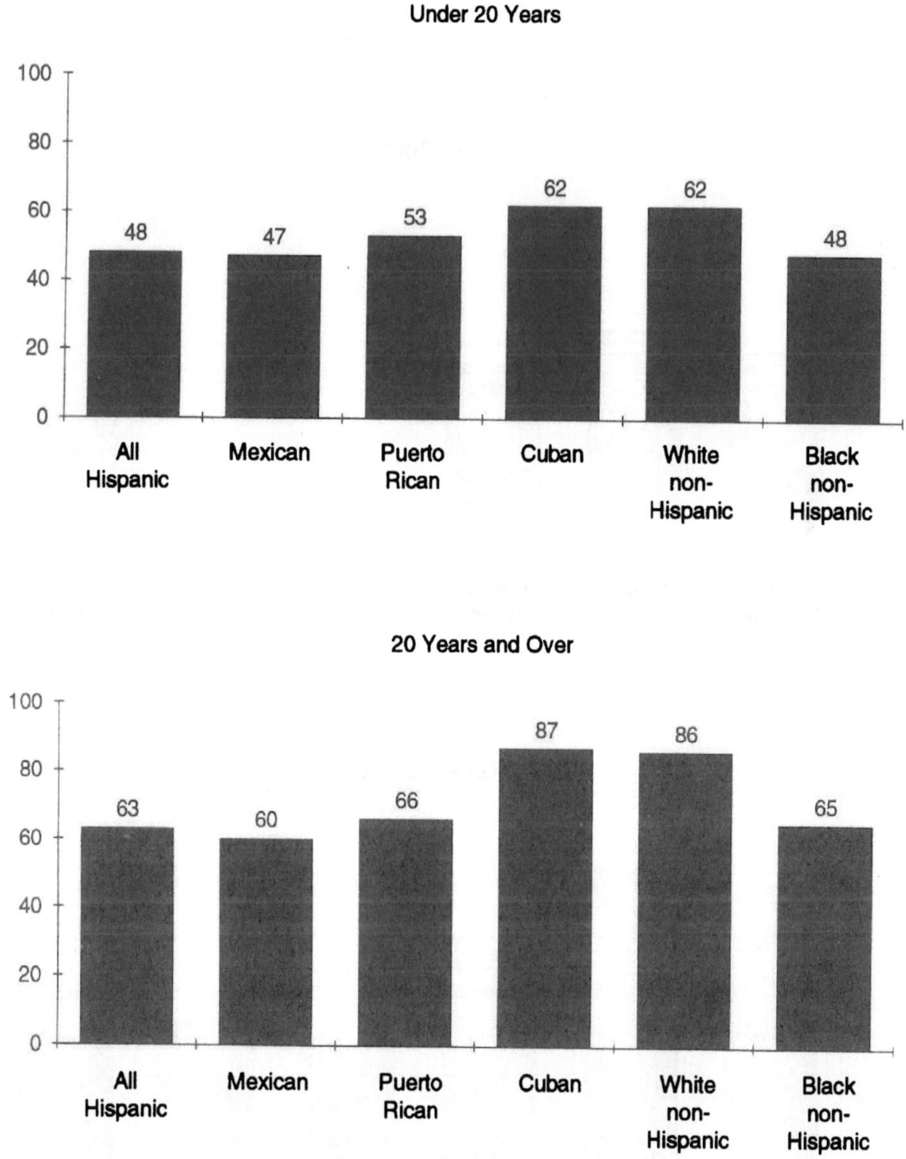

Figure 6. Percent of mothers beginning prenatal care in first trimester, by age, 1990.

Teenagers again are particularly at risk for having delayed or no prenatal care (Figure 7, part b). Among Puerto Rican teenage mothers, about one in seven had late or no prenatal care in 1990, about the same as for African-American non-Hispanic teens, but lower than for Mexican teens.

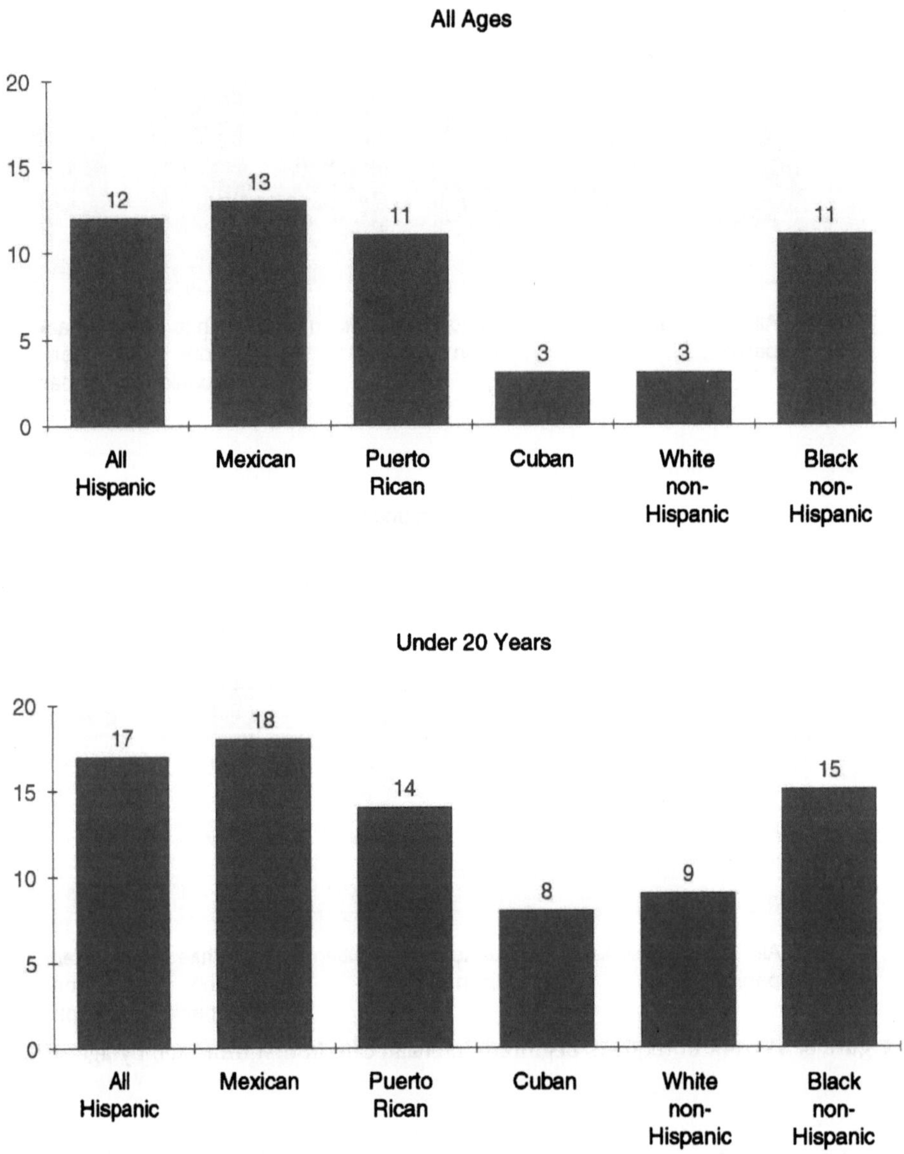

Figure 7. Percent of mothers starting prenatal care in third trimester or having no care, 1990.

WEIGHT AT BIRTH

A critically important measure of birth outcome is the weight of the baby at birth. Babies weighing less than 2500 grams (5½ pounds) have a much higher risk of congenital malformations, mental retardation, and other physical and neurological impairments, and of dying in the first year of life. As a measure of pregnancy outcome, low birth weight has the advantage of being accurately and completely reported on the birth certificate.

Consistent with the high level of teenage childbearing, limited educational attainment, and late or no prenatal care, a relatively high rate of low birth weight would be expected for babies born to Puerto Rican mothers. Indeed, that is the pattern that has been observed over the past decade. In 1990, 9.0% of Puerto Rican infants weighed less than 2500 grams (5½ pounds) at birth, midway between the levels of 5.5 to 5.7% for Mexican-American, Cuban-American, and Caucasian non-Hispanic babies and 13.3% for African-American non-Hispanic babies (Figure 8). Being a teenage mother is in itself a risk factor for low birth weight, and the data show that the incidence of low birth weight is higher among births of Puerto Rican teens than for births to older mothers: 10.1% compared with 8.7%. This pattern is observed for other Hispanic groups as well.

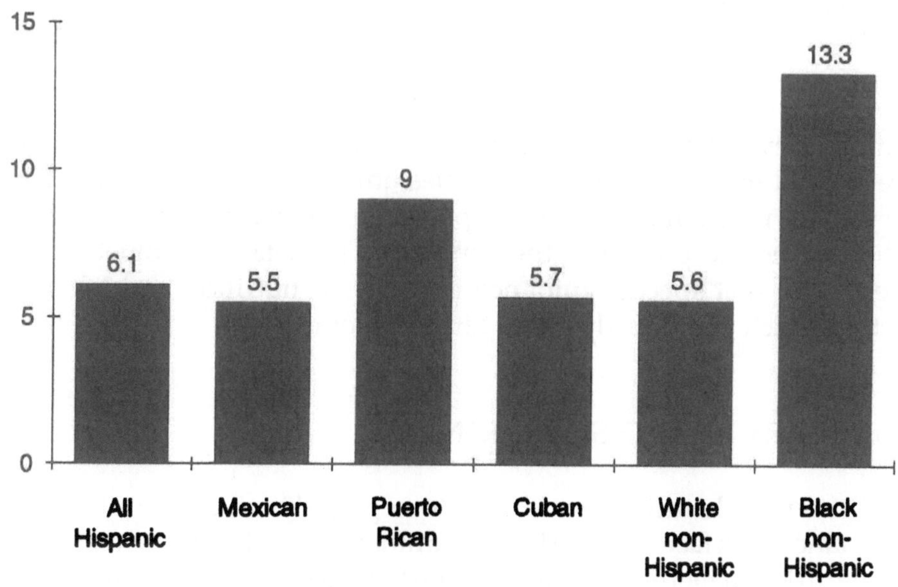

Figure 8. Percent of births weighing less than 2500 grams, 1990.

Infants who are born at very low birth weight (less than 1500 grams or 3 pounds 4 ounces) are at the greatest risk of dying or of being seriously disabled. Although the risk of very low birth weight for Hispanic births in general is similar to that for Caucasian non-Hispanic babies, Puerto Rican infants are at a relatively elevated risk of weighing less than 1500 grams at birth (Figure 9, part a and b).

Some of the high risk for low birth weight observed for Puerto Rican babies is reduced for babies whose mothers began prenatal care in the first trimester. Of those infants, 8.0% weighed less than 2500 grams, compared with 12.9% of those whose mothers received late or no prenatal care. Low-birth-weight levels are also reduced for better educated mothers. In 1990, 8.0% of births of Puerto Rican mothers who were high school graduates were of low birth weight compared to 10.3% of births to mothers who did not complete high school.

The prevalence of low birth weight among Puerto Rican births has been relatively high throughout the 1980s and in 1990. Maternal tobacco and alcohol use and weight gain during pregnancy may account in part for the high prevalence of low birth weight for Puerto Ricans. Data on some of these topics are available for the first time beginning in 1989, with the adoption of a revised birth certificate.[7,8] In 1989, 14.5% of Puerto Rican mothers were reported to have smoked during pregnancy, compared with 3.6 to 6.3% of Mexican-American, Cuban-American, and Central and South American women. Puerto Rican mothers also had higher rates of alcohol use, 3.3% compared with 1.0 to 1.8% for Mexican-American, Cuban-American, and Central and South American mothers. Finally, one-fourth of Puerto Rican mothers gained less than 21 pounds during pregnancy, a weight-gain level that is associated with an elevated risk of low birth weight. It appears that interventions are needed to reduce teen pregnancies among Puerto Ricans residing on the U.S. mainland, especially repeat teen pregnancies, and for those who do become pregnant, the content of prenatal care must be addressed so that specific guidance is given on nutrition and life-style factors which can directly affect birth outcome.

SUMMARY AND DISCUSSION

Maternal characteristics known to negatively affect the outcome of pregnancy (risk factors) have been examined for births occurring in 1990 to Puerto Rican mothers residing on the U.S. mainland and compared to those of other Hispanic, Caucasian, and African-American non-

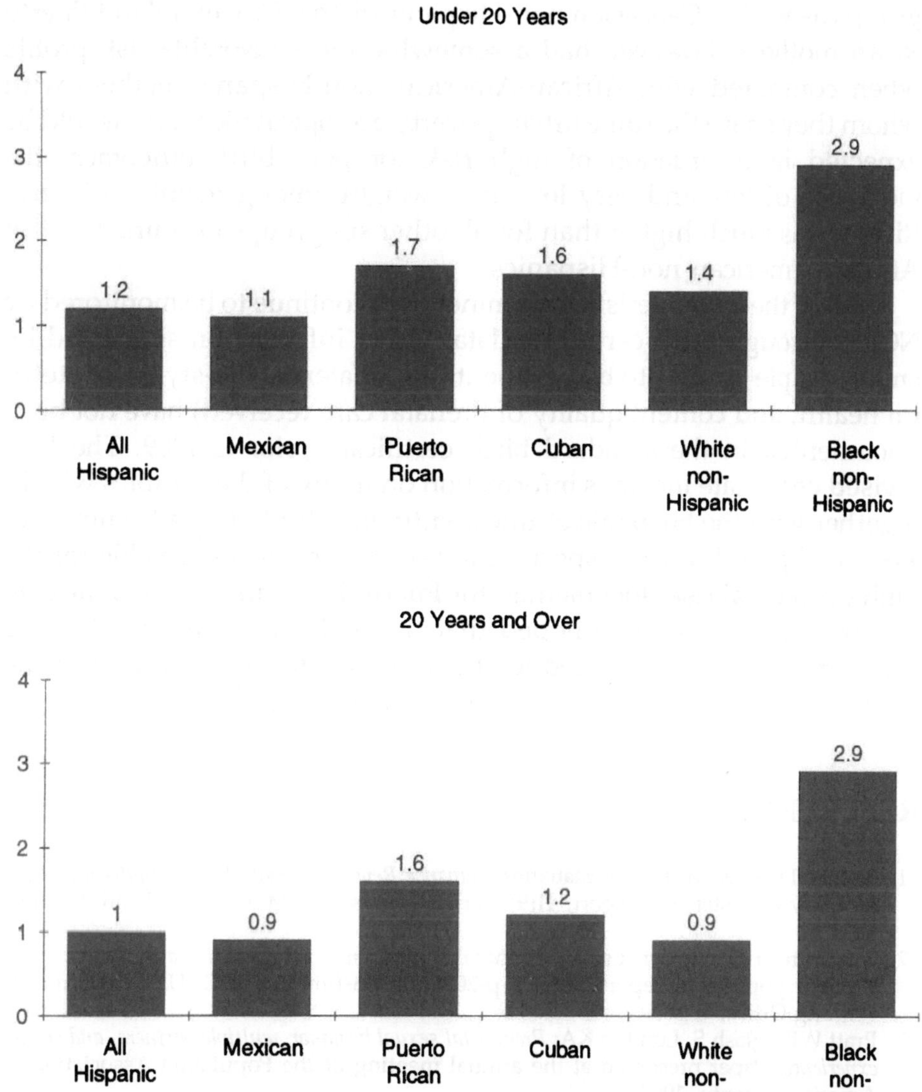

Figure 9. Percent of births weighing less than 1500 grams, by age of mother, 1990.

Hispanic subgroups. A critically important measure of birth outcome related to these maternal characteristics has also been examined and levels for Puerto Rican babies have been compared with other ethnic and racial subgroups comprising the U.S. mainland population. In virtually all the characteristics examined, U.S. mainland Puerto Ricans were at a distinct disadvantage compared with other Hispanic subgroups as well as Caucasian non-Hispanic births. U.S. mainland Puerto Rican mothers, however, had a somewhat more favorable risk profile when compared with African-American non-Hispanic mothers with whom they share the same urban/poverty ecological niche. As would be expected in a situation of high risk for poor birth outcomes, the incidence of low and very low birth weight among mainland Puerto Ricans was much higher than for all other subgroups examined except African-American non-Hispanics.

All of the characteristics examined will continue to be monitored by NCHS through birth certificate data. Other information suggested by small sample studies to be pertinent (i.e., maternal life-styles, obstetrical health, and content/quality of prenatal care received) have not been documented in the standard birth certificate prior to 1989. The 1989 revised certificate includes information on many of these topics which, together with the Hispanic/ethnic identifiers adopted by all states as of 1993, will permit greater specification of the causes responsible for the high obstetrical risk documented for Puerto Rican mothers residing on the mainland. It is to be hoped that this will translate into effective program interventions to reduce the documented risk, at least to the level so far in evidence for the U.S. mainland as a whole.

REFERENCES

1. National Center for Health Statistics: *Advance Report of Final Natality Statistics, 1990.* Monthly vital statistics report, 41(9), suppl. Hyattsville, MD, Public Health Service, 1993
2. U.S. Bureau of the Census: *The Hispanic Population in the United States, March 1990.* Current population reports, series p-20(449). Washington, DC: U.S. Government Printing Office, 1991
3. Pratt WF, Eglash S, London KA: *Premarital sexual behavior, multiple partners, and sexual experience.* Paper presented at the annual meeting of the Population Association of America, Toronto, 1990
4. Joyce T: The social and economic correlates of pregnancy resolution among adolescents in New York City, by race and ethnicity: A multivariate analysis. *Amer. J. Pub. Health*, 78:626–631, 1988
5. Henshaw, SK, Silverman J: The characteristics and prior contraceptive use of U.S. abortion patients. *Fam. Plann. Persp.* 20:158–168, 1988
6. Puerto Rico Department of Health: *Informe Anual de Estadisticas Vitales 1990*. San Juan, Puerto Rico: Commonwealth of Puerto Rico, 1992.
7. National Center for Health Statistics: *Advance Report of New Data from the 1989 Birth Certificate.* Monthly vital statistics report, 40(2), suppl. Hyattsville, MD: Public Health Service, 1992
8. Taffel SM, Ventura SJ, Gay GA: Revised U.S. certificate of live birth—New opportunities for research on birth outcome. *Birth* 16:188–193, 1989

6

Characteristics of Childbearing Hispanic Women in New York City

SALLY ANN LEDERMAN
AND DIANA SIERRA

INTRODUCTION

In studies of Hispanic populations on the U.S. mainland, researchers have generally combined data for diverse Hispanic populations (such as "Central and South American"[1] or "U.S. Mainland-born Hispanics"[2]), or limited their examination to Hispanics from one ethnic group only. Other studies of pregnancy outcome have compared women from different Hispanic groups, but without regard for their place of birth.[3]

In the past decade there has been a growing concern about the

SALLY ANN LEDERMAN and DIANA SIERRA • Center for Population and Family Health, School of Public Health, Columbia University, New York, New York 10032. This chapter was developed from a presentation at the Brown University Conference "The Health and Development of Puerto Rican Mothers and Children on the U.S. Mainland" coauthored by Karla Damus and Wanda Gonzalez.

Puerto Rican Women and Children: Issues in Health, Growth, and Development, edited by Gontran Lamberty and Cynthia Garcia Coll. Plenum Press, New York, 1994.

health needs of the Hispanic population, in part because of their current and projected population growth. According to U.S. mainland census data for 1980, Hispanics totaled 14.5 million.[4] The U.S. Census Bureau also estimated the total Hispanic population for 1989 to be 20.1 million, a 39% increase.[4]

New York City is ranked second of the Hispanic markets on the U.S. mainland, and projections through 1995 show that it will maintain that position. With an estimated population of over 2.3 million Hispanics, New York City accounted for 17.8% of the total mainland Hispanic population in 1985.[4] It is estimated that by 1995 the city's Hispanic population will have increased by 34%, an annual rate of increase of 14.7%, almost double that of African-Americans (8.8%).[4]

With such rapid recent population growth, and the expectation of continued growth in the near future, Hispanic health warrants careful attention. The heterogeneity of the Hispanic population poses a major problem, however, when assessing their health care needs. New York City has a broad, diverse mixture of Hispanics. Although in the Southern and Western U.S. mainland, Mexicans and Cubans are the most numerous Hispanic groups, in New York, Puerto Ricans predominate. In addition, recent immigration waves into New York City have resulted in increasing numbers of births to women of Dominican or Colombian origin.

The impact of this burgeoning population is revealed by an examination of New York City births in the 1980s. From 1985 through 1988, the period covered in this chapter, over 30% of births in New York City were to Hispanics. The percentage of Hispanic births that were to Puerto Rican mothers, however, declined from over 53% in 1985 to 48% in 1988 (although total births to Puerto Ricans rose by 5%).

As these numbers suggest, total births rose between 1985 and 1988. In the same period, the number of births to Dominicans rose by 28%, constituting 22.6% of Hispanic births in 1985 and 25.2% in 1988.

Although different Hispanic groups share a basic common language, there are significant differences in their cultures and migration patterns, differences that could greatly influence the life-style factors that determine birth outcome. According to the National Center for Health Statistics (NCHS) 1988 National Natality Survey,[5] there are significant differences in the health needs and outcomes of different Hispanic groups, particularly in pregnancy outcomes. Factors contributing to these differences have been presented by Ventura in chapter 5.

Furthermore, the differences in birth outcomes of mainland-born and foreign-born mothers, which have been demonstrated in some ethnic groups,[6,7] have not been studied in a setting where such comparisons can be made across several different Hispanic groups. Because of the large and diverse Hispanic population in New York City, it is of interest to examine similar factors in this setting, where comparison can be made of different Hispanic groups residing and working in similar conditions.

The Hispanic data for this study were obtained from the New York City Department of Health as bivariate tables produced from the New York City computerized birth records for 1985 to 1988.* Much of the data for African-Americans and Caucasians were obtained from the *Summary of Vital Statistics* published each year by the New York City Department of Health. These data were used to explore the relationship of birthplace to several maternal characteristics known to be associated with pregnancy outcome.

Our primary goal was to develop some understanding of the differences among Puerto Ricans, Dominicans, and Colombians, the groups most heavily represented in Hispanic births in New York City and to evaluate the magnitude of differences between their mainland-born and foreign-born women. Most earlier studies of Hispanics residing on the mainland have examined Cubans and Mexicans. Although there are relatively few births to Cubans and Mexicans in New York City, we examined their characteristics and pregnancy outcomes as well, for comparative purposes. Thus, we will show data on maternal characteristics and birth outcomes for five different Hispanic groups, as well as for non-Hispanic African-Americans and non-Hispanic Caucasians, to provide a description of the current situation of Hispanics in New York City. The broad nature of these comparisons will limit the discussion to only a few major maternal characteristics and pregnancy outcomes. Note that for African-Americans and non-Hispanic Caucasians, the vital statistics summary data used did not distinguish foreign-born women.

*Some tables were inadvertently omitted for certain years. Due to major staff changes at the Department of Health, attempts to obtain the missing data were not fully successful. Therefore for some variables fewer years are included, as noted.

METHODS

In the following discussion, data from the birth records have been averaged over 3 to 4 years (from 1985 or 1986 through 1988). In this manner the number of births obtained for each group was sufficiently large to draw limited conclusions even for those groups with few births each year. Nevertheless, there were fewer than 400 births per year to Hispanic women born on the mainland ("native born") in all but the Puerto Rican group (where there were over 14 000 per year; see Table 1). Among Hispanic women born elsewhere than the mainland, births ranged from a low of 400 per year for Cubans to a high of 8000 per year for Puerto Ricans and for Dominicans.

Maternal characteristics examined included: maternal age at delivery; marital status (as imputed by the Department of Health); education

Table 1 Number of Births in New York City, 1985 to 1988

Group	1985	1986	1987	1988
Non-Hispanic African-American	38 420	39 781	40 634	42 100
Non-Hispanic Causasian	40 001	40 632	40 582	41 683
All Hispanics	33 719	34 827	37 997	38 967
Puerto Ricans				
Island born	8298	7926	7756	7303
U.S. mainland born	9663	10 212	10 896	11 519
Total	17 961	18 138	18 652	18 822
Colombian				
Foreign born	1179	1312	1727	1893
U.S. mainland born	19	20	30	39
Total	1198	1332	1757	1932
Cuban				
Foreign born	421	409	374	357
U.S. mainland born	98	107	129	145
Total	529	516	503	502
Mexican				
Foreign born	760	916	1160	1493
U.S. mainland born	39	41	36	59
Total	799	957	1196	1552
Dominican				
Foreign born	7430	7954	8609	9345
U.S. mainland born	214	221	322	471
Total	7644	8175	8931	9816

Source: New York City Department of Health Summary of Vital Statistics.

attained; timing of prenatal care; and reported drug use. Two pregnancy outcomes were examined: birth weight and infant mortality.

MATERNAL CHARACTERISTICS

Maternal Age

Extremes of maternal age have been associated with a variety of perinatal problems.[8,9] Recent studies do suggest, however, that child-bearing after age 35 may carry little or no additional risk in women who initiate prenatal care early and who terminate pregnancy when chromosomal abnormalities are documented.[10,11] However, this lowered risk may apply to populations that are largely mainland born, Caucasian, and middle class. In New York City Hispanics, older maternal age may still represent a high-risk situation because of factors such as high parity, and inadequate treatment of medical conditions developing with age. In fact it has been shown that Hispanics are at increased risk for certain medical conditions that affect pregnancy; specifically, diabetes, hypertension, HIV infection, and alcoholism.[12] Therefore, we examined both births to teen mothers (either <20 years or <15 years) and births to women over 34 years of age. It should be noted, however, that observed outcome differences of the various ethnic groups may reflect different age distributions within these age groups, as well as differences in the fraction of births to women of these more extreme ages.

The proportion of births to foreign-born teens under 20 (Figure 1) shows substantial variation among the groups from a low of 2.4% among foreign-born Cubans to a high of 18.4% among foreign-born Mexicans. The teen (<20 years) pregnancy rate among mainland born Hispanic women is generally substantially higher than among foreign-born women, ranging from 13.7% among mainland born Mexicans to almost 43% in mainland-born Dominicans. Only the Mexican group has a lower teen pregnancy rate among mainland-born mothers than among their foreign-born counterparts. Also, only foreign-born Cubans showed lower rates of pregnancy at <20 years than Caucasians (2.4% vs. 3.7%, respectively). More generally, these figures show that there is little correspondence between teen pregnancy rates in mainland-born and foreign-born women in any of the ethnic groups.* Puerto

*For Puerto Ricans, "foreign born" includes those women born in Puerto Rico.

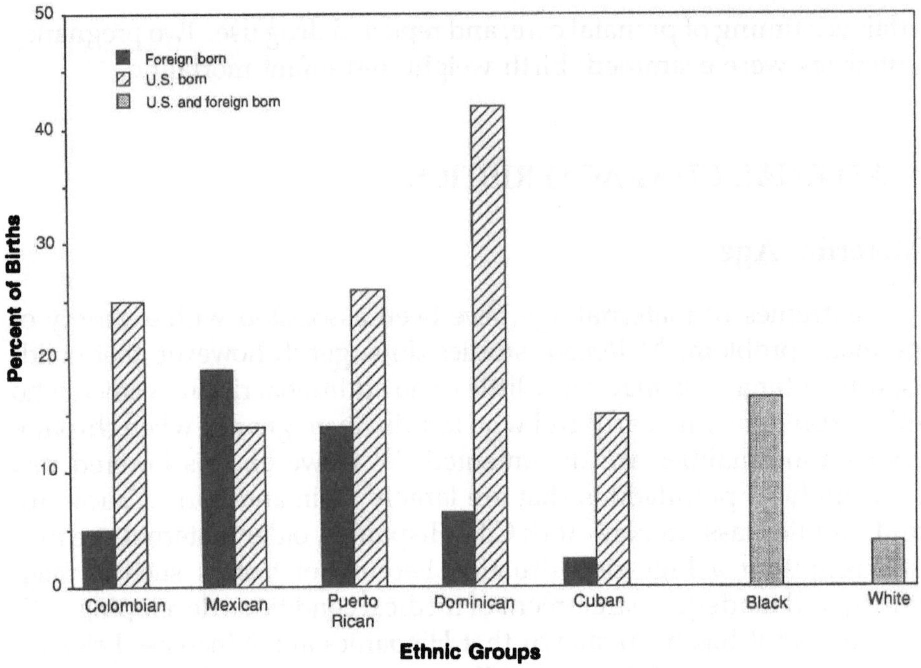

Figure 1. Maternal age <20 years.

Ricans have the second highest teen pregnancy rates of all groups for both mainland- and foreign-born women.

Figure 2 combines births to teens and to women 35 or older, to identify total births at extremes of maternal age. Among foreign-born women, Puerto Ricans had the highest rate, 25.7%. Among the mainland-born, only Dominicans and Colombians (who each have fewer than 400 births per year) have higher rates than Puerto Ricans. Because of their much greater number of births, Puerto Ricans provide the bulk of births at extremes of maternal age.

Marital Status

The percent of unmarried mothers is shown in Figure 3. Mainland-born mothers were more likely to be unmarried than foreign-born others, except for Mexicans. Puerto Ricans had the highest percent of unmarried mothers; for both mainland- and island-born Puerto Ricans over 60% of mothers were unmarried. Among the foreign-born mothers, Cubans had the lowest rates of births to unmarried mothers,

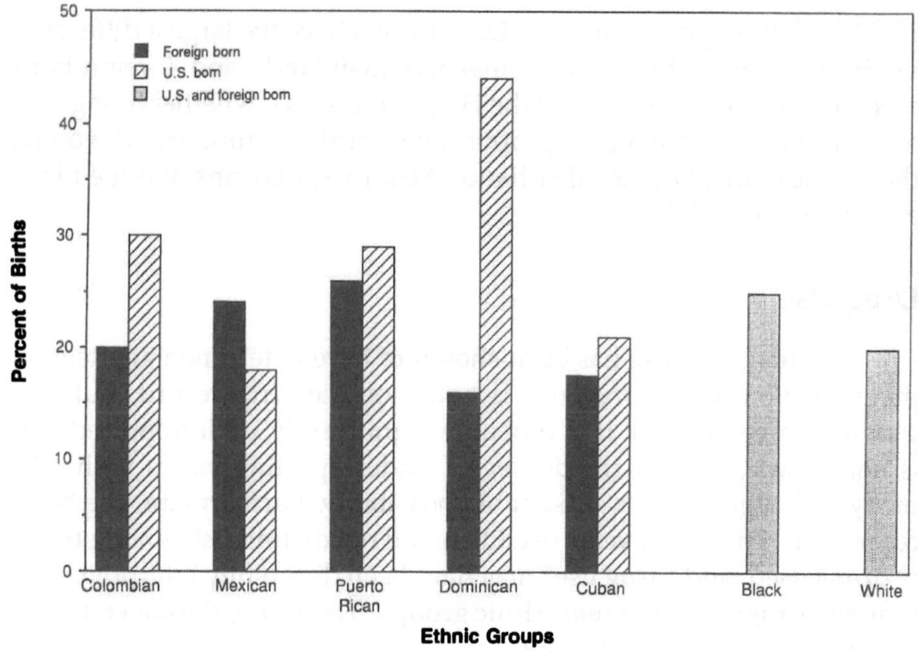

Figure 2. Maternal age <20 and >34 years.

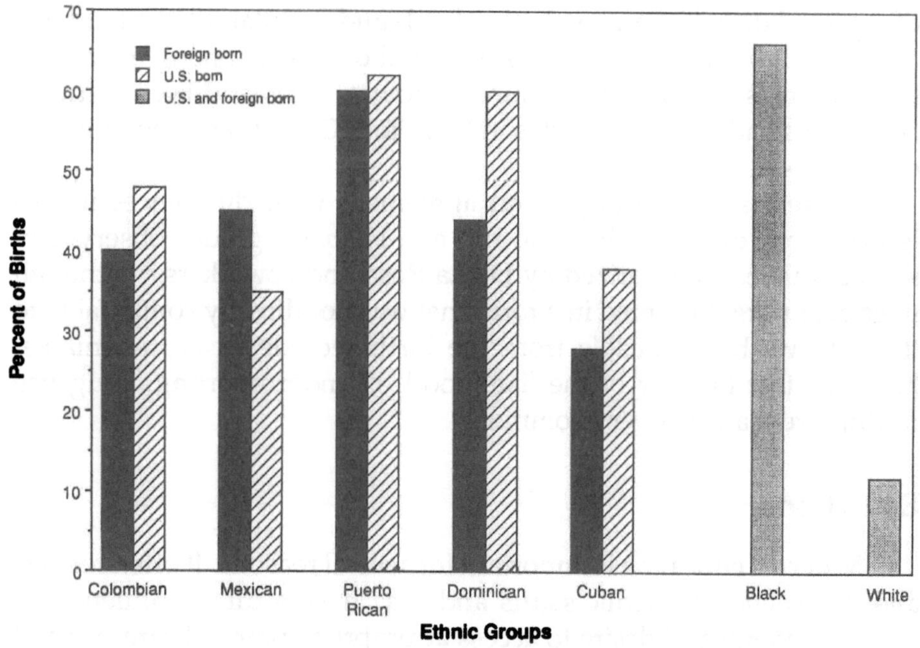

Figure 3. Births to unmarried women.

29.5%. Within a given ethnicity, Dominicans have the largest difference in the percent of births to unmarried mainland- and foreign-born mothers (41.9% vs. 59.8%). All the Hispanic groups, whether foreign- or mainland-born had a higher proportion of births to unmarried women than Caucasians. On the other hand, African-Americans had the highest rate overall, 65.4%.

Drug Use

Maternal drug use has been shown to have a detrimental effect on pregnancy outcome. Drug use is noted on the birth record, but it is generally accepted that it is probably significantly underreported.[13] It is not known whether the degree of underreporting varies with ethnicity, although this is a reasonable possibility. Furthermore, the birth records for some of the years used here did not distinguish among types of drugs used, and "drug use" may have been differently interpreted for different drugs and different ethnic groups. Therefore, the data on drug use must be viewed cautiously.

For all groups, drug use was considerably less common among foreign-born mothers, with Cubans having the lowest rate (Figure 4). Among the Hispanic groups, Puerto Ricans had the highest percentage of reported drug use among both island- and mainland-born mothers. Mexicans have the lowest rate of maternal drug use among mainland-born mothers. Across all examined groups, mainland-born African-Americans had the highest rates in New York City of reported maternal drug use—12.5%.

These results are in general agreement with differences in use levels among different Hispanic and non-Hispanic groups observed in several studies summarized by De La Rosa and coworkers,[14] although their data were presented in a form that was not directly comparable to the data we had available from the birth records. It is undeniable, however, that in view of the likelihood of underreporting, drug use during pregnancy is very common.

Education

Maternal education is important for several reasons. It often reflects and determines economic status and may have a direct influence on maternal ability and desire to access appropriate prenatal care. Several

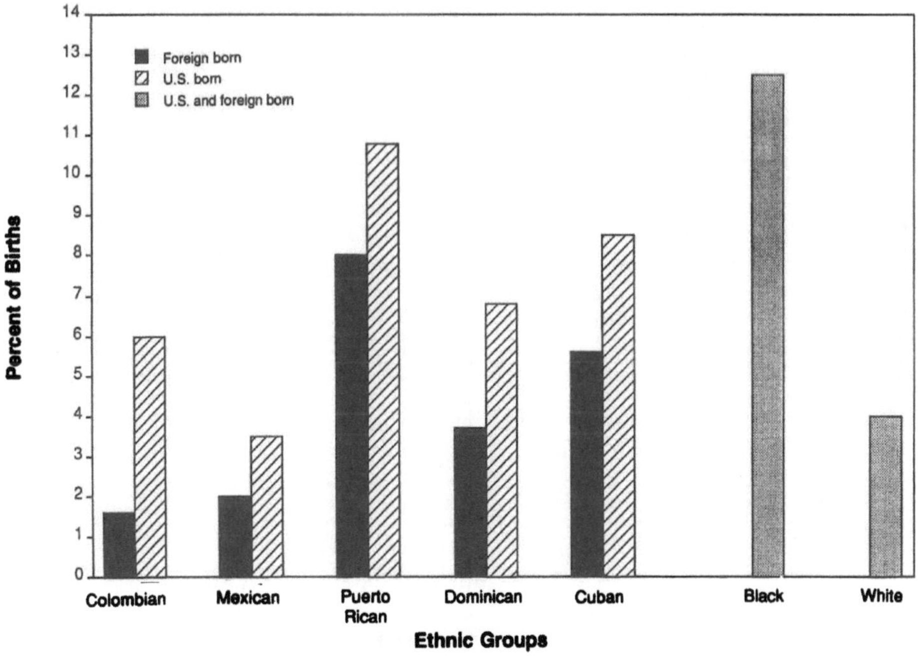

Figure 4. Maternal drug use reported.

aspects of education were reviewed in the Hispanic data. (Since the *Vital Statistic Summary* did not have comparable data for African-Americans and Caucasians, only data for Hispanics are shown.)

The proportion of mothers with only an elementary school education varied widely, ranging from a low of 1% in mainland-born Colombians to nearly 50% in foreign-born Mexicans (Figure 5). In all ethnic groups, foreign-born mothers were at least twice as likely to have had only elementary school education, but in some cases the differences were much larger. The disparity between mainland-born and foreign-born mothers was greatest for Mexicans (6.9% vs. 49.4% having only an elementary school education).

Higher education (i.e., any education after high school) also indicates the educational attainment of an ethnic group. Post-high-school education was most common for mainland-born Mexicans and Cubans and least common for foreign-born Mexicans (Figure 6). Puerto Ricans show little difference whether mainland born or foreign born, whereas the differences are large for Mexican women.

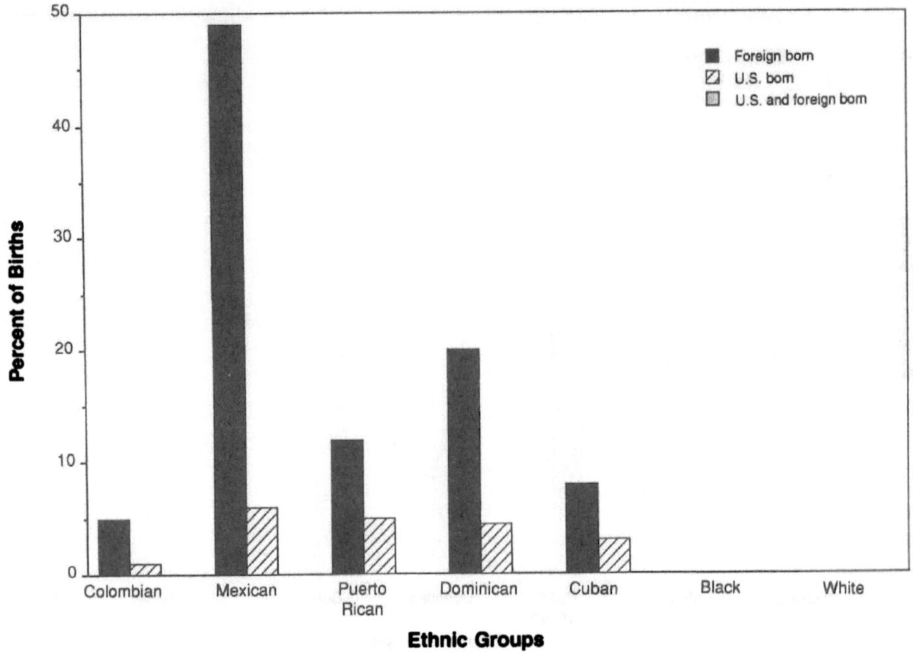

Figure 5. Elementary education only.

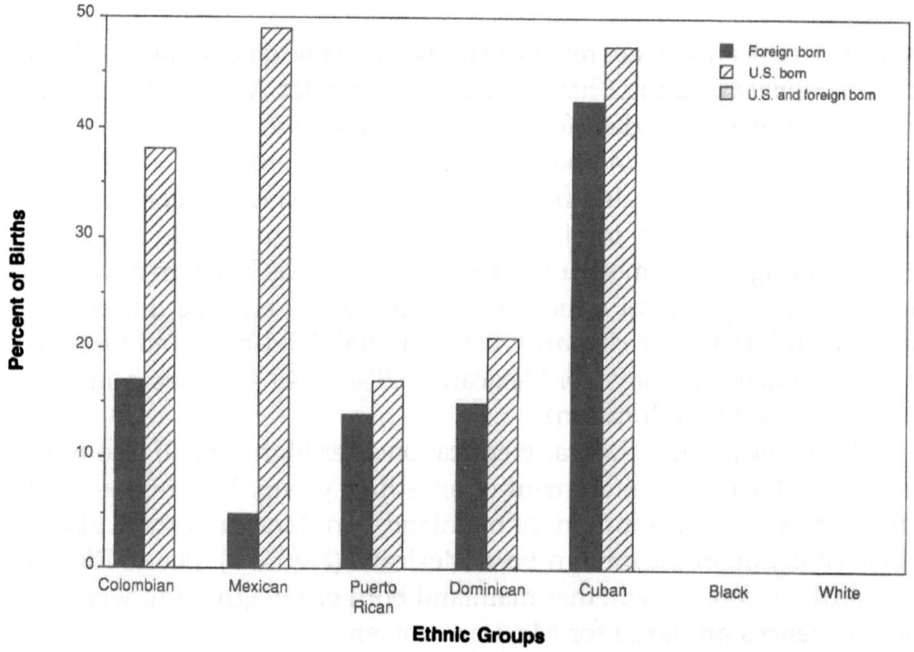

Figure 6. Post-high-school education.

Employment

Figure 7 shows employment status during pregnancy for the Hispanic mothers. More than 40% of all groups were unemployed. Except among Cubans, foreign-born women generally had higher levels of unemployment. The greatest differences between mainland-born and foreign-born groups of the same ethnicity were among Colombians and Mexicans where 70% or more of the foreign-born women were unemployed.

Employment does seem to parallel education level; the groups with high rates of higher education (mainland-born Colombians, Mexicans, and Cubans) also have high employment rates.

Prenatal Care

Inadequate prenatal care may be viewed either as a marker for high-risk pregnancies, or a contributing cause. Alexander and Cornely[15] have shown, using almost half a million birth records, that risk factors associated with marital status, education, age/pregnancy history, and

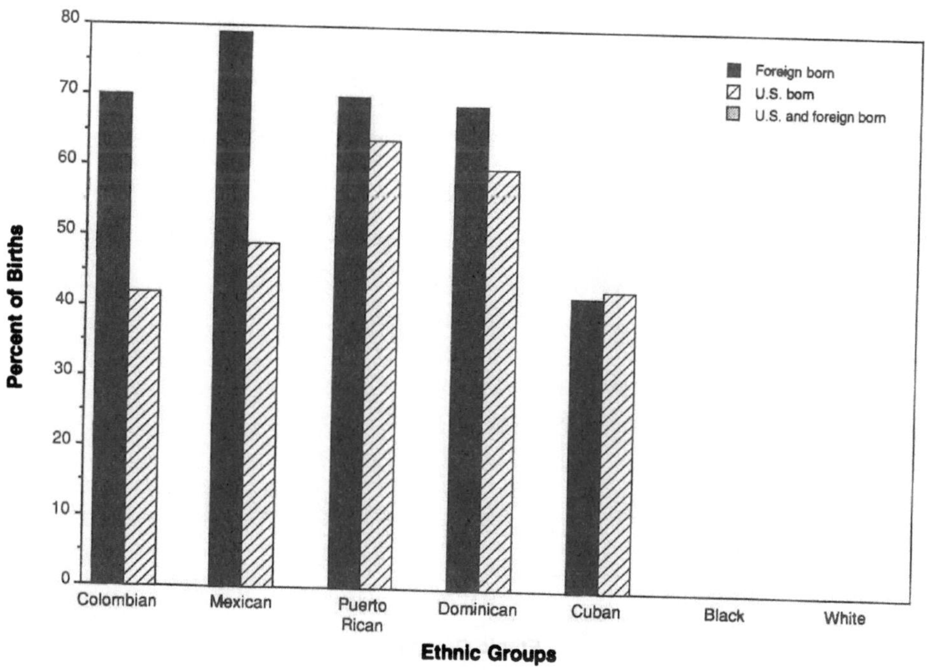

Figure 7. Women unemployed during pregnancy.

previous pregnancy terminations, all increase as the level of use of prenatal care declines. Despite higher levels of risk, however, women with "intensive" prenatal care (i.e., exceeding recommendations) had better outcomes than women with lesser levels of care, suggesting a beneficial effect of care itself. Others[16] have reported that over 70% of pregnant women over 40 (a high risk group) were in the late or no prenatal care group.

Not surprisingly, in our data the information on *early* (first trimester) prenatal care shows a pattern with a marked consistency with education levels (similar data were not available for African-Americans and Caucasians). In fact, the highest rates of use of early prenatal care (Figure 8) are in the three groups with high percentages of higher education (specifically, mainland born and foreign born Cubans and mainland born Mexicans). Foreign born Mexicans have the lowest rates of early care as well as the lowest rate of higher education.

The proportion of *late or no* prenatal care ranges from 20 to 25% (Figure 9) among Puerto Ricans, Dominicans, Colombians, and non-Hispanic African-Americans. Foreign born Mexicans have the highest rate of inadequate care of all the groups, nearly one-third having late or

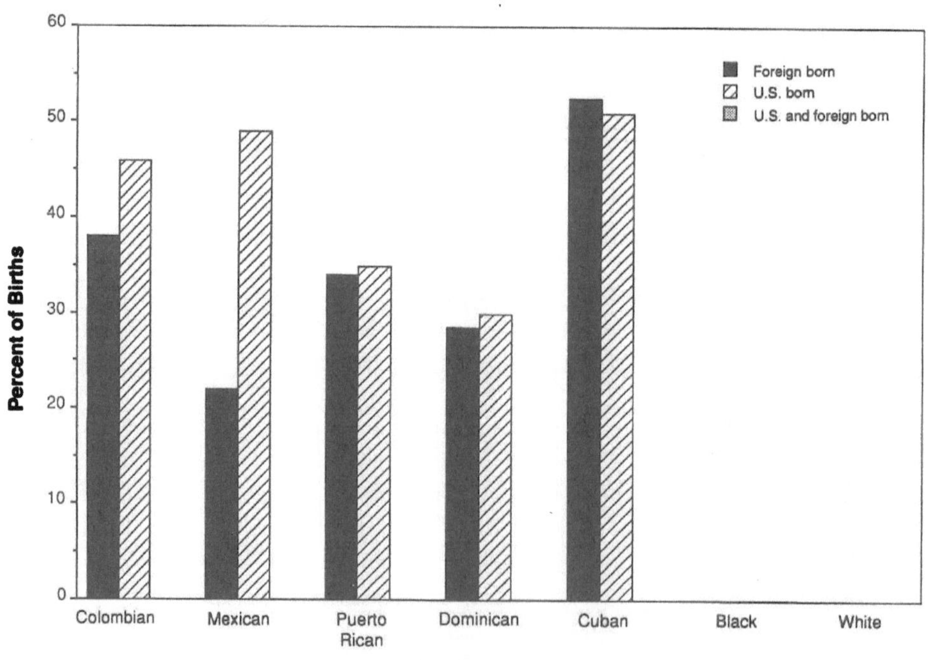

Figure 8. First trimester prenatal care.

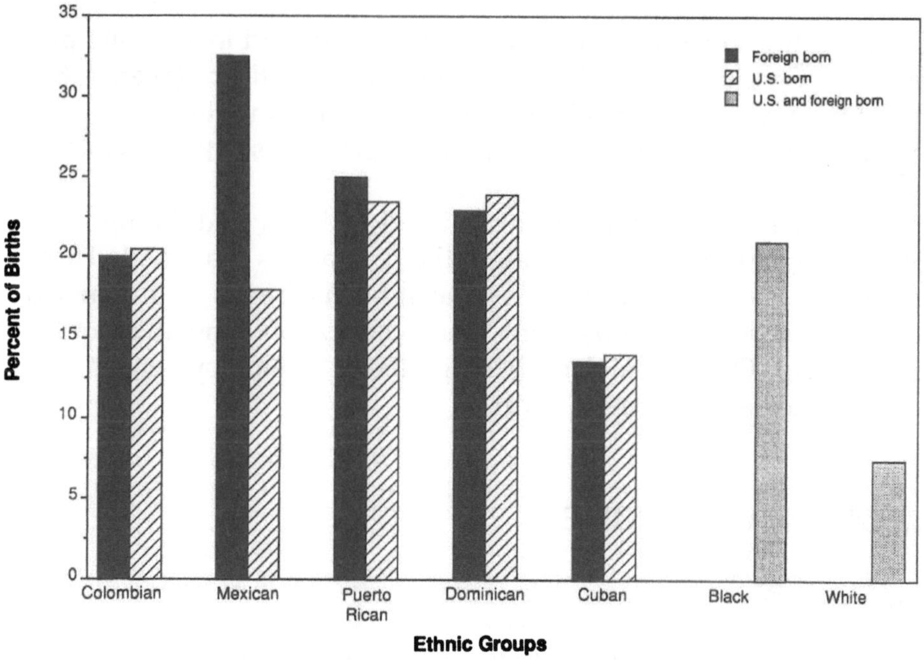

Figure 9. Late or no prenatal care.

no care. As a result, they show the biggest difference in their mainland-born and foreign-born groups, as they did for education. Cubans have the lowest rates of all Hispanics, whether mainland or foreign born (13.9% and 13.6%, respectively), but their rate is still more than double that of non-Hispanic Caucasians. A recent report[17] indicates that between 1977 and 1987 there was no significant increase in the percentage of pregnant women in New York State receiving prenatal care in the first trimester. Considering the many reasons for early use of prenatal care, the frequency of late or no care in our data (even considering possible misclassification) is disturbing.

If we were to rank the mother's risk in each of these factors (age, education, marital status, employment, and prenatal care), the following pattern would emerge. Among foreign-born mothers, Mexican mothers have the most disadvantageous conditions regarding teen pregnancy, lack of education and employment, and inadequate prenatal care. Island-born Puerto Ricans, a very much larger group of mothers in New York City (31 000 vs. 4300 Mexicans, 1985–1988; see Table 1) have the largest proportion of unmarried mothers and the second worst rates of teen births, higher education, unemployment, and inadequate prenatal care. Considering that Puerto Ricans are U.S. citizens (even if they are not born on the mainland), it is perhaps surprising that among the foreign-born, only Mexican women show higher levels of the risk factors studied.

Among mainland-born women, Puerto Ricans and Dominicans show the highest frequencies of all of the risk factors examined. These two groups have the highest rates of teen births, births to unmarried mothers, low levels of post-high-school education, and inadequate prenatal care. Of the mainland-born mothers, unemployment is also most common among Puerto Ricans.

PREGNANCY OUTCOME

Low Birth Weight

Many of the maternal characteristics reviewed are known associates of poor pregnancy outcome. Low-birth-weight rates are one index of pregnancy success. Of the five foreign-born Hispanic groups, Puerto Rican women have the highest rate of low birth weight (Figure 10), in accordance with their distribution of risk factors. For the foreign born, low birth weight was least among Colombian mothers. This is in accord with their low rates of births to teen and unmarried women, and the relatively low rates of inadequate prenatal care among foreign-born Colombian women.

Among the mainland born, low-birth-weight rates are generally higher than for the corresponding foreign born, except for Mexicans. Although the rates of low birth weight *are* somewhat lower for U.S. mainland-born Mexicans than for their corresponding foreign-born mothers, it should be noted that there were fewer than 60 births per year (number of low-weight births = 8) in this group and the low-birth weight rate may not be reliable. The same consideration applies to mainland-born Colombians, with fewer than 40 births each year. Previous studies have also found that infants of foreign-born women often manifest an advantage in birth weight. In a New York City population, this advantage has been credited to advantages in childhood social status, income, and educational attainment of the baby's father among the foreign born.[6]

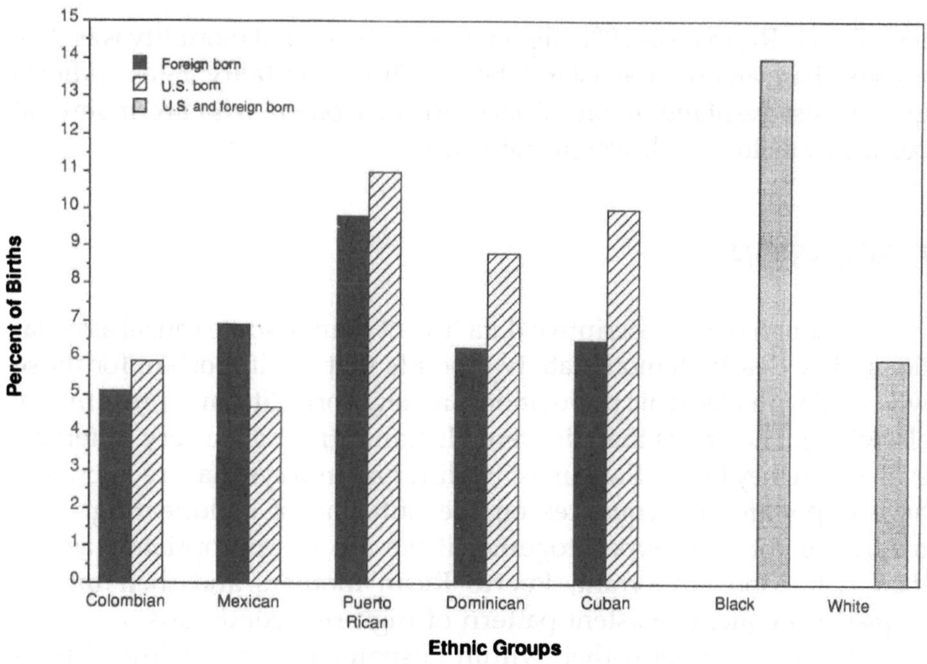

Figure 10. Birth weight <2500 grams.

Mortality

It is difficult to estimate neonatal and postneonatal mortality rates, because of the small number of births and deaths in some groups, even when averaged over several years. The available data suggest that Puerto Ricans have the second highest rate of neonatal mortality in both the mainland-born and foreign-born groups. Only Cubans have higher rates but deaths average only about three per year, making rate estimates unreliable.

Both mainland- and island-born Puerto Ricans also have the second highest level of postneonatal mortality. Among the foreign born, Mexicans fare worse. Among the mainland born, Cubans fare worse. However, the rates for Cubans and Mexicans are derived from only one to three deaths per year and probably also do not represent reliable mortality rates. Thus overall, Puerto Rican deaths, which represent a major fraction of all infant deaths because of the high number of births, are both reliably estimated and unacceptably frequent.

It should be further noted that neonatal mortality among mainland-born Puerto Ricans was 20% higher and postneonatal mortality was 10% higher than among the island born. Thus, mortality rates indicate greater disadvantage among Puerto Rican women who are mainland born, just as low-birth-weight rates do.

DISCUSSION

Although these descriptive data do not demonstrate causal associations, they clearly demonstrate two points that are important for those who deal with Hispanic populations in New York City, and presumably elsewhere. The first is that different Hispanic groups are very different, even when they live in the same city, differing in ways that are known to have important consequences on the outcome of childbearing. Hispanics cannot be grouped together if we are to appropriately assess their risk. More important, Puerto Rican mothers and their infants display a unique, consistent pattern of high-risk conditions.

The second point is that, within Hispanic groups, mainland-born and foreign-born mothers may evidence important differences in maternal characteristics associated with poor pregnancy outcome. Thus, the fraction of the population that is mainland born in a given area may influence the overall risk. It is important to also note that different Hispanic groups are not comparably affected by being foreign born. For example, educational levels are very different for mainland- and foreign-born Mexicans, but much less so for Puerto Ricans.

With respect to specific variables examined here, some overall observations can be made. In general, mainland-born Hispanic mothers were less likely to be married than foreign-born mothers (only Mexicans were an exception). African-Americans had the highest portion of unwed mothers, but Puerto Ricans were a close second. Use of drugs followed a similar pattern, being highest among African-Americans and second highest among Puerto Ricans. Ahmed[18] used vital registration data for Washington, D.C. to study the significance of childbearing in unmarried women. Adverse conditions associated with being unmarried included narcotic addiction and early first delivery. The effect of marital status also varied with age; unwed mothers over 19 years of age were at higher risk than younger unwed mothers. Numerous factors, probably differing in different subpopulations contribute to this variation. Multivariate analyses can reveal some of the factors underlying such differences.

The high rate of births to Hispanic mothers less than 20 years of age (clearly the highest risk age group) is disturbing. Despite the attention given to teen births among African-Americans, rates in this age range were higher among three of the mainland-born Hispanic groups—Puerto Ricans, Dominicans, and Colombians. These groups constitute a significant and growing proportion of the child-bearing population in New York City, and the trend to single parenting creates significant strain on the city's social services. This is likely to be particularly true since these three mainland-born groups also have high rates of reported drug use and of low birth weight (although African-Americans have higher rates in both cases).

It is a sad commentary that mainland-born Hispanic women generally have worse pregnancy outcomes than their foreign-born counterparts. Examination of data collected over a longer period, and including a wider array of variables with a complex analytical approach will probably be necessary if we are to understand fully the roles that teen childbearing, lack of education, inadequate care, and other factors play in determining the observed differences in pregnancy outcome both across and within these Hispanic groups.

However, even the descriptive data shown here have important policy implications. To improve pregnancy outcome, women need to seek prenatal care early, avoid use of illicit drugs, and avoid unwanted and unplanned pregnancies. Reversing the trend toward increasing rates of births to unmarried women would benefit women and children, and reduce the strain on medical and social services as well. All these changes are likely to be encouraged by education. This education would have to have two distinct components. First, we must provide ongoing education for women of reproductive age to improve self-care, and encourage responsible reproduction and family planning. Second, educational opportunities for upcoming generations should be available. This will encourage personal and economic development which will increase women's life options and their ability to take care of themselves and their families. The low rates of employment reported here are no doubt influenced by the low levels of education.

Development of multifaceted, culturally appropriate programs will require a long-term commitment. Unless we can change the circumstances currently surrounding child-bearing, however, we will see increasing numbers of uneducated women, living in impoverished female-headed households, with increasing rates of low birth weight and infant mortality.

REFERENCES

1. Ventura SJ: Births of Hispanic parentage, 1982. *Monthly Vital Statistics Report*; 34(4 Suppl), 1–16, 1985
2. Binkin NJ, Rust KR, Williams RL: Racial differences in neonatal mortality. *Amer. J. Dis. Child* 142:434–440, 1988
3. Stroup-Benham CA, Trevino FM: Reproductive characteristics of Mexican-American, mainland Puerto Rican, and Cuban-American women, *JAMA* 265:222–226, 1991
4. Hispanic Policy Development, Inc: *The Hispanic Almanac*, 2nd ed. New York, Hispanic Policy Development Project, Inc., Publishers, 1990, p. 8
5. National Center for Health Statistics: Advance Report of Final Natality Statistics, 1988. Monthly *Vital Statistics Report* 39(4, suppl.): 1–20, Hyattsville, MD, Public Health Service, 1990
6. Valanis BM, Rush D: A partial explanation of superior birth weights among foreign-born women. *Soc. Biol.* 26:198–210, 1979
7. Kleinman JC, Fingerhut LA, Prager K: Differences in infant mortality by race, nativity status, and other maternal characteristics. *Amer. J. Dis. Child* 144:194–199, 1990
8. Kiely JL, Paneth N, Susser M: An assessment of the effects of maternal age and parity in different components of perinatal mortality. *Amer. J. Epidemiol.* 123:444–454, 1986
9. Sweeney P: A comparison of low birth weight, perinatal mortality, and infant mortality between first and second births to women 17 years old and younger. *Amer. J. Obstet. Gynecol.* 160:1361–1370, 1989
10. Ales KL, Druzin ML, Santini DL: Impact of advanced maternal age on the outcome of pregnancy. *Gynecol. & Obstet.* 171:209–216, 1990
11. Kirz DS, Dorchester W, Freeman RK: Advanced maternal age: The mature gravida. *Amer. J. Obstet. Gynecol.* 152:7–12, 1985
12. Council on Scientific Affairs: Hispanic health in the United States. *JAMA* 265:248–252, 1991
13. McLean DE, Paneth N: *The Reliability of Birth Certificate Information: 1. Completion Processes and Completeness Rates in New York City*. Unpublished study manuscript; 1986
14. De La Rosa MR, Khalsa JH, Rouse BA: Hispanics and illicit drug use: A review of recent findings. *Internat. J. Addict.* 25:665–691, 1990
15. Alexander GR, Cornely DA: Prenatal care utilization: Its measurement and relationships to pregnancy outcome. *Amer. J. Prev. Med.* 3:243–53, 1987
16. Ryan GM, Sweeney PJ, Solola AS: Prenatal care and pregnancy outcome. *Amer. J. Obstet. Gynecol.* 137:876–881, 1980
17. Anonymous: Birth outcomes in New York State (Part II). *NY State J. Med.* 90(12):619–620, 1990
18. Ahmed F: Unmarried mothers as a high-risk group for adverse pregnancy outcomes. *J. Commun. Health*, 15:35–44, 1990

7

HIV Infection and AIDS among Women: Impact on Hispanic Women and Children Residing in the United States

BARBARA W. KILBOURNE, MARTA GWINN, KEN G. CASTRO, AND MARGARET J. OXTOBY

INTRODUCTION

The first case of acquired immunodeficiency syndrome (AIDS) in a Hispanic woman was diagnosed in 1981.[1] This case represented the first recognition of a problem that has since grown to substantial proportions in this population. By mid-1991, over 3700 AIDS cases occurring

BARBARA W. KILBOURNE, MARTA GWINN, KEN G. CASTRO, and MARGARET J. OXTOBY • Division of HIV/AIDS, National Center for Infectious Diseases, Centers for Disease Control and Prevention, Atlanta, Georgia 30333.

Puerto Rican Women and Children: Issues in Health, Growth, and Development, edited by Gontran Lamberty and Cynthia Garcia Coll. Plenum Press, New York, 1994.

among Hispanic women had been reported to the Centers for Disease Control (CDC), and in those geographic areas with highest human immune virus (HIV)/AIDS prevalence, over 1% of Hispanic women of reproductive age were estimated to be infected with HIV.[2] This chapter describes the epidemiology and sociobehavioral aspects of the HIV/AIDS epidemic in Hispanic women and their children.

ANTHROPOLOGY AND DEMOGRAPHY OF HISPANIC POPULATIONS IN THE UNITED STATES

Hispanics currently comprise the second largest minority group in the United States. The U.S. Census Bureau estimated that 20 million Hispanics resided in the United States in 1989, representing 8.2% of the total population. During 1980–1987, the U.S. Hispanic population is estimated to have grown by 34%, whereas the non-Hispanic population grew by only about 7%.[3] If current population growth trends continue, Hispanics will represent the largest minority population in the United States by the early 21st century.

The U.S. Hispanic population is concentrated in specific areas. More than 85% reside in Arizona, California, Colorado, Florida, Illinois, New Jersey, New Mexico, New York, and Texas. Most live in the nation's largest metropolitan areas.[3]

Classification and subclassification of U.S. Hispanic populations hold important implications for population-based research. The term *Hispanic* is used broadly to refer to populations with ancestral ties to Spain, Latin America, or the Spanish-speaking Caribbean (e.g., Puerto Rico). The use of this term constitutes a demographic oversimplification, since there are substantial differences between Hispanic subgroups of different origins. For example, Hispanics living on the Pacific Coast or in the Southwest are predominantly linked to Mexico, whereas Hispanics living in the Northeast tend to have ties to Puerto Rico. Many Hispanics living in Florida and nearby regions are from Cuba. Therefore, studies using different definitions of "Hispanic" may not be comparable.[4] This may result in the misclassification of groups in a community and provide programs that do not respond to actual needs or cultural sensitivities.[5] Researchers need to recognize the complexity of this issue and make informed decisions regarding the use of "Hispanic" terminology.[6]

INCIDENCE OF HIV/AIDS IN HISPANICS

High prevalences of HIV infection and AIDS have been observed among African-Americans and Hispanics in the United States. African-Americans make up 12% of the U.S. population, but account for 28% of reported AIDS cases. Similarly, Hispanics make up 8% of the U.S. population,[7] but account for 16% of reported AIDS cases (Table 1).

Trends in the HIV/AIDS epidemic suggest that Hispanics, specifically those of Puerto Rican descent, bear a disproportionate burden of this public health problem. Data on cumulative AIDS incidence rates by place of birth indicate that Puerto Ricans are the single ethnic group most disproportionately affected by AIDS in the United States when compared with Hispanic AIDS cases amongst those of Latin American descent.[8] Persons of Puerto Rican descent were the only Hispanic subgroup in whom most cases were in heterosexual injection drug users (IDU). In the Northeast, 61% of Puerto Ricans with AIDS were heterosexual IDUs.[8] The impact of AIDS among Puerto Ricans is further reflected in mortality statistics. A study of AIDS mortality among Puerto Ricans and other Hispanics in New York City during 1981–1987 found that Puerto Ricans represented the racial/ethnic group most severely affected by the AIDS epidemic, with 362 deaths from AIDS per 100 000 population for Puerto Rico-born males and 182 per 100 000 for Caucasian males.[9] The cumulative age-adjusted AIDS mortality rates were higher for Puerto Rico-born males in every age group. For 1987, the proportion of deaths in New York City due to AIDS was 10% among Puerto Rican-born persons, 12% among other Hispanics (50% of whom are mainland-born Puerto Ricans), 6% among African-Americans and 2% among Caucasians.

AIDS AND HIV INFECTION IN WOMEN

The number of new AIDS cases among adolescent and adult females has increased remarkably since 1981. Although only about 10% of the approximately 180 000 AIDS cases reported to CDC by the end of 1990 had occurred in women, over 60% of these cases in women had been reported since the beginning of 1989. This growth in the number of AIDS cases in adolescent and adult females is reflected in the increasing proportion of women with AIDS; from 6% of reported AIDS cases in

Table 1 Comparison of AIDS in Men and Women Reported to the CDC in 1990 with 1990 U.S. Population Estimates, by Race/Ethnicity

	Men				Women			
	AIDS		1990 population estimates		AIDS		1990 population estimates	
Race/Ethnicity	Number	Percent	Number	Percent	Number	Percent	Number	Percent
Caucasian	20 943	56	73 893 021	76	1236	25	80 020 971	77
African-American	10 263	27	11 296 959	12	2539	52	12 597 131	12
Hispanic	6026	16	8 425 152	9	1069	22	8 123 662	8
Other/Unknown	433	1	3 591 339	4	46	1	3 812 681	4
Total	37 665	100	97 206 471	100	4890	100	104 554 445	100

1984 to approximately 10% by 1990. Intravenous drug use accounted for 47% of all AIDS cases among women, but the proportion due to heterosexual transmission has increased over time. In 1984, heterosexual transmission accounted for less than 25% of AIDS cases in women; by the end of 1990, this risk category accounted for 34% of all AIDS cases in women and 38% of cases in Hispanic women (Table 2). The numbers of AIDS cases due to heterosexual transmission are higher for women than for men (Figure 1).

Over 80% of women who were diagnosed with AIDS were of childbearing age (15–44 years). Further, adolescent and adult females represented a disproportionate share of AIDS cases in younger persons. As of 1990, women accounted for 9% of AIDS cases among persons older than 30 years, but for 35% of cases among persons aged 13 to 19 years. Thus, AIDS cases in women were concentrated among those of childbearing age, contributing to the potential for perinatal transmission of HIV. Mortality statistics reflect the impact AIDS has had on this age group. In 1987, AIDS was the eighth leading cause of death for women of childbearing age; by 1991, it was expected to become one of the five leading causes of death in this population (Figure 2).[10] Furthermore, in Puerto Rico, in 1987, AIDS was the leading cause of death in women 25–29 years of age.[11]

Incidence of AIDS in Hispanic Women

From 1986 through 1990, the absolute number of women with AIDS increased in all racial/ethnic groups. The proportion of African-American women with AIDS did not change significantly during that time (from 54 to 56%), however, while the proportion of Hispanics increased from 18 to 22%, and the proportion of Caucasians decreased from 28 to 25%.[12]

From 1989 through 1990, the number of AIDS cases in female Hispanics living in the United States increased by 49%. In contrast, increases of 30 and 33% were observed during the same time period for cases in Caucasian and African-American females, respectively.

Of the 3766 Hispanic women with AIDS reported to CDC by mid-1991, 1901 (51%) acquired AIDS through IDU, 1412 (38%) through heterosexual contact (often with a male partner infected by IDU), 201 (5%) through transfusion of blood or blood products, while for 252 (7%) the mode of transmission category was undetermined. The undetermined category includes persons whose mode of exposure is still

Table 2 AIDS in Women, by Transmission Category and Race/Ethnicity, United States and U.S. Territories, Reported in 1990

	African-American		Hispanic		Caucasian		Total[a]	
Transmission category	Number	Percent	Number	Percent	Number	Percent	Number	Percent
Injection drug use	1351	53	495	46	471	38	2329	48
Heterosexual contact	823	32	407	38	416	34	1657	34
Transfusion	88	4	70	7	211	17	376	8
Other/undetermined[b]	277	11	97	9	138	11	528	11
Total	2539	100	1069	100	1236	100	4890	100

[a]Total includes 19 Asian/Pacific Islanders, 9 American Indian/Alaskan Natives, and 18 cases whose race/ethnicity was not reported.
[b]Cases under investigation; cases lost to follow-up, and cases whose mode of exposure to HIV remains undetermined after investigation.

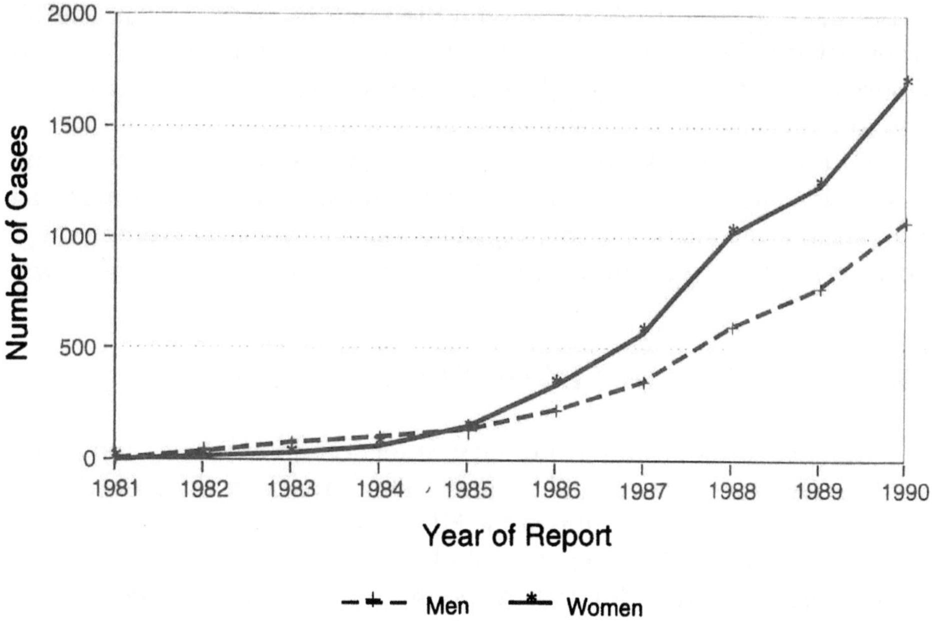

Figure 1. Heterosexual transmission (AIDS): Trends by gender.

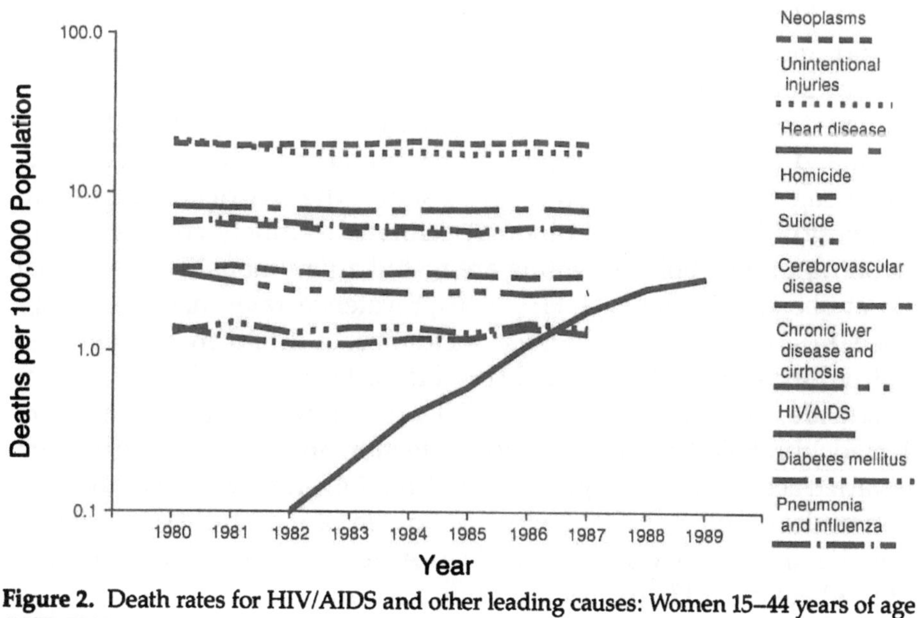

Figure 2. Death rates for HIV/AIDS and other leading causes: Women 15–44 years of age (1980–1989).

under investigation (5%); those who died before investigation (0.9%), were lost to follow-up (0.1%), or declined to be interviewed (0.2%); and whose mode of exposure to HIV remains undetermined after investigation (0.2%).

By the end of 1990, the cumulative incidence rate of AIDS among Hispanic women from heterosexual transmission was eight times that for Caucasian women.[12] Eighty-eight percent of Hispanic women diagnosed with AIDS were in the childbearing age-group of 15 to 44 years.

PREVALENCE OF HIV IN HISPANIC WOMEN

Because progression from HIV infection to AIDS is long and variable (average 7–10 years),[13] women who have been diagnosed with AIDS represent only a portion of the HIV epidemic. Based on AIDS case projections done in 1989, as estimated 1 million persons in the United States were infected with HIV.[14] Although it is not known how many of these were women, the following HIV seroprevalence studies indicate the magnitude of HIV infection in this population.[15]

Since 1985, the Department of Defense has performed routine HIV antibody testing of all applicants for military service. For female applicants, the highest HIV seropositive rates were found in Puerto Rico (0.37%), New Jersey (0.28%), Washington, D.C. (0.28%), New York (0.25%), and Maryland (0.18%). Hispanic women had a seroprevalence rate four times that of Caucasian women.[16]

The Centers for Disease Control and the National Institute of Child Health and Human Development maintain surveillance of HIV infection among childbearing women in 44 states, the District of Columbia, and Puerto Rico.[2] Residual blood specimens routinely collected from newborns for metabolic screening are tested anonymously for maternal HIV antibody. The highest HIV seroprevalence rates have been observed in areas with the highest incidence of AIDS in women and children, including New York, New Jersey, Florida, and Puerto Rico. Nationwide, an estimated 1.5 per 1000 women delivering in 1989 were infected with HIV. Prevalence of HIV infection among Hispanic women has varied according to geographic location. During 1988–1990, the HIV seroprevalence rate per 1000 Hispanic women ranged from 0.5 in Texas, where the most Hispanics are Mexican-American, to 10.8 in New York State, where most Hispanics are Puerto Rican.

Based on these results, an estimated 6000 infants were born to HIV-infected mothers in the United States in 1989; approximately 30% of these births occurred in New York State. Hispanic women living in New York City, again most of whom are of Puerto Rican descent, accounted for over 500, or nearly 10%, of all births of HIV-infected women in the United States.[17,18]

AIDS AND HIV IN HISPANIC CHILDREN

Of the over 3000 children (12 years of age and younger) with AIDS reported to CDC as of mid-1991, 53% were African-American and 25% were Hispanic. Nineteen percent of all pediatric cases have been diagnosed in Hispanic children living in the contiguous United States; another 6% of cases occurred among children in Puerto Rico. New York City has reported almost half of the Hispanic children with AIDS residing in the United States. Thirty-eight percent of all children with AIDS reported in New York City are Hispanic.

The impact of HIV/AIDS on mortality for children younger than 15 years of age was reviewed using national mortality statistics for 1988.[19,20] The impact of HIV/AIDS is most striking in the 1- to 4-year-old age group and in African-American and Hispanic children, particularly in the Northeast. By 1988, HIV/AIDS was the leading cause of death in Hispanic children 1 through 4 years of age in New York State, accounting for 15% of all deaths in Hispanics.

PERINATAL TRANSMISSION

Perinatal HIV infection is the result of transmission of HIV from an infected mother to her infant during pregnancy or delivery and rarely through breast-feeding. The perinatal transmission rate for HIV infection is estimated to be 25 to 35%.[21] Eighty-four percent of all pediatric AIDS cases and 87% of Hispanic pediatric cases reported through 1990 resulted from perinatal transmission (Table 3). Of all perinatal cases, 26% occurred among Hispanics living in the contiguous United States, while 6% were residents of Puerto Rico. New York City reported 10% of all perinatal cases and over half (53%) of the Hispanic perinatal cases, excluding those reported from Puerto Rico. The increased numbers of Hispanic women who have acquired HIV have been accompanied by increased numbers of infected Hispanic children (Figure 3).

Table 3 AIDS in Children (<13 years of age) by Transmission Category and Race/Ethnicity, United States and U.S. Territories, Reported through June 30, 1991

	African-American		Hispanic		White		Total[a]	
Transmission category	Number	Percent	Number	Percent	Number	Percent	Number	Percent
Perinatal	1530	93	683	87	410	61	2645	84
Transfusion	59	4	61	8	146	22	271	9
Hemophilia	20	1	24	3	102	15	149	5
Other/undetermined[b]	45	3	20	3	10	1	75	2
Total	1654	100	788	100	668	100	3140	100

[a]Total includes 16 Asian/Pacific Islanders, 7 American Indian/Alaskan Natives, and 7 cases whose race/ethnicity was not reported.
[b]Cases under investigation; cases lost to follow-up, and cases whose mode of exposure to HIV remains undetermined after investigation.

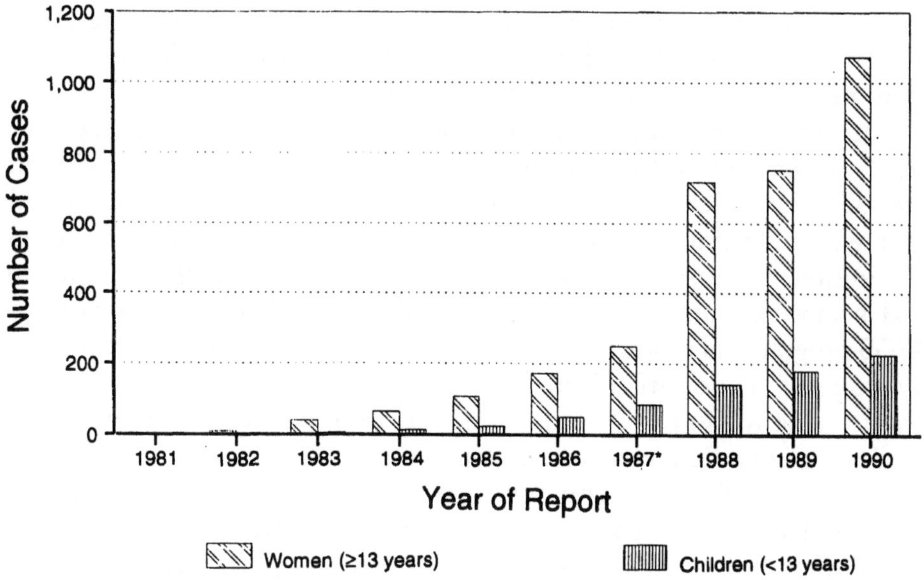

Figure 3. AIDS in Hispanic women and children: United States and Puerto Rico (Reported 1981–1990).

SOCIAL AND BEHAVIORAL ASPECTS

In addition to devastating the immune systems of persons infected with HIV, the epidemic is also devastating the life-styles and social milieu of affected persons and their significant others. Several behaviors relate to a person's risk for acquiring HIV. While these behaviors result from individual choices, many are influenced by established beliefs and behavioral and cultural norms that have evolved over long periods. For example, studies of Hispanic women indicate that, compared with Mexican-American women, Puerto Rican and Cuban-American women may be at greater risk for unintended pregnancies. This same unprotected sex may also place these women at greater risk for HIV if their partners are infected. This observed difference may directly reflect differences in patterns of contraceptive and protective sexual practices among these women.[22]

Other studies have suggested that there are fundamental differences in life-style practices among the different Hispanic communities. Among less acculturated women attending an urban family planning clinic in Los Angeles, Spanish-speaking (Mexican-American) women reported fewer traditional risk factors for AIDS than English-speaking women. That is, Spanish-speaking women were less likely to report a history of drug or alcohol use or sexually transmitted diseases, and were more likely to have had fewer sex partners.[23]

In 1988, a symposium was held to develop a national strategy for AIDS prevention and control in Hispanic communities in the United States.[24] Several characteristics of these communities were identified that were thought to hinder Hispanics' response to effective AIDS prevention. Because the Hispanic community is so diverse in culture and socioeconomic characteristics, a diverse approach to preventive AIDS programs is required. The provision of health care and preventive messages is made difficult because many Hispanics are recent immigrants; some are in the United States only temporarily, and some arrive as illegal aliens. Behaviors associated with HIV infection (i.e., IDU and homosexual activity among men) are stigmatizing and not openly discussed in Hispanic communities. Many Hispanic communities have also suffered other health problems with disproportionate morbidity and mortality. Traditionally, the health care delivery system has been less accessible to Hispanics than it has been to Caucasians. This is thought to reflect multiple problems, including limited knowledge of the means to appropriately access the health care system and fear of insensitivity.

Some characteristics of the Hispanic communities that may facilitate effective responses to AIDS prevention programs were also identified during this symposium. Hispanic communities have very strong family bonds that provide social support for affected persons. Family and children are central concerns for Hispanic communities, and these concerns can be elicited to encourage preventive behavior. Programs that take these characteristics into consideration are being developed by community, regional, and national Hispanic organizations to confront the problem of AIDS among Hispanics.[24]

The effects of poverty, homelessness, and drugs on Hispanic women at risk for HIV infection have been studied through the use of focus groups.[25] The dominant concern reported by these women was overcoming threats to their provider role and caring for their families, particularly children. In the East Harlem section of New York City an ethnographic study found that IDU women could actually increase their risk of HIV infection by attempting to create a "conventional" family, because the men they chose to be monogamous with were often HIV-infected IDUs who were unwilling to take precautions necessary to protect their female partners.[26] For those women who are aware of their personal risk of HIV/AIDS, the most important intervention may be to assist them to translate this knowledge and awareness into appropriate behavioral changes.[27]

FUTURE TRENDS/RECOMMENDATIONS

The national AIDS case surveillance reporting system contains only reports of HIV-infected women and children who have been diagnosed with AIDS. The seroprevalence study of HIV infection among women of childbearing age, as described above, and other seroprevalence surveys will be crucial to identify populations and areas with the greatest needs during the course of the HIV/AIDS epidemic.

Public health surveillance shows that the primary routes of HIV transmission among Hispanic women are IDU and sexual intercourse, often with a male partner infected through IDU. Therefore, programs for preventing HIV infection among Hispanic women and men should focus on drug-treatment and prevention of needle-sharing in addition to stressing precautions for heterosexual contact. Existing drug prevention and drug rehabilitation programs should include HIV prevention services, including HIV-antibody testing and counseling, information about early interventions for HIV-positive persons, access to these early interventions, and referral for social services and medical management of HIV infection.[28] In addition, programs and services should address the needs of the many children that will become orphaned once their infected mothers have died.

The development of culturally sensitive HIV prevention programs that utilize the recognized characteristics of the Hispanic communities are clearly warranted to effectively halt the spread of HIV transmission among women, children, and adolescents.

REFERENCES

1. Centers for Disease Control: Update on Kaposi's sarcoma and opportunistic infections in previously healthy persons–United States. *Morbidity and Mortality Weekly Report* 31:294, 300–301, 1982
2. Gwinn M, Pappaioanou M, George JR: Prevalence of HIV infection in childbearing women in the United States: Surveillance using newborn blood samples. *JAMA* 265:1704–1708, 1991

3. U.S. Bureau of the Census: The Hispanic population in the United States: March, 1988. *Current Population Reports*, Population characteristics, Series P-20, No. 431. Washington, DC, U.S. Government Printing Office, 1988
4. Hayes-Bautista DE: Identifying "Hispanic" populations: The influence of research methodology upon public policy. *Amer. J. Pub. Health.* 70:353–356, 1980
5. Hayes-Bautista DE, Chapa J: Latino terminology: Conceptual bases for standardized terminology. *Amer. J. Pub. Health* 77:61–68, 1987
6. Novello AC, Wise PH, Kleinman DV: Hispanic health: Time for data, time for action. (editorial) *JAMA* 265:253–255, 1991
7. U.S. Bureau of the Census: *Current Population Reports*, Series P-25, No. 1040-RD-1. Population estimates by race and Hispanic origin for states, metropolitan areas, and selected counties; 1980 to 1985. Washington, D.C., U.S. Government Printing Office, 1986
8. Selik RM, Castro KG, Pappaioanou M, Buehler JW: Birthplace and the risk of AIDS among Hispanics in the United States. *Amer. J. Pub. Health* 9:836–839, 1989
9. Menendez BS, Drucker E, Vermund SH, Castano RR, Perez-Agosto RR, Parga FJ, Blum S: AIDS mortality among Puerto Ricans and other Hispanics in New York City, 1981–1987. *AIDS* 3:644–648, 1990
10. Chu SY, Buehler JW, Berkleman RL: Impact of the human immunodeficiency virus epidemic on mortality in women of reproductive age, United States. *JAMA* 264:225–229, 1990
11. Puerto Rico Health Department: *Informacíon Anual de Estadisticas Vitales.* (Annual Summary of Vital Statistics), 1987
12. Ellerbrock TV, Bush TJ, Chamberland ME, Oxtoby MJ: Epidemiology of women with AIDS in the United States, 1981 through 1990. *JAMA* 265:2971–2975, 1991
13. Hessol HA, Lifson AR, O'Malley PM, Doll LS, Jaffe HW, Rutherford GW: Prevalence, incidence, and progression of human immunodeficiency virus infection in homosexual and bisexual men in hepatitis B vaccine trials, 1978–1988. *Amer. J. Epid.* 130:1167–1175, 1989
14. Centers for Disease Control: HIV prevalence estimates and AIDS case projections for the United States: Report based upon a workshop. *MMWR* 39(No.RR-16):1–31, 1990
15. Centers for Disease Control: *National HIV Seroprevalence Surveys Report.* Summary of Results, Data from serosurveillance activities through 1989. U.S. Department of Health and Human Services, Atlanta, 1990
16. Department of Defense: *Prevalence of HIV-1 Antibody in Civilian Applicants for Military Service, October 1985–September 1990.* Selected tables prepared by the Division of HIV/AIDS, Centers for Disease Control. Atlanta, GA: Centers for Disease Control; 1990.
17. Novick LF, Berns D, Stricof R, Stevens R, Pass K, Wethers J: HIV seroprevalence in newborns in New York State. *JAMA* 261:1745–1750, 1989
18. Novick LF, Glebatis DM, Stricof RL: II. Newborn seroprevalence study: Methods and results. New York State HIV seroprevalence project. *Amer. J. Pub. Health* 81 (supplement):15–21, 1991
19. Kilbourne BW, Buehler JW, Rogers MF: AIDS as a cause of death in children, adolescents, and young adults. (Letter) *Amer. J. Pub. Health* 80:499–500, 1990
20. Chu SY, Buehler JW, Oxtoby MJ, Kilbourne BW: Impact of the human immunodeficiency virus epidemic on mortality in children, United States. *Pediatrics* 87:806–810, 1991
21. Oxtoby M: Perinatally acquired human immunodeficiency virus infection. *Ped. Infect. Dis. J.* 9:609–619, 1990
22. Stroup-Benham CA, Trevino FM: Reproductive characteristics of Mexican-American, mainland Puerto Rican, and Cuban-American women. *JAMA* 265:222–226, 1991
23. Rapkin AJ, Erickson PI: Differences in knowledge of and risk factors for AIDS between Hispanic and non-Hispanic women attending an urban family planning clinic. *AIDS* 4:889–899, 1990

24. Hahn RA, Castro KG: The health and health care status of Latino populations in the U.S.: A brief review, in *Latinos and AIDS: Monographs*, UCLA Press, Los Angeles, 1989.
25. Nyamathi A, Vasquez R: Impact of poverty, homelessness, and drugs on Hispanic women at risk for HIV infection. *Hispanic J. Behav. Sciences* 11:299–314, 1989
26. Suffet F, Lefshitz M: Women addicts and the threat of AIDS risk and risk reduction activities by black and Hispanic/Latina women. *Amer. Psychologist* 23:949–957, 1988
27. Gayle JA, Selik RM, Chu SY: Surveillance for AIDS and HIV infection among black and Hispanic children and women of childbearing age, 1981–1989. *MMWR Surveillance Summaries* 89:(SS-3)23–30, 1990

8

Physical Growth, Sexual Maturation, and Obesity in Puerto Rican Children

REYNALDO MARTORELL, FERNANDO S. MENDOZA, KATHERINE BAISDEN, AND IVAN G. PAWSON

INTRODUCTION

Bean and Tienda[1] emphasize three features in assessing demographic and socioeconomic changes in the U.S. Hispanic population over the last two decades: rapid growth, regional concentration, and extensive demographic and socioeconomic variation according to national origin.

The Hispanic Health and Nutrition Examination Survey (HHANES), conducted between 1982 and 1984, was the first large-scale assessment of the health and nutritional status of the U.S. Hispanic population.[2] Its

---

REYNALDO MARTORELL • Center for International Health, Emory University School of Public Health, Atlanta, Georgia 30329. FERNANDO S. MENDOZA • Department of Pediatrics, Lucile Salter Packard Children's Hospital at Stanford University, Stanford, California 94305. KATHERINE BAISDEN • Center for Chicano Research, Stanford University, Stanford, California 94305. IVAN G. PAWSON • Koret Center for Human Nutrition, San Francisco General Hospital, San Francisco, California 94110.

Puerto Rican Women and Children: Issues in Health, Growth, and Development, edited by Gontran Lamberty and Cynthia Garcia Coll. Plenum Press, New York, 1994.

undertaking was no doubt motivated by the rising visibility of the Hispanic presence in the United States, a phenomenon described by Bean and Tienda,[1] and by the recognition that not enough was known about health and nutrition in this growing segment of the U.S. population. HHANES recognized in its design the marked regional concentration of Hispanics, and focused data collection on Mexican-Americans in the Southwest, Puerto Ricans in the New York area, and Cuban-Americans in Dade County, Florida.

The Stanford Center for Chicano Research, with funds from the Maternal and Child Health Bureau, has carried out research to quantify the nature and extent of health and nutrition problems in the U.S. Hispanic population. The present study is part of this effort. Its emphasis is on the physical growth, maturation, and body composition of the New York area Puerto Rican population. Specifically, the objectives are to describe the growth patterns in height and the rate of sexual development in children and to assess the prevalence of overweight and obesity in children and adults.

METHODS

Data Sources

Hispanic Health and Nutrition Examination Survey was carried out by the National Center for Health Statistics and was designed to provide specific information on designated target populations rather than on the Hispanic population as a whole. The Puerto Rican component was sampled from the New York City area which represented 54% of the 1980 U.S. mainland Puerto Rican population. Individual households were selected and a clustering sampling technique was used to collect data from the sampled households. The sampling methods are described in detail elsewhere.[2]

Data collected during NHANES I (1971–1974) and II (1976–1980) on the general U.S. population are used as reference standards. These data include all subjects measured in these surveys and are reported by Frisancho.[3] Data on height, weight, triceps skinfold thickness, and subscapular skinfold thickness are used in this analysis. Unpublished reference data for the subscapular-to-triceps skinfold-thickness ratio were supplied by Frisancho (personal communication).

Indicators of Growth and Body Composition

The anthropometric variables selected for analyses (height, weight, and triceps and subscapular skinfolds) were collected by trained technicians using standardized procedures and highly calibrated equipment. Height was measured to the nearest 0.1 centimeter in children 2 years of age and older. Weight was measured to the nearest 0.01 kilogram, including the weight of light clothing. Skinfold thicknesses were measured on the right hand side of the body to the nearest 0.5 millimeter. Two derived indicators were used: the body mass index (kg/m^2) and the ratio of subscapular to triceps skinfold thicknesses. These are used as indicators of overweight/obesity and of centralized fat distribution respectively. Only individuals with complete data for height, weight, and triceps and subscapular skinfold thicknesses were selected for study. These criteria resulted in the exclusion of a small percentage of sampled individuals (sample sizes are given in Table 1).

An individual was defined as overweight if the particular anthropometric variable was ≥85th percentile of the reference population and obese if it was ≥95th percentile. For individuals younger than 18 years of age, this comparison was made yearly between Puerto Rican and U.S. populations, which were grouped, for the purposes of presentation, into the following categories: 2 to 4.9, 5 to 11.9, and 12 to 17.9 years of age. Subjects aged older than 18 years were defined as overweight or

Table 1 Sample Sizes for Anthropometry for the Puerto Rican Subsample

Age (years)	Males	Females
2–4.9	113	100
5–11.9	246	256
12–17.9	241	243
18–24.9	131	204
25–29.9	63	101
30–39.9	106	191
40–49.9	94	183
50–59.9	114	148
60+	54	102
Total	1162	1528

Source: Hispanic Health and Nutrition Examination Survey (HHANES), 1982–1984.

obese if they met or exceeded the 85th or 95th percentiles for 18- to 24.9-year-olds in the reference population; this is the youngest adult group for which data are provided by Frisancho.[3] The rationale for using young adults as the reference group is that they are leaner than older adults. A similar rationale was followed by Najjar and Rowland,[4] but these authors used a 20- to 29-year age group.

To clarify the role of socioeconomic and cultural factors in linear growth retardation, poverty, language, and education variables were included in multiple regression analyses. "Poverty" is expressed by the poverty index ratio and is based on household income, composition, and the consumer price index. Values less than 1 indicate that household income falls below the currently defined poverty level for households of similar size. Language preference is a general indicator of an individual's overall level of acculturation or integration into the culture of the host country. Hispanic Health and Nutrition Examination Survey provides data on household language preference for subjects less than 12 years of age and for the specific individual after this age. Two language variables were created: "Spanish" distinguished a preference for Spanish (1 = Spanish, 0 = other) and "Biling" one for bilingualism (1 = bilingual, 0 = others). The reference group is made up of subjects who prefer English or who live in households that do. Information about the education of the head of the household was coded as a single indicator variable. "Gradesch" distinguished those with 8 or fewer years of schooling from the rest (1 = grade school; 0 = others).

Sexual Maturation

Tanner[6] described the most widely used method for rating the development of secondary sexual characteristics. Children are assigned to any of five stages of development from the prepubertal to the adult condition. This is done for pubic hair development in both sexes, for breast development in females, and for changes in the size and appearance of the genitalia in males. The stages are described in detail elsewhere.[5,6] Complete data about secondary sexual characteristics were available for 585 Puerto Rican adolescents: 292 males and 293 females.

SAS probit procedures were used to estimate mean ages at entry and their 95% fiducial limits as described by Villarreal, Martorell, and Mendoza[6] who analyzed the data for the Mexican-American component of HHANES. These statistics can be interpreted as the average age at which children enter a stage. There is, of course, no possible value for stage 1, the prepubertal stage.

There are no national reference data for sexual maturation to use for comparison. The Puerto Rican results are compared to Mexican-Americans from HHANES[6] and to cross-sectional data from a recent study carried out in the Netherlands.[7]

ANALYSES

Tables of means and standard deviations for all anthropometric variables are given elsewhere.[4] Medians were estimated at each age and compared to reference curves for the U.S. population (75th, 50th, and 25th percentiles). Sample weights were used in estimating medians.

Prevalence rates for overweight and obesity are displayed in charts illustrating the proportion of individuals in each age and gender who met or exceeded the 85th (overweight) and 95th (obese) percentiles of the U.S. reference population. Prevalences were estimated taking into account the sample weights.

For analyses of the predictors of height, multiple regressions were carried out with adjustments for sample weights. The design effect of the HHANES survey was incorporated by calculating adjusted t statistics. These were computed after inflating the standard errors by $\sqrt{2}$ (i.e., the average design effect was assumed to equal 2). This approach is recommended by Delgado et al.[8]

Sample weights were not used in estimating median ages of entry for the sexual maturation data; this is because SAS does not make this option available in its probit subroutine. It is unlikely, however, that the consideration of sample weights and design effects in the estimation of ages at entry would have resulted in significantly different values. Still, readers should evaluate these results with caution.

RESULTS

Height

Median values for height for Puerto Ricans are plotted in Figures 1 (males) and 2 (females) and compared with 75th, 50th, and 25th percentile curves for the U.S. reference population. Differences between medians are insignificant during early and middle childhood. In males,

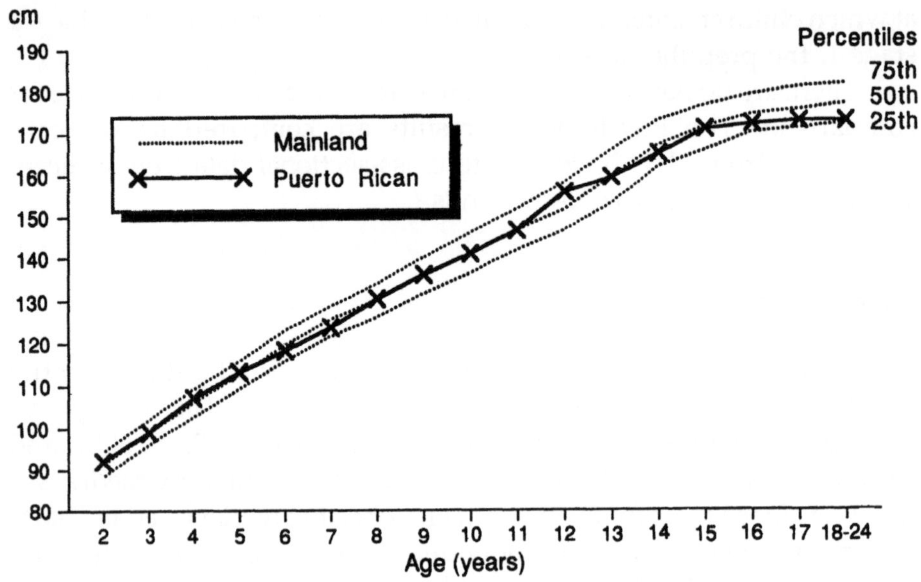

Figure 1. Height medians for Puerto Rican males compared to U.S. reference curves.[3]

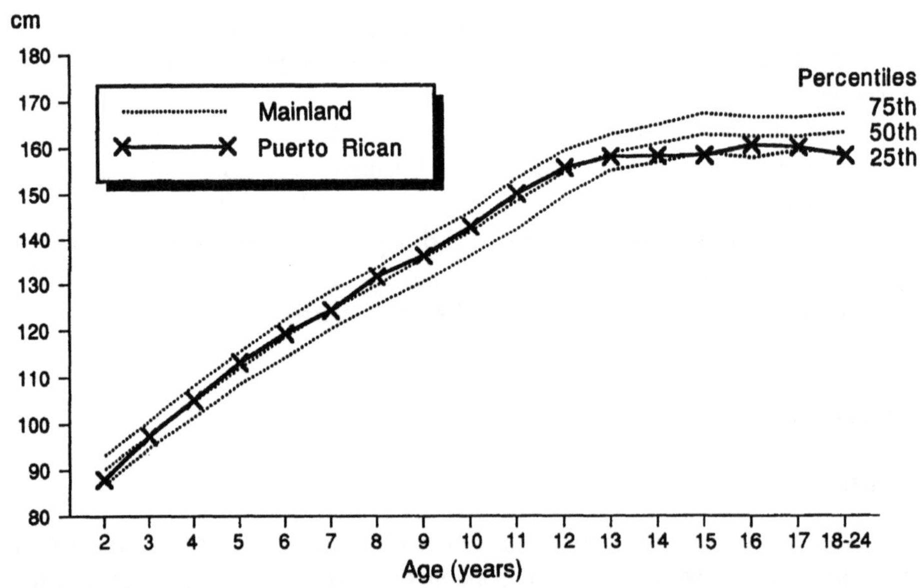

Figure 2. Height medians for Puerto Rican females compared to U.S. reference curves.[3]

differences surface late in adolescence, and by adulthood, the median heights of Puerto Ricans are near the 25th percentile of the U.S. reference population. The pattern in females is similar except that the differences appear earlier in adolescence.

Multiple regression analyses of economic, cultural, and educational predictors of height were conducted separately for 2 to 11 (n = 596), 12 to 17 (n = 380), and 18 to 24.9 (n = 242) years, as shown in Table 2. Few predictors are statistically significant. At 2 to 11 years, older children and children living in homes with greater relative incomes are taller (t = 3.0, p<.005); also, relative to children from English-speaking homes, subjects from Spanish-speaking and bilingual homes tend to be shorter, but the probability statistic exceeds the conventional value of 0.05. Gender (males are taller) is significant in the analysis of subjects 12 to 17 years (t = 6.8, p<.001) and in subjects 18 to 24.9 years (t = 7.8, p<.001).

Sexual Maturation

In Figures 3 to 6, the data in Table 3 are compared to data from a cross-sectional survey of Dutch children and to estimates for Mexican-Americans obtained from HHANES. United States reference data for sexual maturation are not available. Estimates for pubic hair stage 2 (PH2) in females are unstable and are not provided. This is due to the fact that the youngest subjects examined were already 10 years of age and many of the Puerto Rican girls reached PH2 at younger ages.

Relative to Mexican-Americans, Puerto Ricans reach the various stages of sexual maturation at younger ages. Relative to Dutch children, Puerto Ricans reach sexual development stages a few months later in the case of pubic hair stages in both sexes and in the case of the breast stages. In terms of male genitalia stages, values are almost identical for stages 2 and 3 and favor Puerto Ricans slightly in the case of stages 4 and 5.

Body Composition

Body mass index (BMI) medians for Puerto Ricans are compared to the U.S. 75th, 50th, and 25th percentile curves for males (Figure 7) and females (Figure 8). Values for Puerto Ricans exceed the 50th percentile of the reference population at almost all ages.

Table 2 Predictors of Height in Puerto Ricans[a]

	2–11 years (n = 596)				12–17 years (n = 380)				18–24.9 years (n = 242)			
Variable	Parameter	S.E.	t	p	Parameter	S.E.	t	p	Parameter	S.E.	t	p
Intercept	80.117	1.255	63.859	<.001	128.227	4.482	28.609	<.001	161.194	9.097	17.719	<.001
Age	6.204	0.132	47.000	<.001	2.043	0.299	6.833	<.001	−0.158	0.433	0.365	N.S.
Sex	−0.817	0.730	−1.119	N.S.	6.833	1.011	6.759	<.001	13.038	1.662	7.844	<.001
Poverty	0.012	0.004	3.000	<.005	0.006	0.005	1.200	N.S.	0.011	0.008	1.375	N.S.
Gradesch	0.440	1.066	0.413	N.S.	−0.379	1.677	−0.226	N.S.	2.087	2.483	0.841	N.S.
Primary	1.200	0.869	1.381	N.S.	0.902	1.107	0.815	N.S.	0.561	1.747	0.321	N.S.
Biling	−1.709	0.989	−1.728	<.10	−0.739	1.077	−0.686	N.S.	−1.702	1.711	0.995	N.S.
Spanish	−1.395	0.850	−1.641	<.10	−1.361	2.162	−0.630	N.S.	−0.394	2.794	0.014	N.S.

[a]Weighted regressions; standard errors were inflated by a factor of $\sqrt{2}$ to adjust for an average design effect of 2.

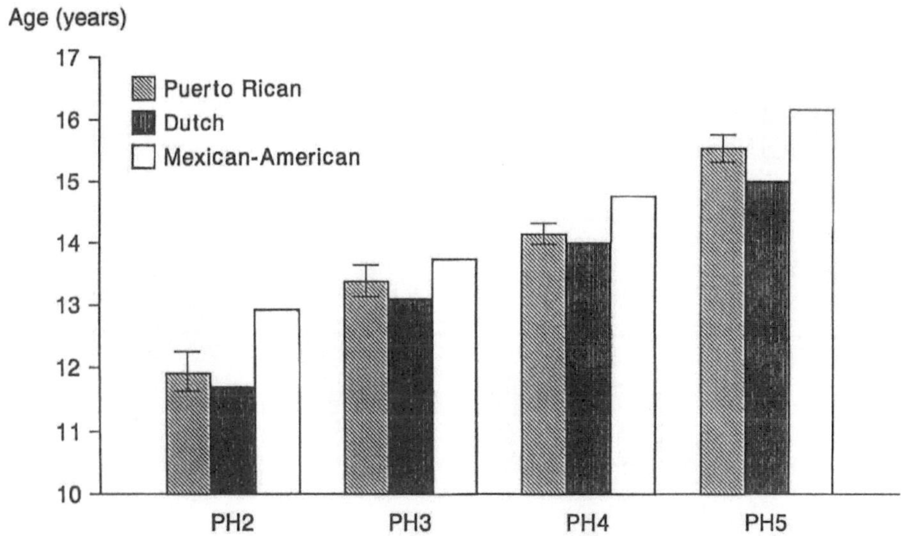

Figure 3. Mean ages at entry for Puerto Rican males (with 95% fiducial limits) compared to Dutch[8] and Mexican-American children[7]: Males: Pubic Hair Stages (n = 292).

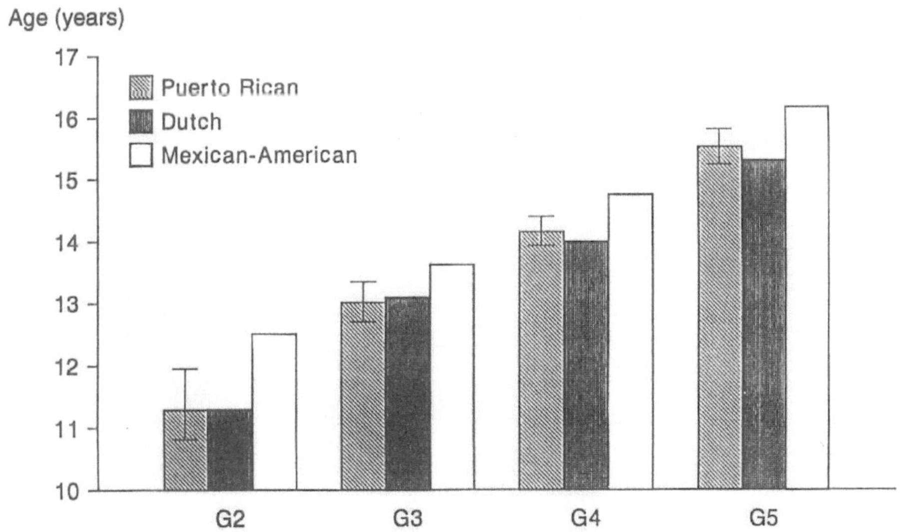

Figure 4. Mean ages at entry for Puerto Ricans (with 95% fiducial limits) compared to Dutch[8] and Mexican-American children[7]: Males: genitalia stages (n = 292).

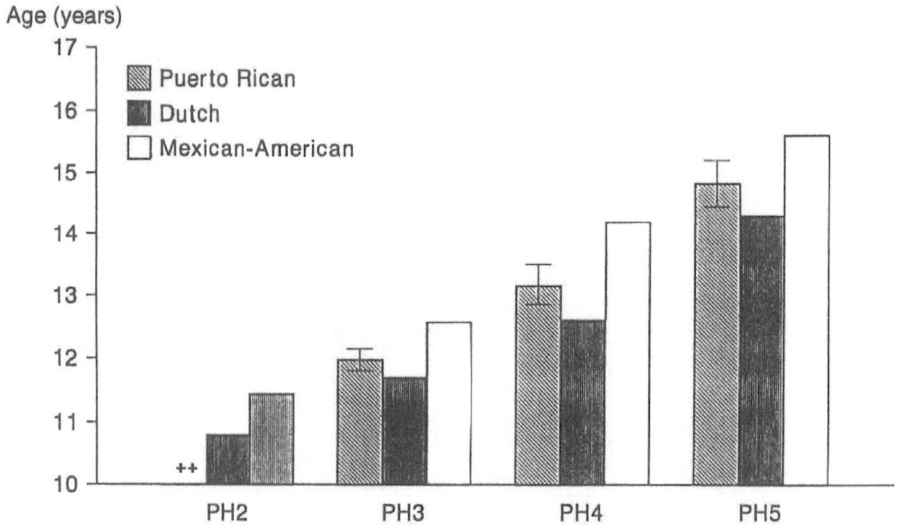

Figure 5. Mean ages at entry for Puerto Ricans (with 95% fiducial limits) compared to Dutch[8] and Mexican-American children[7]: Females: pubic hair stages (n = 293). **Estimate for PH2 in Puerto Ricans is unreliable.

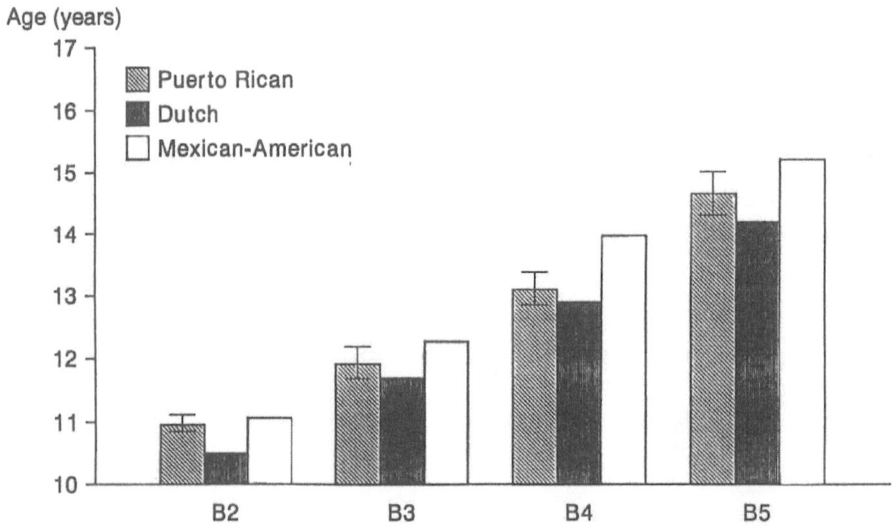

Figure 6. Mean ages at entry for Puerto Ricans (with 95% fiducial limits) compared to Dutch[8] and Mexican-American children[7]: Females: breast stages (n = 293).

Table 3 Mean Ages (Years) at Entry for Puerto Ricans (with 95% Fiducial Limits)

	Males (n = 292)		Females (n = 293)	
Stage	Pubic hair	Genitalia	Pubic hair	Breast
2	11.91 (11.57–12.19)	11.29 (10.62–11.76)	[a]	10.96 (10.80–11.07)
3	13.38 (13.12–13.63)	13.01 (12.67–13.32)	11.97 (11.80–12.14)	11.92 (11.65–12.16)
4	14.14 (13.96–14.30)	14.16 (13.92–14.39)	13.15 (12.80–13.45)	13.10 (12.82–13.35)
5	15.53 (15.31–15.75)	15.52 (15.23–15.81)	14.83 (14.45–15.21)	14.66 (14.30–15.01)

[a]Unstable estimates.

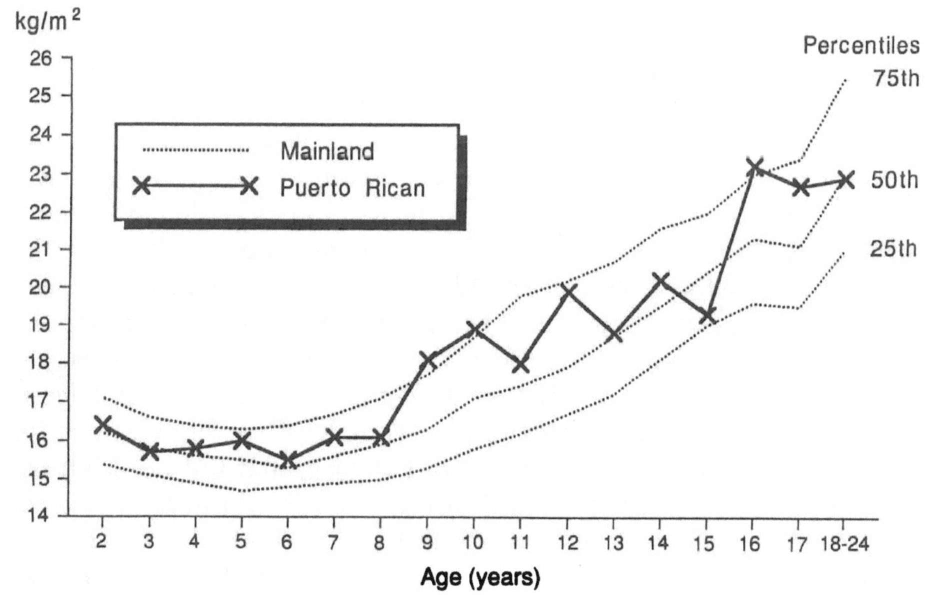

Figure 7. Body mass index medians for Puerto Rican males compared to U.S. reference curves.[3]

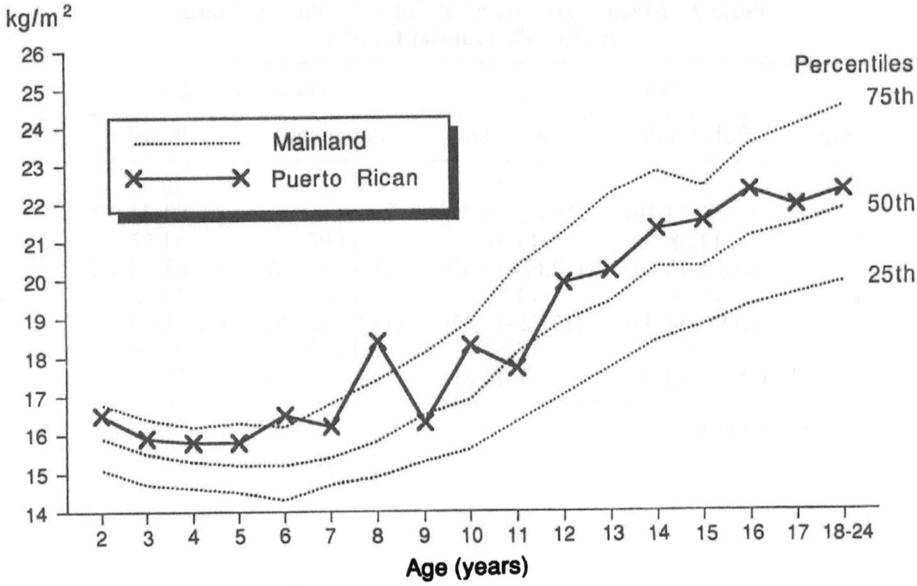

Figure 8. Body mass index medians for Puerto Rican females compared to U.S. reference curves.[3]

The percent of subjects with BMI values greater than the 85th percentile (overweight) and the 95th percentile (obese) are given in Figure 9 for children and adults. The horizontal lines depict the values of overweight and obese (e.g., 15 and 5% respectively) that a population identical to the U.S. reference population would be expected to have. Values for Puerto Ricans exceed the expected values at almost all ages, particularly among older adults and to a greater extent in females. For example, among those 60 years or older, over 30% of the males and over 60% of the females are overweight. These values are over twice the expected prevalence in males and over four times that in females.

A similar analysis is shown in Figures 10 and 11 for triceps and subscapular skinfold thicknesses. Females have high values for both variables whereas males have high subscapular but not high triceps values in older children and adults. Finally, an analysis of the percentage of Puerto Ricans exceeding the 85th and 95th percentiles of the subscapular/triceps ratio is shown in Figure 12. Especially as adults, Puerto Ricans have a pronounced tendency to deposit fat in the trunk.

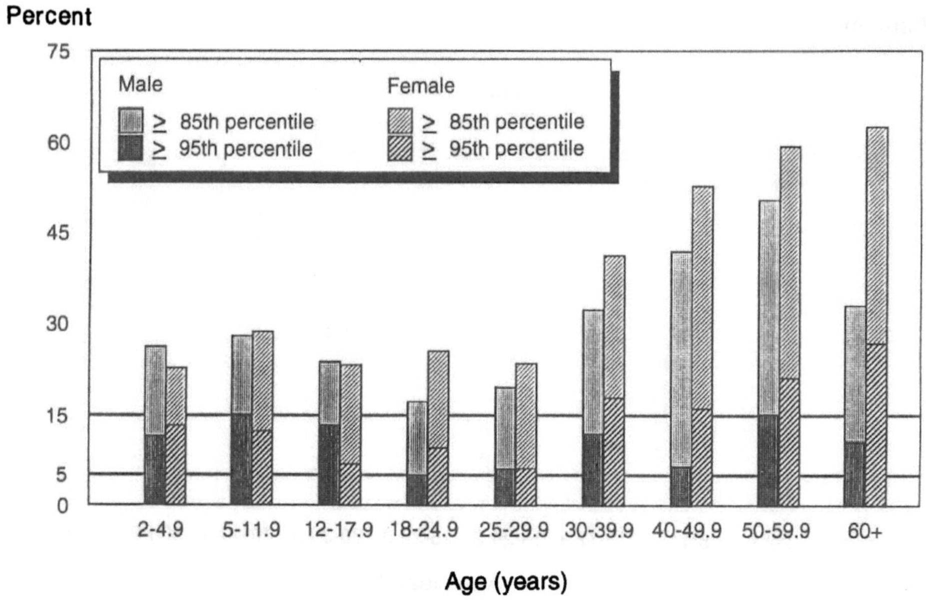

Figure 9. Percent of Puerto Ricans with high BMI values relative to U.S. reference values.[3]

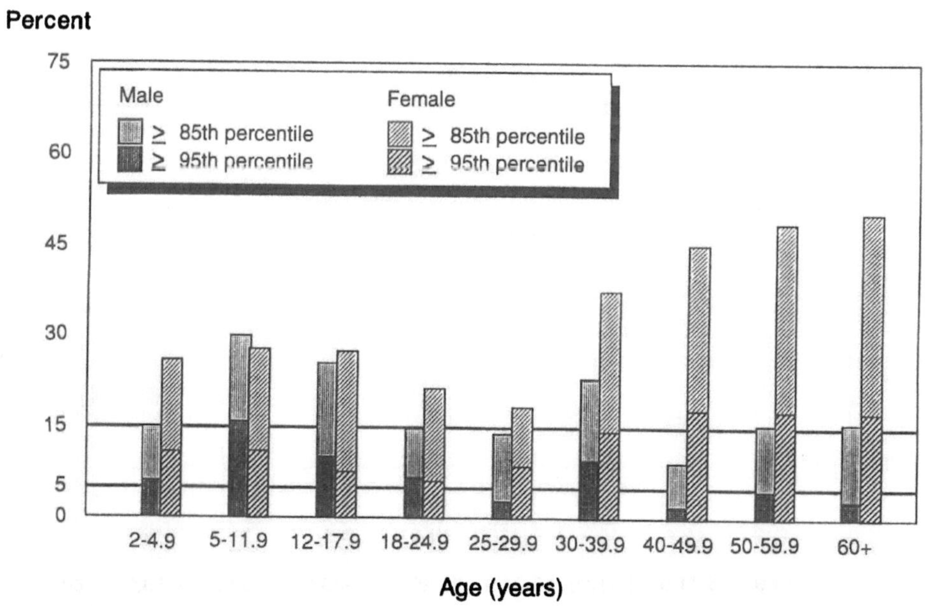

Figure 10. Percent of Puerto Ricans with high triceps skinfold thicknesses relative to U.S. reference values.[3]

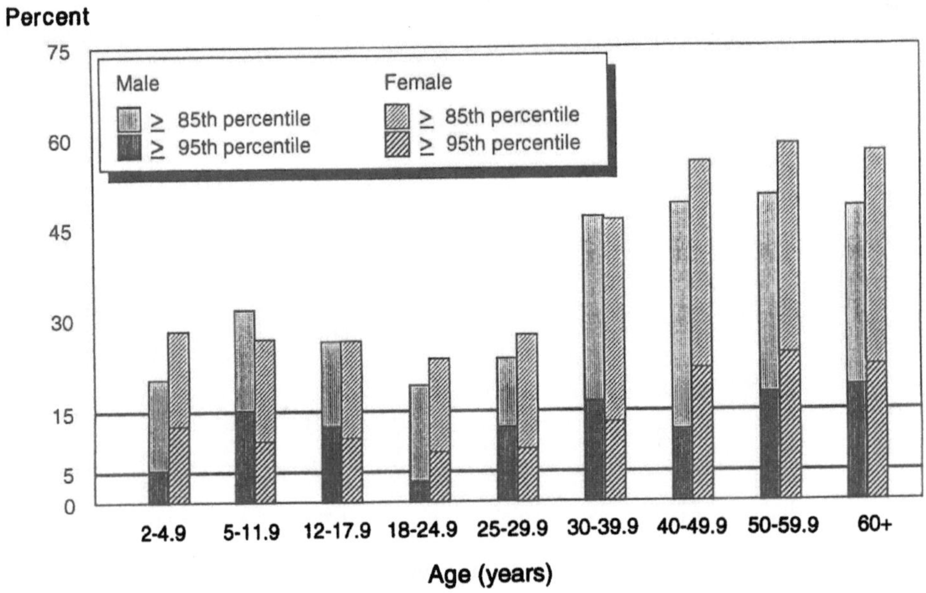

Figure 11. Percent of Puerto Ricans with high subscapular skinfold thicknesses relative to U.S. reference values.[3]

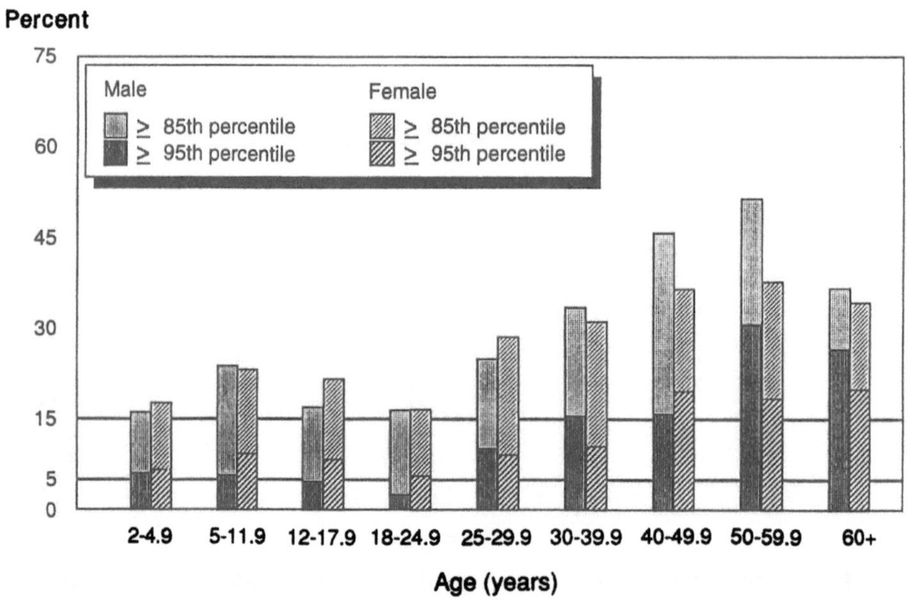

Figure 12. Percent of Puerto Ricans with high ratio of subscapular to triceps skinfold thicknesses relative to U.S. reference values.[3]

DISCUSSION

Anthropometric data for Puerto Ricans are compared to U.S. national reference data derived from all subjects measured in NHANES I and II.[3] This allows for direct comparisons of the size and body composition of the Puerto Rican population to national averages and distributions. Whether this is an appropriate reference population to use is an open question. All ethnic groups of the United States should, in theory, be represented in the NHANES surveys in proportion to their numbers (after adjusting for sample weights). As such, the subjects of NHANES I and II are predominately non-Hispanic Caucasian and African-American in origin. Hispanics and a few other ethnic groups are represented but in small numbers.

Puerto Ricans are as tall as the general population prior to adolescence but appear to fall significantly behind during adolescence. By the time they are young adults, Puerto Ricans have median heights that are near the 25th percentile of the U.S. distribution. A similar pattern has been described by Martorell, Mendoza, and Castillo[9] for Mexican-Americans for HHANES. Cubans measured in HHANES are also similar. Is this characteristic influenced by genetic as opposed to environmental factors (e.g., health, nutrition)? Perhaps, but other answers are possible. Martorell, Mendoza, and Castillo[9] point out that cross-sectional data may make it appear that growth is impaired in adolescence when, in fact, the retardation in height in the adolescents may have actually occurred earlier in childhood. Strong secular increases in height have been documented for the Mexican-American population[10] which could cause the statistical artifact described above. Undoubtedly, a similar phenomenon of improvement over time has occurred among Puerto Ricans. Only future surveys of the size of Puerto Rican children will settle the issue of when Puerto Ricans become smaller than the general population. Of great interest is the eventual size (i.e., as adolescents and adults) of the cohorts of preadolescent children who, at the time of HHANES (1982–1984), were as tall as the general U.S. population. Though uncertainty remains about the cause of the short stature of adolescents, growth potential in early childhood in the Puerto Rican population is similar to that of the general U.S. population. Pediatricians examining young children should feel assured of the general appropriateness of U.S. reference curves in use; these are provided by NCHS and are based on data from NHANES I and earlier surveys for children 2 years or older and on data from the Fels longitudinal study for younger subjects.[11]

The multivariate analysis of the predictors of height uncovered few significant variables. Other than sex, only poverty was associated with height and only in children 2 to 11 years of age. This is partly due to the fact that standard errors were inflated to adjusted them for an average design effect of two; this, of course, lowers the estimated *t* values and the corresponding level of statistical significance. Whether this adjustment is necessary or desirable in exploring relationships is subject to discussion. If adjustments for the design effect had not been made, the language-use variables (i.e., Spanish and Biling) would have been statistically significant at ages 2 to 11 years and poverty and Spanish would have also been significant in the 18 to 24.9 year group. Thus, there are hints that poorer children and children who are Spanish or bilingual speakers (relative to those who prefer English) are shorter. Relationships are weak, however, even in the absence of adjustments for the design effect. This should not be surprising. As a population approaches a state of unconstrained growth, and this is clearly the case in the Puerto Rican population prior to adolescence, relationships between socioeconomic and cultural factors should weaken or disappear.

Data were also presented on sexual maturation. The method used requires an observer to rate each individual according to five stages.[5] Observers are trained by means of drawings and photographs and shown what to look for in each stage. Though reproducibility can be good in well-trained subjects, cross-study comparisons must be done with caution. Methods of assessment in HHANES can be assumed to be similar for Mexican-Americans and Puerto Ricans. Therefore, the finding of earlier maturation in Puerto Ricans relative to Mexican-Americans can be considered to be valid. Caution should be exercised, however, in comparing HHANES results to those of other studies, including these of the recent survey of Dutch children used in this study.[7] This last comparison suggests similar or only minor delays in sexual maturation in Puerto Ricans compared to Europeans. Marked deviations in sexual development among Puerto Ricans, whether in acceleration or retardation, can be discarded.

A serious public health problem is clearly evident. Significant proportions of Puerto Rican adults are overweight (≥ 85th percentile) or obese (≥ 95th percentile) regardless of the anthropometric indicator selected (i.e., body mass index, triceps skinfold thickness, subscapular skinfold thickness). Also clear is the greater tendency among Puerto Ricans for fat to be deposited in the trunk. Most disturbing is the finding that children are also fatter than the general population. Similarly, Mexican-Americans and Cubans are just as fat as Puerto Ricans.[2] The consistency of these findings across these groups suggests that overweight and obesity is a widespread phenomenon amongst Hispanics on the U.S. mainland and a clear public health concern. The need for vigorous public health programs to confront this potential health problem is urgent.

ACKNOWLEDGMENT. Supported by grant MCJ-060518, Maternal and Child Health Bureau, HRSA, DHHS.

REFERENCES

1. Bean FD, Tienda M: *The Hispanic Population of the United States.* New York, Russell Sage Foundation, 1987
2. National Center for Health Statistics: Plan and operation of the Hispanic Health and Nutrition Examination Survey, 1982–84. *Vital Health Statistics,*DHHS publication (PHS) 85-1321, 1(19), 1985
3. Frisancho AR: *Anthropometric Standards for the Assessment of Growth and Nutritional Status.* Ann Arbor, MI, University of Michigan Press, 1990
4. Najjar MF, Rowland M: Anthropometric reference data and prevalence of overweight, United States, 1976–80. *Vital Health Statistics* [11] 1987;238 [DHHS publication (PHS) 87-1688]
5. Tanner JM: *Growth at Adolescence.* 2nd ed. Oxford: Blackwell Scientific Publication; 1962
6. Villarreal SF, Martorell R, Mendoza F: Sexual maturation in Mexican-American adolescents. *Amer. J. Hum. Bio.* 1:87–95, 1989
7. Roede JJ, Van Wieringen JC: Growth diagrams 1980: Netherlands Third Nationwide Survey. *Tijdschr Soc Gezondheitsz* 63(suppl):1–34, 1985
8. Delgado JL, Johnson, CL, Ila R, Treviño F: Hispanic health and nutrition examination survey: Methodological considerations. *Amer. J. Pub. Health* 30(suppl):6–10, 1990
9. Martorell R, Mendoza FS, Castillo RO: Genetic and environmental determinants of growth of Mexican-Americans. *Pediatrics* 84(5):864–871, 1989
10. Malina R, Martorell R, Mendoza F: Growth status of Mexican-American children and youth: Historical trends and contemporary issues. *Yearbook Phys. Anthropol.* 29:45–79, 1986
11. Hamill PVV, Drizd TA, Johnson CL, et al: Physical growth: National Center for Health Statistics. *Amer. J. Clin. Nutr.* 32:607–629, 1979
12. Pawson IG, Martorell R, Mendoza F: Prevalence of overweight and obesity in U.S. Hispanic populations. *Amer. J. Clin. Nutr.* 53(Suppl.)(6):1522S–1528S, 1991

9

The Cultural Context of Adolescent Childrearing in Three Groups of Urban Minority Mothers

GAIL A. WASSERMAN, SUSAN A. BRUNELLI, VIRGINIA A. RAUH, AND LUZ E. ALVARADO

INTRODUCTION

In order to examine the role of cultural and family differences in parenting attitudes and practices in the development of inner-city children, we have been following a sample of urban minority mothers and children from the birth of the children through age 3 years. In well-matched groups of Puerto Rican, Dominican, and African-American adolescent and adult mothers, we have regularly assessed indices of

GAIL A. WASSERMAN and SUSAN A. BRUNELLI • College of Physicians and Surgeons, Columbia University and New York State Psychiatric Institute, New York, New York 10032. VIRGINIA A. RAUH • Center for Population and Family Health, Columbia University School of Public Health, New York, New York 10032. LUZ E. ALVARADO • New York State Psychiatric Institute, New York, New York 10032.

Puerto Rican Women and Children: Issues in Health, Growth, and Development, edited by Gontran Lamberty and Cynthia Garcia Coll. Plenum Press, New York, 1994.

maternal psychosocial functioning, parenting attitudes and practices, and child cognitive and behavioral outcomes.

BACKGROUND

Early studies of the consequences of teenage parenting often compared adolescent mothers (who were, most commonly, young minority women from impoverished families) with more affluent samples of adult mothers. To a large degree, what appeared as age differences in earlier reports of parenting quality and child outcome can thus be accounted for by socioeconomic factors.[1] For example, many indicators of adverse perinatal outcome, including low birth weight and short gestation age, reflect, to a large degree, the lower socioeconomic status and lower utilization of antenatal care in pregnant adolescents more than maternal age,[2,3] although birth weight is adversely affected by the nutritional needs of the growing teenager.[4]

With regard to maternal and child behavior, even in more recent studies with some socioeconomic control, group differences in parenting and child outcome do remain, and these generally favor adult mothers and their children.[5,6,7] These results suggest, for example, that adult mothers are more verbal with their infants. Comparable results have been reported in studies examining samples of minority and nonminority women; thus, compared to those of adults, infants of Mexican-American adolescents show less ability to cope with stress and their mothers show less effective verbal and affective behavior when interacting with them.[8]

Beyond the possibility of infant developmental risk as a consequence of maternal perinatal/behavioral factors, adolescent childbearing may represent added hazard to the mother, in terms of disrupted education and continued economic disadvantage. On the other hand, early childbearing may be adaptive for the disadvantaged minority adolescent, who has objectively limited options for employment but has an available social network to assist with childcare responsibility. Thus, Furstenberg, Brooks-Gunn, and Morgan report that, over a span of years, many African-American adolescent mothers go on to finish high school and find employment.

The consequences of adolescent childbearing for mother and child are therefore deeply rooted in a particular social context and must be viewed from the perspective of cultural factors, including (sub)cultural acceptance and economic disadvantage. The strains often attributable to maternal youth are likely related more to other mediators of child and maternal outcome which covary with adolescent childbearing, such as minority status, poverty, and differences across age and subcultures in residence patterns and in childrearing.

Childrearing attitudes and practices vary across subcultures.[10,11] What is acceptable or even optimal may be specific to one's subcultural group.[12–14] The confounding of ethnicity and social class creates further confusion, because social class in and of itself is thought to influence parenting practices and attitude.[14]

Not only are there likely to be great differences between African-American and Hispanic women in factors which influence parenting, such as measures of life-style, attitudes, and personality, but there is also considerable diversity among the various cultural groups on the U.S. mainland considered together to make up the category of Hispanics. Little information is available in general about child-care patterns and developmental outcome among Hispanics[15] although they make up the second largest U.S. minority group. The origins of groups of Hispanics in such studies are not specified, or groups originating from different countries, with different histories and values, are often combined. Variations within the Hispanic population are largely unexplored.

Garcia Coll, in a series of comparisons of island Puerto Ricans with mainland African-Americans,[16,17] and with mainland Caucasians[16] reported effects of both maternal age and "culture" on various perinatal indicators. More optimal outcome was reported among island (Puerto Rican) as opposed to mainland African-American infants and in infants of adult mothers. Since the reliability of many such perinatal measures (including Apgar, gestation age determination, and even head circumference) is low, however, and likely to differ substantially from hospital to hospital, comparisons within one setting are more meaningful. In that respect, maternal age differences were more marked within the African-American sample than they were in the Puerto Rican sample, suggesting culture-specific patterns of adolescent health-care utilization. These patterns, in turn, may reflect greater acceptance for early marriage and childbearing within the Puerto Rican sample. In the newborn period, compared to Caucasian mothers, Puerto Ricans reported more perceived stress, less maternal satisfaction, less flexibility, fewer concerns about the maternal role, and less encouragement of positive interactions with the child. Puerto Rican mothers reported more acceptance of teenage childbearing, highlighting again "the supportive cultural context of teenage childbearing within this population."[16]

Field and Widmayer[18] compared the interactions of four groups of women of low socioeconomic status (SES) and their 4-month-old infants. Three of the four groups were women of Hispanic origin: Puerto Rican, Cuban, and South American; the fourth group was made up of African-Americans. While considering all women of South American origin as a single group, again confusing the issue of specificity, comparisons among the other three groups are interesting. During free play, Puerto Rican mothers showed more positive interactive behavior (contingent responsivity, game playing) than did Cuban women, who showed more than did the African-American mothers. Cuban mothers' interactions were characterized more by their educational tone than by playfulness. During feeding, Puerto Rican mothers were more alert and attentive than Cubans, who were more alert/attentive than African-Americans. Puerto Rican mothers showed more overall optimal feeding behavior than did Cubans, who did not differ from African-Americans. These authors interpreted their findings as demonstrating, for Hispanics, a relationship between length of residence on the U.S. mainland and more optimal interactive behavior, although this relationship clearly did not hold up for African-Americans who had been in "mainland residence" the longest. Thus, subcultural factors among the three groups may have accounted for these differences.

As described by Rodriguez in chapter 1, economic pressure and lack of restrictions on movement led to a "massive influx" of Puerto Rican migrants into New York City between 1950 and 1970, such that by the 1980s one-third of all persons of Puerto Rican ancestry were living in the mainland United States (with two-thirds living in Puerto Rico), and 55% of all mainland Puerto Ricans were living in New York City.[19] In contrast to certain other immigrant Hispanic groups, such as Cubans, the largest proportion of immigrants from Puerto Rico were the rural poor, with few years of education. The Puerto Rican population in New York remains younger due to large family size than the general population [20] and Puerto Rican mothers are younger[21] than are other Hispanic mothers (probably due to higher rates of adolescent pregnancy). This population also reflects the educational, occupational, and socioeconomic disadvantages described by Rodriguez for all mainland Puerto Ricans. For example, in 1980 in the Bronx, where there is the heaviest concentration of Puerto Ricans in New York City, average family income for female-headed Hispanic families was $6581, as compared to $15 872 for male-headed Hispanic families.[22] Despite gains over the last several years in other ethnic groups (and even in other groups of Hispanic immigrants), "the situation of the Puerto Ricans has become more tenuous."[20]

Until 1965, the largest proportion of Hispanic immigration into New York City was by Puerto Ricans. Since then, immigration from Puerto Rico has diminished, and, to some extent, reversed[20] while that from other Caribbean and South American countries has increased. Initially, as a result of political changes in the Dominican Republic in the early 1960s, and continuing as economic conditions there have worsened, immigration of Dominicans into New York City has increased substantially. Dominicans are now the second largest Hispanic group in New York City. Up to 50% of these may be illegal residents, which may compromise access to social and health-care benefits.[23] Reflecting their more recent arrival, relative to Puerto Ricans, Dominicans are less likely to speak English or to be high school graduates[24] despite higher median household income. Perhaps reflecting their more recent arrival and their more limited opportunities for family survival in father-absent homes, Dominican families are less likely to be headed by single mothers or to receive public assistance. Dominican mothers miss fewer prenatal visits and deliver fewer babies with low birth weight or perinatal complications, despite more difficult access to health-care benefits.[23]

Comparisons between Dominican and Puerto Rican samples are interesting because of similarities and differences between these groups. Both groups have settled into a New York City niche of urban poverty. Both immigration waves were primarily comprised of individuals from rural areas, of low economic and educational attainment in their places of origin. Individuals in both groups regularly travel back and forth between the Caribbean and New York. The groups differ substantially in length of U.S. residence and in ease of access to such social and health-care benefits as assistance for dependent children (AFDC) or Medicaid.

Both Hispanic migration cohorts came into a niche already occupied by African-Americans, some of whom were already long-term residents of the urban Northeast, and some of whom migrated from the South during and immediately after the Second World War.[25]

Group differences in length of U.S. urban residence are likely to be reflected in degree of acculturation and access to mainstream U.S. cultural values.[26] These historical differences in the timing of arrival of each group onto the urban scene may reflect, to a degree, cohort effects. Such differences in acculturation and in demographics may interact with maternal age to influence childrearing patterns and, in turn, child outcome. From another perspective, if length of U.S. residence entails longer contact with U.S. urban poverty, it should be associated with increasingly poor health and social outcomes for mothers and children.[27] These two opposing processes are complicated even further by differences attributable to educational/economic differences in the immigrant's country of origin, and by differential access to health and welfare benefits as a function of U.S. citizenship.

METHOD

Subjects

This paper reports on data from a sample of African-American and Hispanic adolescent and adult mothers and their infants, who were primarily of Puerto Rican or Dominican origin. This sample, as described more fully below, was recruited in the postpartum period, and is currently being followed yearly through age 3 years.

Selection

All African-American and Hispanic adolescent mothers (age <19 years) giving birth on the service ward of Columbia-Presbyterian Hospital, New York City, during a 12-month period in 1987–1988 were invited to participate in the study. The population served by the ward reflects the ethnic makeup of the neighborhood, and is largely African-American and Hispanic. For each adolescent recruited, we selected an African-American or Hispanic adult control (age ⩾20 years) from the same ward.

Infants or mothers with certain perinatal conditions which might impact on either maternal adjustment or child development were excluded. These conditions included: birth weight <2400 grams, gestation age <35 weeks, Apgar <7, congenital anomalies, multiple births, and maternal drug abuse. Forty-two teens were excluded for these reasons, leaving a sample of 144 adolescent mothers.

After recruiting an adolescent mother, we attempted to enlist the next adult mother delivering at the hospital, who met the above exclusionary criteria. Because all teens were having either their first or second child, we restricted adult recruitment to women of similarly low parity. Finally, because we wanted to compare adolescent mothers with women who had delayed childbearing beyond their teens, we excluded adult women who had had their first child before the age of 19. A sample of 139 adult mothers was selected in this fashion.

Each subject was asked to designate herself as "African-American" or "Hispanic"; in order to examine subgroups of Hispanic mothers of either Puerto Rican or Dominican origin, we divided the sample of Hispanic women into two groups, based on their report of their mother's and/or father's country of birth (Puerto Rico or the Dominican Republic). This excluded a small group (n = 21) of Hispanic women whose parents were Hispanics of Cuban or South American ancestry. Based on these designations, the postnatal sample included, for adolescents, 33 Puerto Ricans, 51 Dominicans, and 47 African-American; for adults, the sample included 24 Puerto Ricans, 79 Dominicans, and 28 African-Americans. Further details of subject selection are available elsewhere.[28]

Procedure

All instruments not already available in Spanish were translated from English to Spanish by a bilingual team member and translated back into English by another. Discrepancies between Puerto Rican and Dominican idioms were resolved by providing both alternatives for each mother.

Postnatal Interview

Each mother was interviewed in her hospital room by a bilingual interviewer in the language of her choice. Because of literacy problems, all questions were read aloud to the mother, and she selected response options from index cards.

Assessment at 12 Months

Home and laboratory visits were conducted for 90 adolescent and 90 adult mothers and children, although numbers vary somewhat on certain measures, as noted below. Retrieved and nonretrieved cases did not differ in any demographic measures, including maternal age, country of origin, ethnicity, education, language, public assistance, parity or social class; there were no differences in paternal age or education. Finally, retrieved and nonretrieved subjects did not differ in measures of postnatal support, depression, or childrearing attitudes. During the home visit we repeated the postnatal interview and assessed the quality of the home environment. During the laboratory visit, we assessed infant developmental status, maternal intelligence, and videotaped a 30-minute structured interaction between mother and infant, in a comfortable room equipped with age-appropriate toys. For the behavioral data, we report here only findings from coding of the Free Play segment of the interaction, a 10-minute period during which mother was asked to play with the baby as she might "if she had some free time at home."

Measures

The postnatal interview collected demographic information, as well as data concerning depressive symptoms,[29] and childrearing attitudes (warmth, encouragement of independence, strictness and aggravation subscales of the Parental Attitudes Toward Child Rearing Questionnaire: PACR).[30] Social support was measured by the Inventory of Socially Supportive Behaviors,[31] which yields four subscales (tangible, emotional, guidance, and social interaction support). For each Inventory of Socially Supportive Behaviors item, we collected information regarding the source of the provided support: subjects were asked to designate the individual most likely to provide that particular aspect of support, from a predetermined set of alternatives. Most commonly, mothers reported support from their own mother, a partner, friends, or no one. This interview was repeated at 12 months postpartum.

Mothers' reports of their own contributions and those of fathers and maternal grandmothers to 15 routine household and childcare tasks at 12 months were assessed by means of the Division of Household Responsibilities Scale.[32] Maternal ratings are made on a Likert-type scale consisting of: 2 = most of the time; 1 = some of the time; and 0 = never. Separate and reliable Childcare and Housework scores for mothers, fathers, and maternal grandmothers were computed by summing item scores across the two domains.

Quality of the home environment was assessed during the 12-month home visit using the Home Observation for Measurement of the Environment.[33] This instrument examines environmental characteristics shown to foster early development, such as parental responsivity to child demands.

Maternal IQ was estimated by the Broad Cognitive Ability Full Scale of the Woodcock-Johnson Psychoeducational Battery. Spanish-speaking mothers were tested on the Spanish version of this test. Infant developmental level was measured by the Bayley MDI, administered by bilingual staff.

Maternal interactive behavior was scored by bilingual coders, using the Maternal Style Scale,[34] for minutes 2–7 of the 10-minute free play period. Coders viewed each videotape repeatedly, scoring presence/absence of a set of predetermined behaviors within each 10-second interval. Previous work has identified seven internally consistent and developmentally stable subscales: Attention-Management, Verbal Teaching, Physical Teaching, Orders, Distractions, Encouragement, and Negative Behavior. Additionally, for each 10-second interval, coders classified the mother as either Ignoring, Initiating, or Responsive. Further details of the scoring procedure, including reliability information, are available elsewhere.[35,36] Prompted by both theoretical and empirical justification, a single composite variable was created, reflecting Positive Maternal Style. This reliable composite measure summed the scores for Verbal Teaching, Positive Affect, Encouragement, Physical Teaching, and Attention Management.

Data Analysis

Across both time points, for continuous data, repeated measures, Analyses of Variance examined the effects of maternal Age (adolescent/adult) and Ethnicity (Puerto Rican, Dominican, African-American). For data available only at birth or 12 months (e.g., birth weight, behavioral coding, MDI), Analyses of Variance examined Age and Ethnicity differences. Because residence patterns are an important mediator of many of our home-based measures[43] separate analyses at 12 months covaried out the contribution of mother's living situation. In either case, planned contrasts allowed comparisons between African-American and Hispanics, as well as between Puerto Ricans and Dominicans. Categorical data were tested by means of a series of Chi-Square analyses, comparing first African-Americans and Hispanics, and then examining subgroups of Hispanics.

RESULTS

Sample

Sample characteristics, for subjects available at both time points, are presented in Table 1, although there are no differences between the

Table 1 Sample Characteristics

	Adolescent			Adult		
	Puerto Rican (n = 19)	Dominican (n = 34)	African-American (n = 26)	Puerto Rican (n = 14)	Dominican (n = 54)	African-American (n = 17)
	$\bar{X}$	$\bar{X}$	$\bar{X}$	$\bar{X}$	$\bar{X}$	$\bar{X}$
Infant						
Birthweight (grams)	3334	3348	3157	3513	3440	3306
Maternal						
Age	17.37	17.62	17.31	25.43	26.52	24.82
Education[a]	9.26	9.58	10.29	11.86	11.83	12.59
Occupational status	31.62	25.29	23.48	30.75	27.27	27.15
Intelligence	62.52	69.96	66.06	67.00	61.29	68.35
Parity	1.21	1.08	1.24	1.50	1.50	1.29
Age at menarche (years)[a,c]	11.18	12.04	12.40	12.82	13.22	12.23
Age at first birth	16.45	16.62	16.53	22.93	24.22	22.71
Number of grades repeated[a,b]	1.10	.58	.79	.43	.22	.53
	%	%	%	%	%	%
Marital status[a,b]						
Married	26.3	11.5	—	42.9	42.6	23.5
Divorced/Separated/Widowed	—	3.8	—	7.1	31.5	5.9
Never married	73.7	84.6	100.0	50.0	25.9	70.6
Postnatal living situation[a,b]						
With husband/partner	42.1	26.9	17.6	42.9	38.9	47.1
With family other than partner	52.6	73.1	79.4	28.6	31.5	52.9
Alone	5.3	—	—	28.6	24.1	—
Other	—	—	2.9	—	5.6	—

[a]Significant Age Effects
[b]Significant Ethnic Effects
[c]Significant Age × Ethnicity Interaction
Note. See text for F-values and X^2-values.

present sample and the larger complete sample on which we reported earlier.[34] Despite parity restrictions in sampling, adolescent mothers had had significantly fewer prior children [$F(1,163) = 13.04$, $p < .0001$]. Adolescents reported earlier menarche [$F(1,162) = 10.40$, $p < .001$], and there was a significant Age by Ethnicity interaction [$F(2,162) = 3.48$, $p < .05$], such that, among teenagers, Puerto Ricans reported earlier menarche than did either African-Americans ($t_{(36,82)} = 2.84$, $p < .01$) or Dominicans ($t_{(41,54)} = 1.78$, $p < .08$). As expected, birth weight was somewhat lower in infants born to adolescents [$F(1,163) = 3.66$, $p < .06$], and adolescents had fewer completed years of education [$F(1,163) = 61.27$, $p < .0001$] and had repeated significantly more grades in school [$F(1,163) = 16.85$, $p < .001$]. Mothers of Puerto Rican origin and African-American mothers had repeated significantly more years of school than had mothers from the Dominican Republic: for Ethnicity, $F(2,163) = 5.25$, $p < .01$; for Puerto Rican/Dominican and African-American/Dominican comparisons, respectively, $t_{(111)} = 3.83$, and $t_{(91,45)} = 3.43$, both p's $< .001$. There were no Age differences in either maternal intelligence, or in the socioeconomic status of mother's family of origin. There were no other significant differences across Ethnicity, or in interactions between Age and Ethnicity, for these measures, nor were there ethnicity-associated differences in maternal age.

As shown in Table 1, teen mothers were significantly less likely to be married than adults [$\chi^2_{(1)} = 29.05$, $p < .00001$]. African-American mothers in both age groups were also less likely to be married than were mothers in either of the Hispanic groups [$\chi^2_{(2)} = 16.35$, $p < .0003$]. Not one African-American adolescent was married [$\chi^2_{(2)} = 9.29$, $p < .01$], and Puerto Rican teens were more than twice as likely as Dominican teens to be married (though this latter difference was not significant).[2] In a larger sample, the apparent increased likelihood of Puerto Rican, as opposed to Dominican, teens to be married was not found. African-American adult mothers were twice as likely to have never married as were Puerto Rican and Dominican adult mothers combined [$\chi^2_{(2)} = 6.27$, $p < .05$]; in individual comparisons, Dominican adults were more likely to have been married compared with African-American adults [$\chi^2_{(1)} = 4.77$, $p < .05$]. Puerto Rican women were midway between the two other groups, and did not differ significantly from either. Similarly, as seen in Table 1, residence patterns varied both by maternal Age and Ethnicity [$\chi^2_{(3)} = 29.35$ and 15.59, p's $< .00001$ and $.02$]. While African-Americans in general were more likely to remain in their families of origin, this is particularly the case for adolescents. And although adolescents were generally more likely than adults to remain in their families of origin, Puerto Rican teens were more likely than either Dominican or African-American teenagers to live with a partner.

Measures Available at both Postnatal and 12-Month Assessments

Longitudinal Changes (see Table 2)

The significant multivariate effects of Age (teen/adult), $F(4,155) = 2.43$, $p < .05$; Ethnicity $F(8,308) = 6.19$, $p < .0001$ and Time (postnatal/12 months) on support subscales were followed by univariate Age by Ethnicity by Time Repeated Measures ANOVAs. For most support measures (Guidance, Social Interaction, and Emotional), levels declined significantly between the postnatal and 12-month assessments [$F(1,158) = 14.79$, 11.57 and 29.59, respectively, all p's $< .001$].

Similarly, although the level of depressive symptoms is high for all groups of mothers (at the postnatal and 12-month assessments, approximately 65 and 50% are above the clinical cutoff on the CES-D), there is a significant decline in reported symptoms across the first postnatal year [$F(1,158) = 8.45$, $p < .01$].

As for Childrearing Attitudes, there were significant multivariate effects for maternal age [$F(4,155) = 2.45$, $p < .05$) and ethnicity ($F(8,308) = 4.02$, $p < .001$). Univariate anovas showed that there are significant decreases over the first postpartum year in mothers' reported Strictness and Encouragement of Independence [$F(1,158) = 11.45$ and 11.86, p's $<$ .01]. There is also a significant Ethnicity by time Interaction for Aggravation [$F(2,158) = 3.49$, $p < .05$] such that, while there are no longitudinal changes for either African-American or Puerto Rican mothers, Dominican mothers report significant decreases across the first postpartum year ($t_{(79)} = 2.38$, $p < .02$).

Teen/Adult Differences (see Table 2)

Across assessment waves, adolescents reported significantly more instrumental (Guidance and Tangible) support than did adults [$F(1,158) = 7.28$ and 3.80, p's $< .01$ and .05, respectively]. As for Childrearing Attitudes, maternal Warmth was significantly higher among adults [$F(1,158) = 6.26$, $p < .05$]. With respect to depressive symptoms, at 12 months, more teens scored above the cut-off (60 vs. 45%; $p < .05$). These levels remain remarkably high, suggesting a chronic and clini-

Table 2 Mothers' Support, Depressive Symptoms, and Childrearing Attitudes, Averaged across Assessments

	Adolescent			Adult		
	Puerto Rican (n = 19)	Dominican (n = 34)	African-American (n = 26)	Puerto Rican (n = 14)	Dominican (n = 54)	African-American (n = 17)
	$\overline{X}$	$\overline{X}$	$\overline{X}$	$\overline{X}$	$\overline{X}$	$\overline{X}$
Social Support[a]						
Guidance	59.74	56.44	68.44	55.00	43.66	64.94
Tangible	40.32	37.60	48.90	39.39	31.60	46.12
Social interaction	23.76	21.69	26.46	22.96	19.90	26.38
Emotional	57.92	51.77	61.15	55.75	48.14	61.94
Depressive Symptoms	33.29	32.37	29.44	29.82	30.51	29.47
Childrearing Attitudes[b]						
Strictness	69.16	74.02	62.38	63.18	71.56	63.65
Aggravation	106.97	113.27	99.81	·102.79	109.61	96.85
Independence	67.68	71.04	68.63	67.07	67.90	72.12
Warmth	80.61	82.90	80.61	83.57	83.53	82.68

[a]Multivariate F (Age: 4,155) = 2.43, p = .05; F (Ethnic: 8,308) = 6.19, p < .0001.
[b]Multivariate F (Age: 4,155) = 2.45, p = .05; F (Ethnic: 8,308) = 4.02, p < .0001.
Note. See text for univariate F-values and significance.

cally meaningful level of depressive symptoms in the inner-city mothers of young children.

Ethnic Differences

A priori contrasts were used to examine all measures for which there was a significant main effect of Ethnicity (or interactions with Ethnicity); these first compared African-American and Hispanic mothers, and then examined differences between Puerto Ricans and Dominicans. Results are consistent across all types of Social Support; as Table 2 shows, there is a significant main effect of Ethnicity for Guidance, Tangible, Social Interaction and Emotional support [$F(2,158) = 20.45$, 28.34, 13.32 and 17.87, all p's $< .001$, respectively]. For each type of support, across assessment waves, African-American mothers reported significantly more support than did Hispanic mothers [$t_{(161)} = 5.37$, 6.34, 4.20 and 4.23, all p's $< .0001$, for Guidance, Tangible, Social Interaction, and Emotional Support, respectively]. Puerto Rican mothers reported significantly more of each support type than did Dominican mothers [$t_{(161)} = 3.09$, 3.03, 2.32, and 3.31, p's $= .002$, .003, .02 and .001, respectively]. Childrearing attitudes reflective of Strictness and Aggravation showed a similar pattern of differences. That is, there were significant main effects of Ethnicity for both Strictness and Aggravation [$F(2,158) = 7.86$ and 9.14, p's $< .001$ and .01, respectively]. These associations reflected the greater tendency of Hispanic, as opposed to African-American, mothers to report both types of negative childrearing attitudes [$t_{(161)} = 3.05$ and 3.40, p's $< .005$, respectively]. Among Hispanics, mothers from the Dominican Republic were significantly more likely than were Puerto Rican mothers to endorse attitudes reflecting Strictness [$t_{(161)} = 2.20$, $p < .05$], and were marginally more likely to express Aggravation [$t_{(161)} = 1.75$, $p < .08$]. Finally, there was a significant Age by Ethnicity interaction [$F(2,158) = 4.22$, $p < .05$] for Encouragement of Independence: among adults, African-Americans were significantly more likely to endorse such attitudes than were Hispanics [$t_{(83)} = 2.50$, $p < .02$], while there were no differences among adolescents.

Measures Available Only at 12 Months

Teen/Adult Differences

As can be seen in Tables 3 and 4, adolescent mothers, in many ways, provide a less adequate childrearing environment for their in-

Table 3 Childrearing Environment and Child Outcome at 12 Months

	Adolescent			Adult		
	Puerto Rican (n = 19)	Dominican (n = 34)	African-American (n = 26)	Puerto Rican (n = 14)	Dominican (n = 54)	African-American (n = 17)
	$\overline{X}$	$\overline{X}$	$\overline{X}$	$\overline{X}$	$\overline{X}$	$\overline{X}$
Environmental measures						
Home scale total score[a,d]	31.89	31.92	29.74	35.57	32.90	34.94
Positive maternal style[c]	−36.94	−41.73	−37.83	−46.77	−34.19	−44.33
Number of resident children[c,d]	1.42	1.11	2.05	1.50	1.70	1.23
Number of resident adults	2.63	3.03	2.15	1.14	2.00	1.59
MDI	105.00	100.74	101.16	114.69	102.90	105.61

[a]Significant Age Effects; [b]Significant Ethnic Effects; [c]Significant Age × Ethnic Interaction; [d]Significant with Residence Covaried.
Note. See text for significant F-values and X^2-values.

Table 4 Support Measures at 12 Months

	Adolescent			Adult		
	Puerto Rican (n = 19)	Dominican (n = 34)	African-American (n = 26)	Puerto Rican (n = 14)	Dominican (n = 54)	African-American (n = 17)
	$\overline{X}$	$\overline{X}$	$\overline{X}$	$\overline{X}$	$\overline{X}$	$\overline{X}$
Father's participation in childcare[a,d]	2.62	2.31	3.85	4.14	2.66	4.41
Father's participation in housework[a,b,d]	.71	.69	.68	2.21	.98	1.82
Father's emotional support[a,b,d]	9.52	3.54	10.97	10.79	3.31	17.59
Grandmother's participation in childcare	4.77	4.32	4.77	3.33	3.78	4.00
Grandmother's participation in housework[d]	4.07	3.00	4.42	3.33	3.22	2.85
Mother's participation in childcare[a]	9.62	9.07	9.26	9.50	9.72	9.47
Mother's participation in housework[a]	3.47	3.54	3.32	4.29	4.29	4.13

[a]Significant Age Effects; [b]Significant Ethnic Effects; [c]Significant Age × Ethnic Interaction; [d]Significant with Residence Covaried.
Note. See text for significant F-values and X^2-values.

fants. HOME Scale Total scores are significantly lower for adolescents [$F(1,162) = 11.37$, $p < .001$]. They live in more crowded households overall, with significantly more other adults [$F(1,163) = 7.56$, $p < .007$]. Table 4 shows that adolescents received significantly less help from their partners in housework [$F(1,163) = 10.87$, $p < .001$], and less emotional support from them as well [$F(1,161) = 3.09$, $p < .10$]. Adolescent mothers do less housework and childcare than other mothers [$F(1,165) = 19.40$ and 4.19, p's $< .0001$ and .03 respectively]. To some degree, these differences reflect differences in marital status and residence patterns noted above.[34] In fact, with residence pattern covaried out, Age differences in HOME Scale scores and in Father's Contribution to Housework remain significant [$F(1,164) = 9.136$, $p < .003$, and $F(1,165) = 6.66$, $p < .02$]. Not surprisingly, Age differences in the number of other resident adults in the home are attenuated when residence pattern is controlled [$F(1,165) = 3.12$, $p < .08$]. Age differences in the amount of Emotional Support received from Partner disappear once mother's living situation is taken into account. Maternal age differences in the amount of housework (but not childcare) remain even after covarying out the contribution of residence pattern [$F(1,180) = 15.26$, $p < .0001$]. With residence pattern covaried, maternal grandmothers in teen households are shown to perform more housework than those in adult households [$F(1,94) = 11.78$, $p < .05$]. Finally, maternal age differences are reflected in the somewhat poorer MDI performance seen in infants of adolescents [$F(1,137) = 2.86$, $p < .10$], although this difference is not statistically significant.

Ethnic Differences

The significant Ethnic effect for Father's Participation in Childcare [$F(2,163) = 5.37$, $p < .01$] reflects the higher levels of paternal involvement in African-American families ($t_{(162)} = 2.58$, $p < .01$) and the relatively greater involvement in Puerto Rican, as opposed to Dominican, families ($t_{(111)} = 1.67$, $p < .10$). In comparable fashion, there is a significant main effect of Ethnicity on Father's Emotional Support [$F(2,163) = 13.97$, $p < .0001$], with scores higher in African-American, as compared to Hispanic, families ($t_{(160)} = 4.79$, $p < .000$) and also higher in Puerto Rican, as compared to Dominican, families ($t_{(109)} = 3.63$, $p < .0001$). There is a significant Age by Ethnicity Interaction for Positive Maternal Style [$F(2,135) = 4.43$, $p < .02$]: while African-American and Puerto Rican teens are somewhat less positive in interaction (though not significantly so), there are no age differences among Dominicans, largely because Dominican adults' scores are even lower than those for Dominican teens. Dominican adults are significantly less positive during interaction than are either African-American adults ($t_{(58)} = 2.12$, $p < .05$) or Puerto Ricans adults ($t_{(59)} = 2.51$, $p < .02$). There is a significant Age by Ethnicity interaction for Number of Children resident in the household, [$F(2,163) = 8.68$, $p < .0001$] reflecting the greater number of children residing the households of African-American teens as opposed to African-American adults ($t_{(49)} = 2.24$, $p < .03$), with the reverse pattern among Dominicans, such that adults live with more children than do teens ($t_{(78)} = 3.63$, $p < .001$). Following ANCOVAs to remove the effect of residence pattern on these home-based measures, all ethnic differences remain significant. For Father's Contribution to Childcare and Partner's Emotional Support, respectively, $F(2,165) = 5.93$, $p = .003$ and $F(2,163) = 14.89$, $p = .0001$. Similarly, the Age by Ethnicity interaction for Number of Children in the Home remains significant [$F(2,165) = 8.84$, $p = .0001$]. Finally, with residence covaried out, there is a significant effect of Ethnicity on Father's Contribution to Housework [$F(2,165) = 3.71$, $p < .03$], although contrasts showed that none of the Ethnic groups differ significantly from the others. There are no significant ethnic differences (either before or after removal of the contribution of residence pattern) in either housework or childcare of either mother or maternal grandmother.

Again these environmental differences appear to be reflected in infant performance, such that there is a significant effect of Ethnicity on MDI [$F(2,137) = 3.09$, $p < .05$], reflecting enhanced scores of Puerto Rican, as compared to Dominican, infants ($t_{(98)} = 2.18$, $p < .05$), with no differences between African-American and Puerto Rican infants.

DISCUSSION

As noted above, in many ways adolescent mothers are able to provide a somewhat less than optimal childrearing environment. They live in less child-oriented households, with more other adults in residence, and they receive less emotional support and less help with housework from their partners. To an extent, some, if not all, of these results are mediated by age differences in living arrangements, in that adolescents are more likely to remain with their families of origin, rather than to create a new nuclear family structure with partners. If the baby's father is not present in the household, he is less likely to provide either emotional or instrumental support to the mother.[37] In an earlier study, we reported that the increased likelihood of adolescents to reside in non-partner-headed households bore a stronger association with lower HOME Scale scores than did maternal youth itself.[38] On the other hand, in agreement with others' findings, we report here that some groups of teens show somewhat less optimal behavior in interaction with their infants, suggesting that, independent of the home setting, there may be additional risk attributable to maternal youth itself. In any event, all of these functional environmental indices are likely to contribute to the observed somewhat lowered developmental scores of infants of adolescent mothers.

As reported earlier,[28] adolescent mothers report earlier menarche than adults, and have repeated more grades in school, although the latter findings likely represent island/mainland differences in statutory educational requirements.

These age-specific profiles must be further clarified by examination of ethnocultural differences among sample groups. For example, despite their greater tendency to be married and/or to reside with a partner, Hispanic women, and particularly, Dominican women, receive substantially less childcare and emotional support from their partners. Childcare and intimate support from partners have been found to be important determinants of a variety of maternal attributes and behaviors, including depressive symptoms,[32] and caregiving attitudes and practices.[37,39–41] Not surprisingly, these differences in support are mirrored by corresponding ethnic differences in childrearing attitudes and behavior, although cultural patterns in childrearing exist independent of support.[37,11] In the present study, Dominican women report more negative childrearing attitudes than do Puerto Rican women, who report more than do African-American women. Similarly, adult Dominican mothers show less positive interactive behavior with their infants than do either Puerto Rican or African-American mothers. This ethnicity difference for parenting does not hold for Dominican teens, who by virtue of their exposure to U.S. schools are probably more rapidly assimilated than are Dominican adult women. And finally, this ordering of ethnic groups is maintained for infant developmental status, with African-American infants and Puerto Rican infants receiving higher scores than do Dominican infants.

As we have noted elsewhere,[28] these findings represent group differences in length of residence. We would expect that longer-term

U.S. mainland residents, such as Puerto Ricans, would show attitudes, values, and practices more similar to the local culture (i.e., African-Americans) than would newer residents (i.e., Dominicans). In general, Puerto Rican scores on many measures fall between those of Dominicans and African-Americans.

That acculturation to urban poverty offers added risk to the immigrant mother and child[27] is demonstrated by the marital status of adult women. That is, the likelihood of raising a child as a single mother is greatest among African-American adults, followed by Puerto Rican adults, and finally by Dominican adult women. These findings reflect group differences in length of mainland U.S. residence, perhaps indicative of a cohort effect, which reflects the temporal order of arrival of the three groups into the urban Northeast. The high proportion of Dominican adults who report themselves as separated, divorced, or widowed may represent unstable migration practices, fed by a marginal economy and by legal constraints on immigration, such that parents and children regularly travel between the Dominican Republic and New York. Furthermore, in the long run, predictions regarding the marital status of Dominican women, based on inferences about the experiences of Puerto Rican women, may not be accurate. In an intergenerational study of Puerto Ricans in New York City in the 1970s, Rogler[22] states that 57% of women in the "1950 migration cohort" (those born approximately in 1920) were currently married, but that only 37% of the next generation of women (those born around 1950) were married. While it is still too soon to tell whether these "second generation effects" will prevail among the more recently arrived Dominican women, they may not follow the Puerto Rican pattern at all because of Dominicans' reduced access to health and welfare benefits. Paradoxically, reduced access may prevent or forestall the disintegration of the nuclear family, as single women find it more difficult to manage without financial and other support of husbands or partners.

The present sample, selected to minimize adverse health outcomes for mother and child, offers few other opportunities to examine the degree to which length of residence is associated with increasingly poor outcome in "second generation" immigrants. On the other hand, the opposing process, whereby longer-term residents show more mainstream values and practices, is amply demonstrated. For example, ethnic differences in father's emotional and childcare support likely reflect group differences in length of U.S. residence. In somewhat comparable measures of household responsibilities and decision making, Rogler[22] reports a significantly more egalitarian marital relationship in second-generation Puerto Ricans as compared to their immigrant parents. Similar to the intergenerational trends toward more mainstream American attitudes and values also reported in the same study,[22] the present study finds that both negative childrearing attitudes and practices are negatively associated with length of mainland U.S. residence.

This composite pattern of less available paternal support, and more harsh childrearing attitudes and practices places the child of the newly immigrated family at increased cognitive/behavioral risk.[30,42] These associations appear in the present study as well, in that Dominican infants have significantly lower MDI scores than do either Puerto Rican or Black infants.

In making sense of the positive trend in these findings, it must be remembered that, in the present study, mothers and infants with the poorest health outcomes were selected out, leaving a sample, not only with fewer adverse perinatal conditions, but also with more adaptive psychosocial functioning. Therefore we cannot shed any light on population trends which might indicate increasingly adverse mother–child consequences the longer the contact with "chronic urban poverty."[27] In fact, it is likely that our sampling criteria ensured only inclusion of "survivors" of this process. It may well be the case that both trends are operating simultaneously; within a given group over time, increasing numbers of vulnerable mothers are lost to conditions which entail high risk to them and their children. On the other hand, over time, the health care and childrearing characteristics of those not lost are probably increasingly reflective of mainstream practices. This second process may explain the cohort effects reported here for African-Americans, Puerto Ricans, and Dominicans in childrearing, support, and child outcome.

Adolescent pregnancy itself is one of the adverse conditions discussed above, presenting both perinatal and developmental risks to the infant consequent to maternal immaturity. On the other hand, our work (see Figure 1) suggests that adolescent childrearing occurs within a particular sociocultural context which may either ameliorate or exacerbate this strain. Examples of such potentially protective factors may be: the greater support offered by the partner of an African-American teen, as opposed to a Hispanic teen; and the greater likelihood that the Hispanic, as compared to African-American adolescent mother will be married. Analogous ethnospecific processes operate as protective fac-

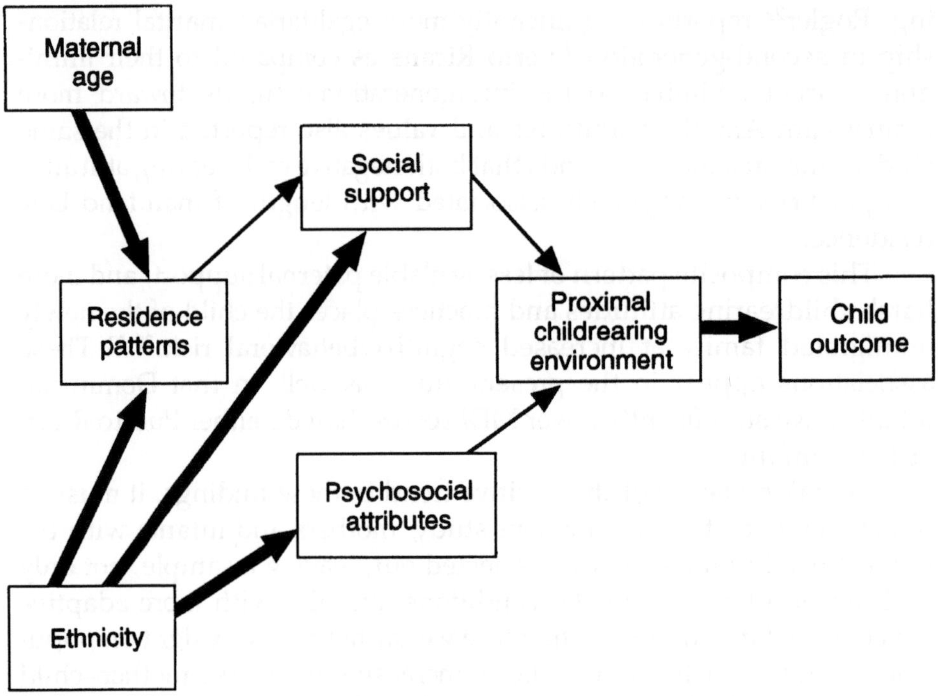

Figure 1. Mother–child system.

tors countering adolescent pregnancy itself.[43] Rather than treating adolescent parenting as a universally negative event, future work should be directed toward identifying the cooccurrence of factors which entail the greatest risk and/or protective factors for mother and child.

ACKNOWLEDGMENT. Supported by grant MCJ-360540, Maternal and Child Health Bureau, HRSA, DHHS.

REFERENCES

1. Baldwin W, Cain VS: The children of teenage parents. *Family Planning Perspectives* 12:34–43, 1980
2. Blum RW, Goldhagen J: Teenage pregnancy in perspective. *Clinical Pediatrics* 20:335–340, 1981
3. Leppert PC, Namerow PB, Barker D: Pregnancy outcomes among adolescent and older women receiving comprehensive prenatal care. *Journal of Adolescent Health Care* 7:112–117, 1986

4. Frisancho AR, Matos J, Bollettino LA: Influence of growth status and placental function on birth wright of infants born to young still-growing teenagers. *American Journal of Clinical Nutrition* 40:801–807, 1984
5. Jones FA, Green V, Krauss DR: Maternal responsiveness of primiparous mothers during the postpartum period: Age differences. *Pediatrics* 65:579–584, 1980
6. Levine L, Garcia Coll CT, Oh W: Determinants of mother-infant interaction in adolescent mothers. *Pediatrics* 75:23–29, 1985
7. Ragozin AS, Basham RB, Crnic KA, Greenberg MT, Robinson NM: Effects of maternal age on parenting role. *Developmental Psychology* 18:627–634, 1982
8. Teberg AJ, Howell VH, Wingert WA: Attachment interaction behavior between young teenage mothers and their infants. *Journal of Adolescent Health Care* 4:61–66, 1983
9. Furstenberg FF Jr, Brooks-Gunn J, Morgan SP: *Adolescent Mothers in Later Life*. New York, Cambridge University Press, 1986
10. Durrett ME, O'Bryant S, Pennebaker JW: Childrearing reports of White, Black and Mexican-American families. *Developmental Psychology* 11:871, 1975
11. Rauh VA, Wasserman GA, Brunelli SA: Determinants of maternal childrearing attitudes. *Journal of the American Academy of Child and Adolescent Psychiatry* 29:375–381, 1990
12. Brooks-Gunn J, Furstenberg FF: Antecedents and consequences of parenting: The case of adolescent motherhood, in A. Fogel, & G.F. Melson (eds): *Origins of Nurturance: Developmental, Biological and Cultural Perspectives on Caregiving*. Hillsdale, NJ, Lawrence Erlbaum Associates, 1986, pp 233–258
13. Furstenberg FF Jr, Brooks-Gunn J: Teenage childbearing: Causes, consequences, and remedies. In L.H. Aiken & D. Mechanic (eds): *Applications of Social Science to Clinical Medicine and Health Policy*. New Brunswick, NJ, Rutgers University Press, 1986, pp 307–333
14. Ramos-McKay JM, Comas-Diaz L, Rivera LA: Puerto Ricans, in Comas-Diaz L, Griffith EEH (eds): *Clinical Guidelines in Cross-Cultural Mental Health*. New York, John Wiley & Sons, 1988, pp 204–232
15. Lancaster JB, Hamburg BA: The biosocial dimensions of school-age pregnancy and parenthood: An introduction, in Lancaster JB, Hamburg BA (eds.): *School-Age Pregnancy and Parenthood*. New York, Aldine, 1986, pp 3–16
16. Garcia Coll CT: The consequences of teenage childbearing in traditional Puerto Rican culture. In J.K. Nugent, B. Lester, & T.B. Brazelton (eds): *The Cultural Context of Infancy, Vol* I. Norwood NJ, Ablex, 1989, pp 111–132
17. Lester B, Garcia Coll CT, Sepkoski C: A cross-cultural study of teenage pregnancy and neonatal behavior, in T.M. Field & A. Sostek (eds): *Infants Born at Risk: Physiological, Perceptual, and Cognitive Processes*. NY, Grune & Stratton, 1983, pp 147–169
18. Field TM, Widmayer SM: Mother-infant interaction among lower SES Black, Cuban, Puerto Rican and South American immigrants, in Field TM, Sostek AM, Vietze P, Liederman PH (eds): *Culture and Early Interactions*. Hillsdale, NJ, Lawrence Erlbaum Associates, 1981, pp 41–62
19. Lash T, Sigal H, Dudzinski D: *Children and Families in New York City: An Analysis of the 1976 Survey of Income and Education*. New York, Foundation for Child Development, 1979
20. Canino IA, Earley BF, Rogler LH: *The Puerto Rican Child in New York City: Stress and Mental Health*. New York, Fordham University Hispanic Research Center, 1988
21. Harrison A, Serafica F, McAdoo H: Ethnic families of color. In R.D. Parke (ed): *Review of Child Development Research, Vol 7*. Chicago, University of Chicago Press, 1984, pp 329–371
22. Rogler LH, Cooney RS: *Puerto Rican Families in New York City: Intergenerational Processes*. Copyright by the Hispanic Research Center, Fordham University, New York. Maplewood, NJ, Waterfront Press, 1984

23. Katz J, Darabi K: *Profile of Dominicans in the United States*. Paper presented at the Columbia University Conference on Hispanic Health Care Approaches in New York: A Focus on Dominicans. October, 1987
24. Bettes BA, Dusenbury L, Kerner J, James-Ortiz S, Botvin GJ: Ethnicity and psychosocial factors in alcohol and tobacco use in adolescence. *Child Development* 61:557–565, 1990
25. Billingsley A: *Black Families in White America*. Englewood Cliffs, NJ, Prentice-Hall, 1968
26. Padilla AM: The role of cultural awareness and ethnic loyalty in acculturation. In Padilla, AM (ed): *Acculturation*. Boulder, CO, Westview, 1980, pp 85–110
27. Garcia Coll CT: Developmental outcome of minority infants: A process-oriented look into our beginnings. *Child Development* 61:270–289, 1990
28. Wasserman GA, Rauh VA, Brunelli SA, Garcia-Castro M, Necos B: Psychosocial attributes and life experiences of minority mothers: Age and ethnic variations. *Child Development* 61:566–580, 1990a
29. Radloff LS: The CES-D scale: A self-report depression scale for research in the general population. *Journal of Applied Psychological Measurement* 1:385–401, 1977
30. Goldberg W, Easterbrooks MA: Role of marital quality of toddler development. *Developmental Psychology* 20:504–514, 1984
31. Barrera M, Ainlay SL: The structure of social support; A conceptual and empirical analysis. *Journal of Community Psychology* 11:133–143, 1983
32. Lennon MC, Wasserman GA, Allen RA: Infant care and wives' depressive symptoms. *Women and Health*, 17:1–23, 1991
33. Caldwell B, Bradley R: *Home Observation for Measurement of the Environment*. Little Rock, University of Arkansas at Little Rock, 1984
34. Wasserman GA, Solomon CR: *The Maternal Style Scale*. Copyrighted, 1980
35. Wasserman GA, Allen R, Solomon CR: At-risk toddlers and their mothers: The special case of physical handicap. *Child Development* 56:73–83, 1985
36. Wasserman GA, Green A, Allen R: Going beyond abuse: Maladaptive patterns of interaction in abusing mother-infant pairs. *Journal of the American Academy of Child Psychiatry* 22:245–252, 1983
37. Brunelli SA, Wasserman GA, Rauh VA, Alvarado LE, Caraballo, LR: *Minority Fathers: Contributions to Paternal and Maternal Childrearing* (in review)
38. Wasserman GA, Brunelli SA, Rauh VA: Social support, adjustment and childrearing attitudes among adolescent and adult mothers. *Journal of Adolescent Research* 5:54–66, 1990b
39. Colletta ND: Social support and risk of rejection by adolescent mothers. *Journal of Psychology* 109:191–197, 1981
40. Crnic KA, Greenberg MT, Robinson MN, Ragozin AS: Maternal stress and social support: Effects on the mother-infant relationship from birth to eighteen months. *American Journal of Orthopsychiatry* 54:224–234, 1984
41. Crockenberg S: Predictors and correlates of anger toward and punitive control of toddlers by adolescent mothers. *Child Development* 58:964–975, 1987
42. Belsky J: The determinants of parenting: A process model. *Child Development* 55: 83–96, 1984
43. Abrahamse AF, Morrison PA, Waite LJ: *Beyond Stereotypes: Who Becomes a Single Teenager Mother*. Santa Monica, CA, The RAND Corporation, 1988

10

The Cognitive, Behavioral, and Health Status of Mainland Puerto Rican Children in the Infant Health and Development Program

CECELIA M. MCCARTON, JEANNE BROOKS-GUNN, AND JAMES TONASCIA

INTRODUCTION

Risk in the context of child development has often been defined as those conditions that adversely affect developmental outcomes.[1–4] Factors that

CECELIA M. MCCARTON • Department of Pediatrics, Rose F. Kennedy Center for Research in Mental Retardation and Human Development, Albert Einstein College of Medicine, Bronx, New York 10461. JEANNE BROOKS-GUNN • Department of Developmental Psychology, Teachers College, Columbia University, New York, New York 10032. JAMES TONASCIA • Department of Biostatistics, Johns Hopkins School of Hygiene and Public Health, Baltimore, Maryland 21205.

Puerto Rican Women and Children: Issues in Health, Growth, and Development, edited by Gontran Lamberty and Cynthia Garcia Coll. Plenum Press, New York, 1994.

have been considered risks include biological (e.g., low birth weight); family structural (e.g., large family size, single parenthood, poverty); parental characteristics (e.g., inadequate social support network, low maternal mental health, maternal illiteracy, punitive parenting practices); and environment (e.g., adverse neighborhoods, economic recession, inadequate health care or educational system). Unfortunately, cultural differences are usually not considered in these models. Most research on risk and child outcomes focuses on a specific risk factor (such as low birth weight, poverty, or low social support) or on a small set of factors.

Just as certain factors render children at risk, others may protect children from adverse outcomes. The process by which protective factors operate may be different from that of risk factors. For example, social support may be protective because it can reduce the occurrence of maternal depression, anxiety, and other problems.[5,6] Other protective factors might be services that families received, such as center-based schooling and home visiting programs.

LOW BIRTH WEIGHT AS A RISK FACTOR

Our work is aimed at understanding the mix of risk and protective factors associated with the health and developmental well-being of low-birth-weight premature children. About 250 000 low-birth-weight infants (2500 grams or less) are born each year in the United States, amounting to 6 to 7% of all births.[7–9] More low-birth-weight births occur for Hispanic-Americans and African Americans than for Caucasians.[10] Puerto Rican infants are at particular high risk for low birth weight among Hispanic groups.[11] Many low birth weight infants face problems such as cognitive delays, school failures, major neurosensory handicapping conditions, and emotional problems.[8,12–14,15–17]

In addition, low-birth-weight births are often associated with poverty and its cofactors, such as parental unemployment or underemployment, early parenthood, single parenthood, low levels of schooling, and residence in poor neighborhoods.[18–20] All of these "poverty cofactors"[21–23] adversely affect children's health and development. Children from poor families, and families characterized by the poverty cofactors listed above, are more likely to have low preschool readiness scores, to be held back in school, to have low achievement test scores, and to drop out of school.[1,24–27] They are more likely to have health problems—to be low birth weight, to be hospitalized in the first years of life, and to be of poor health in the elementary school years.[2,10,24,28,29] Thus, low-birth-weight children are likely to experience multiple risks.

DESCRIPTION OF INFANT HEALTH AND DEVELOPMENT PROGRAM

The Infant Health and Development Program (IHDP) is a multicenter, randomized controlled trial to test the efficacy of an intervention to reduce the incidence of health and developmental problems among low birth weight, premature (37 weeks gestational age or less) young children. The Infant Health and Development Program (IHDP) was developed to determine if the developmental delays seen in low-birth-weight young children could be prevented. The success of early intervention programs for children at environmental risk (e.g., poor) provided the rationale for intervening with children at biological risk. Prior to the IHDP, it was not known whether early interventions, which included center-based schooling, offered for the first three years of life, could modify the higher risk for adverse outcomes in low-birth-weight children (for examples of interventions for low-birth-weight infants in the first year of life[30–34]; for examples of interventions for mothers of low-birth-weight infants[35,36]).

Shortly after hospital discharge in 1985, eligible infants at eight sites across the country were randomly assigned to an Intervention group or a Follow-up only group (n = 985 infants). Eleven percent of the mothers were Hispanic, 52% were African-American, and 37% were Caucasian/Asian/Other. The eight sites included three where at least 10% of the mothers were Hispanic-American: Albert Einstein College of Medicine, the Bronx, New York City (40% were Hispanic and primarily Puerto Rican); University of Miami, Miami, Florida (12% were Hispanic and primarily Cuban-American); and University of Texas, Dallas, Texas (14% were Hispanic and primarily Mexican-American).

In this chapter, the effects of the treatment upon Hispanic-American young low-birth-weight children are presented. This discussion first describes the IHDP and then focuses on findings for the Hispanic sample as a whole and for the Puerto Rican sample at the Bronx site.

METHODS SAMPLE

The sample and subsequent procedures are briefly reviewed here and have been previously described.[37,38] Every infant born at each of the eight participating sites with a birth weight ≤2500 grams and a gestational age ≤37 weeks during the nine-month enrollment period, was screened for inclusion in IHDP. Infants were excluded if they lived outside a defined catchment area for each site, or if they were discharged outside the recruitment time period, or if they exceeded 37 weeks gestational age, or if they died within the first 48 hours of life. Infants were also excluded if their mothers were drug or alcohol abusers, or if they were unable to adequately communicate in English, or if there was a report of a psychiatric hospitalization. Other medical reasons for exclusion were hospitalization longer than 60 days after 40 weeks gestation; oxygen support for more than 90 days; severe neurologic abnormality; severe sensory deficit; or chromosomal/multiple anomaly syndrome. A total of 985 infants were randomized into the research program.

The research design included stratification by eight sites and two birth-weight groups (infants weighing 2001 to 2500 grams, designated heavier, and those weighing ≤2000 grams, designated lighter). Each site was to recruit a minimum of 135 infants. One-third of the sample came from the heavier and two-thirds from the lighter group. To reduce the cost of the study, subjects within each weight group were allocated such that one-third were randomized to the Intervention group (n = 377) and two-thirds to the follow-up only group (n = 608). Randomization occurred immediately after hospitalization and randomization variables included birth weight, sex, maternal education, maternal race, and Neonatal Health Index (NHI). The NHI is based on the length of hospital stay adjusted for birth weight.[39]

PROCEDURES

The IHDP was initiated on discharge from the neonatal nursery and continued until 36 months of age, corrected for prematurity. Infants in the intervention and the follow-up only groups participated in the same pediatric follow-up, which comprised medical, developmental, and social assessments, with referral for pediatric care and other services as indicated. The services exclusively for the intervention group consisted of home visits and child attendance at a child development center.

The protocol specified weekly home visits for the first year, and biweekly visits thereafter. The home visitor provided health and developmental information and family support and implemented two specific curricula. One curriculum emphasized cognitive, linguistic, and social development via a program of games and activities for the parent to use with the child. The second curriculum involved a systematic approach to help parents manage self-identified problems.

Beginning at 12 months and continuing until corrected age 36 months, the intervention children attended the child development center five days a week. The teaching staff continued to implement the curriculum of learning activities used by the home visitors and tailored the program to each child's needs and developmental level. Teacher–child ratios were 1:3 for children aged from 12 to 23 months and 1:4 for those aged 24 to 36 months; class sizes were six and eight children, respectively.

Each child in the two study groups was assessed by the clinical staff in the course of eight clinic visits occurring at 40 weeks conceptional age and at 4, 8, 12, 18, 24, 30, and 36 months corrected age. Ninety-two percent of the 36-month assessments occurred within a specified time window of +2 weeks.

At each clinic visit, data were collected from the mother about the child's health and developmental functioning and about the family's social and demographic characteristics. Growth measurements of the child were gathered at all visits. Cognitive assessments were performed at 12, 24, and 36 months. Behavioral data were obtained at 24 and 36 months. Additionally, at 12 and 36 months, home visits were made to assess the quality of the home environment.

Specially trained assessors were used for cognitive, behavioral, and growth assessments. They were monitored to ensure consistency across sites, and they were unaware of the families' study group status. All assessments in the study were administered in English.

MEASURES

Cognitive status was determined at 1 and 2 years, using the Bayley Scales of Infant Mental Development,[40] and at 3 years with the Stanford Binet Intelligence Scale, third edition.[41]

The mother's report of behavior problems was selected as the measure of behavioral competence at 36 months, using the Child Behavior Checklist for ages 2 to 3 years. Employing the authors' Total

Problem Raw Score, higher scores indicate more reported behavior problems.

Health status was regarded as multidimensional. The dimensions evaluated in this study were: morbidity, defined as the presence or absence of health conditions; functional status, defined by limitations in activities of daily living due to health problems and by alterations in physical growth; and maternal perception of the child's health.

Two measures were developed by the Infant Health and Development Program to ascertain (1) the overall morbidity experienced by the child; and (2) the seriousness of the reported health problems. At each assessment, mothers were asked to recall and report the incidence of each illness and condition that occurred since the last assessment. Their verbatim reports were assigned International Classification of Diseases ICD-Ninth Revision codes at the National Study Office, and all reports corresponding to the same code (using the first three digits) were counted as one illness or condition per assessment period.

Mother's Report: Morbidity Index. This index is a summation over the three years of the number of hospitalizations, outpatient surgeries, injuries not resulting in hospitalization or outpatient surgery, and different (code) illnesses and conditions.

Mother's Report: Serious Morbidity Index. This index consists of the number of years (0 to 3) in which there was one or more of the following: hospitalizations, outpatient surgeries, prolonged or recurrent illnesses totaling 30 days or longer in a given year, and injuries and briefer illnesses that were predefined as serious by a panel of pediatricians.

The Functional Status II (R) Scale, used at 36 months, gauged the mother's view of the limitations in the child's basic daily activities as a result of health problems. Higher scores indicate a more favorable functional status. Growth was assessed by length and body mass index at 36 months.

The General Health Ratings Index from the Rand Corporation Health Insurance Study was used at 36 months. Higher scores indicate better perceived health. All health data were collected by the clinic staff.

RESULTS FOR THE CHILDREN OF HISPANIC MOTHERS IN THE IHDP

Was the treatment effective for the Hispanic sample of the IHDP? To address this question, analyses were conducted using Multiple Linear

Regressions. Independent variables included site (dummy coded with each site being compared to the eighth site); birth weight (in grams); neonatal health index (continuous); gender (1 = male, 2 = female); maternal age (in years); maternal education (1 = no high school graduation, 2 = high school graduation, 3 = post secondary education); and maternal ethnicity (dummy coded to compare African-Americans to the other two groups and Hispanics to the other two groups). Then, the treatment effect was entered. Finally, the interaction of each initial status variable with the treatment was entered to determine whether the effectiveness of the treatment was similar for various subgroups.* Results for six of the eight primary outcomes in the cognitive, behavioral, and health domains are briefly presented here (growth results for length and body mass index are not reported, as no notable differences were found).

Cognitive Domain

The treatment had a significant effect at 3 years for all three ethnic groups (as indicated by no significant treatment by ethnicity interaction in the regressions). Figure 1 shows comparisons of Intervention versus Follow-up only in mean cognitive test scores separately for Hispanic, African-American and Caucasian at 1, 2, and 3 years of age. Mean scores are presented separately for the Hispanics, African-Americans, and Caucasians.

No overall treatment effect was seen at 1 year of age, nor was there a treatment by ethnicity interaction.[42] Hispanic, African-American, and Caucasian children had similar scores on the one-year Bayley IQ and mean scores.

A significant treatment effect was seen at 2 years for the total sample.[42] Hispanic children had lower cognitive test scores than Caucasian children, after controlling for maternal education and age. No treatment by Hispanic interaction was found, suggesting that the intervention was equally effective for Hispanic and Caucasian children.[42] The African-American children benefited more than the other two

*These Multiple Linear Regression analyses are described in an earlier article (Infant Health and Development Program, 1990). While the regressions had two ethnicity variables (one for African-American and one for Hispanic), only a summary ethnicity variable was included in the 1990 article. Consequently, we are reporting the results for the African-American and Hispanics separately in this chapter. Both the main effects and the interactions with treatment are discussed here.

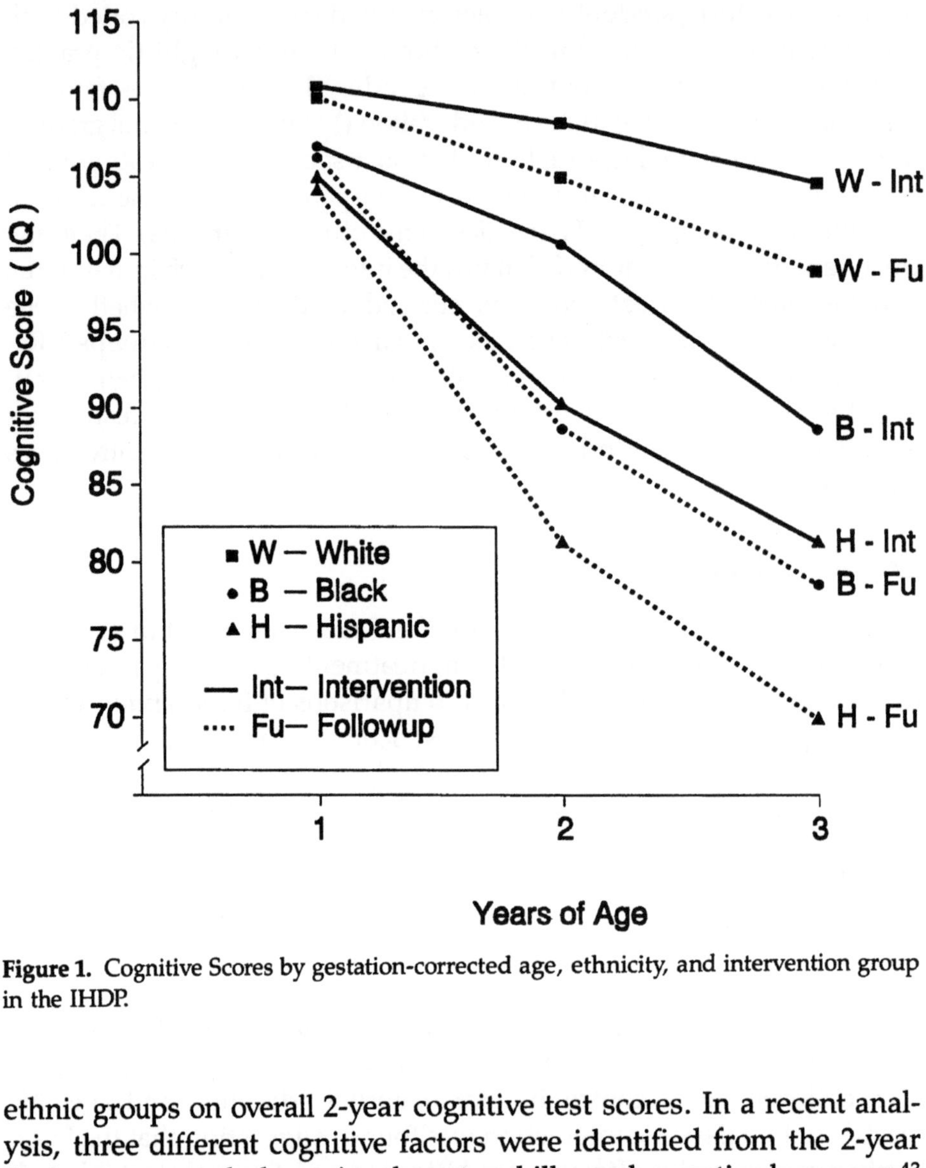

Figure 1. Cognitive Scores by gestation-corrected age, ethnicity, and intervention group in the IHDP.

ethnic groups on overall 2-year cognitive test scores. In a recent analysis, three different cognitive factors were identified from the 2-year Bayley test—vocabulary, visual–motor skills, and receptive language.[43] Significant intervention effects were seen for all three of these cognitive factors. African-American and Hispanic Intervention group children had larger treatment group differences on visual–motor skills than did Caucasian children, and African-American children had larger treatment effects on receptive language than did Caucasian children.

The treatment was efficacious at 3 years for the total sample and for the three ethnic groups.[42] Again, Hispanic children had lower scores than did Caucasian children. At 3 years, four different cognitive factors were identified from the Stanford-Binet Test—receptive language, vocabulary, visual–motor and spatial skills, and reasoning. Hispanic and African-American children benefited from the intervention more than the Caucasian children vis-à-vis visual–motor and receptive language skills.[44]

Over time, cognitive test scores declined in all three ethnic groups. At the same time, children who received the treatment experienced less severe declines over time.[42]. This drop may be explained in part due to the fact that different tests were used (so that normative data are not comparable over time), and that competencies change dramatically over the first three years of life. For example, tests in the first year of life do not tap language or reasoning skills, both of which are represented in the second- and third-year tests.[45–48]

We speculate that these differences among the three ethnic groups are in part due to the fact that African-American and Hispanic children are more disadvantaged. Of the numerous sociodemographic characteristics of the families, only maternal age and education were entered into the regressions. And even within the maternal education variable, many fewer African-American and Hispanic mothers in the "some college" education group had graduated from college, compared to the Caucasian sample.[49] Factors such as single parenthood, differential residential and schooling patterns, persistent poverty, and multigenerational poverty differentiate the African-American and Hispanic children from the Caucasian children in this sample.[44] Other samples show similar differences associated with poverty.[22,26,50] A description of ethnic differences even when controlling for poverty status is presented in Table 1.[42] Characteristics of the poor African-American, Caucasian, and Hispanic children (poverty defined according to Census Bureau definitions using family income and numbers of family members), are presented, with the poor Hispanic and African-American children being more disadvantaged than the poor Caucasian children in the IHDP sample.

Thus, the low-birth-weight premature Hispanic and African-American children are more likely to have low cognitive test scores than the Caucasian children and, in some cases, are more likely to have benefited from the intervention. The two areas in which low-birth-weight children are known to have deficits—visual–motor and receptive language skills—are the domains in which the Hispanic and African-American children had larger treatment effects than the Cauca-

Table 1 Percent of Poor Follow-Up Children Who Experienced Risk Factors in the Infant Health and Development Program

Risk factor	African-American (n = 158)	Hispanic (n = 26)	Caucasian (n = 46)	Total (n = 230)
Maternal characteristics				
Unemployment of head of household	52.5	53.8	19.6	46.1
Low maternal education (<12th grade)	47.5	65.4	39.1	47.8
Low maternal PPVT-R (<81)	77.8	88.5	37.0	70.9
Low birthweight (<1500 grams)	29.7	30.8	21.7	28.3
High depression	25.3	26.9	37.0	27.8
High stressful life events	19.0	23.1	28.3	21.3
Low social support	41.1	53.8	19.6	38.3
Familial structural risks				
Father absence	74.1	53.8	39.1	64.8
High family density (> child-adult ratio >2)	27.8	23.1	19.6	25.7
Low HOME score	38.0	19.2	6.5	29.6
Parenting belief risk				
Categorical view of child development	50.0	50.0	23.9	44.8

Maternal characteristics include maternal education, verbal ability, mental health, stressful life events, and low social support. Mothers who had not completed high school were considered at risk for this sample. Mothers' scores on the Peabody Picture Vocabulary Test-Revised[5] which were lower than the 25 percentile (PPVT-R < 66) were another risk. Mothers' mental health (e.g., depression, highly stressful life events, and low social support) is associated with children's cognitive and social-emotional development.[52–54] Maternal depression was evaluated by the General Health Questionnaire[55] when the child was twelve months of age. The GHQ is a 12-item scale, tapping depression, somatization, and anxiety. A GHQ score was computed, with higher values indicating more psychological distress (range: 0–32). High risk was defined as having a total score higher than the highest 25% (i.e., GHQ > 13), indicating higher depression. Stressful life events reported by the mother were measured at 12 months. A stressful life event score was computed by summing the occurrence of 18 stressful life events, including maternal illness, friend/relative illness or death, change in schooling, work or residence, and need for service (range: 0–9). High risk was defined as the highest 25% on the scale (number of stressful events > 3). Mothers' social support network was measured by six vignettes asking mothers to report sources of monetary, emotional, and child care support.[56–58] An overall score was obtained by summing support across the vignettes (range: 0–12), with higher value indicating more social support. High risk was defined as the lowest 25% scores on the scale (total score < 7).[59]

Family structural risks included teenage motherhood, father absence, and high family density. Teenage mothers have been found in some studies to be less verbal, less responsive, and more punitive in interacting with their children than older mothers.[60–63] Mothers whose age was younger than 18 years when the child was born were considered high risk. Father presence was determined by whether the husband or father of the child lived in the household when the child was 12 months old. Family density was represented by a child-to-adult ratio in the household at 12 months, reflecting not only family size but the availability of human resources in the home. High-risk was defined as a child-to-adult ratio of greater than 2.[59]

Parenting belief risk was reflected by a categorical view of child development. Parental beliefs about child development were measured by the Concepts of Development Questionnaire.[64] The CODQ is a 20-item scale which reflects two levels of parental beliefs about development. At the categorical level, a parent holds a rigid, simplistic view of child behavior. At the perspective level, parents have a more sophisticated views of child behavior, seeing development influenced by multiple factors. A total score was used (range: 1.05–2.65); higher scores indicated a more perspective view, and lower scores a more categorical view. The high-risk group consisted of mothers whose scores were lower than the 25 percentile.[59]

sian children.[8,13,65,66] These findings only emerged when cognitive test scores were broken down into their cognitive components. These results underscore the importance of considering specific cognitive skills, rather than only focusing on overall cognitive test scores.[45,67]

Behavior Domain

Similar analyses have been conducted for behavior problems, measured at 2 and 3 years. The Behavior Checklist (21 items rated on a three-point scale)[68,69] was read to the mothers at the 2- and 3-year visits; the Child Behavior Checklist (99 items rated on a three point scale)[70] at 36 months. A small but significant treatment effect was seen at both ages.[37,42] The treatment effect was seen across ethnic groups.

Hispanic mothers, however, perceive their children as having more problems at 3 years on both behavior problem scales than do mothers in the other two ethnic groups, controlling for maternal age and education.[42] Since these scales rely on maternal report, it is not known whether Hispanic children have more problematic behavior or whether their mothers' perceive 3-year-old behavior differently. We believe that the latter explanation is more likely. Indeed, in an analysis of teacher report of behavior problems in the intervention group children, no ethnic differences appeared.[71] Compliance may be more valued in certain Hispanic cultural groups, rendering the bids for autonomy that characterize the toddler to be rated as more severe.

Health Domain

Over the total sample, children in the treatment group had higher morbidity as reported by their mothers. These results did not differ by ethnicity. African-American and Hispanic mothers, however, reported that their children had less morbidity than did Caucasian mothers, controlling for maternal education and age as well as neonatal status.

When focusing only on serious morbidity, no treatment effect was found, either for the total sample or the three ethnic groups separately. Mothers from all three ethnic groups reported the same levels of serious morbidity.

Perceived health was also similar across treatment group. African-American mothers reported that their children were healthier than Caucasian mothers, in keeping with the finding of less reported morbidity. Hispanic mothers did not differ from Caucasian mothers on the Rand health rating.

No treatment effects were seen for functional status. African-American mothers whose children were in the treatment group, however, reported higher functional status than those mothers whose children were in the follow-up only group. No such differences were seen for Hispanic mothers' reports. Hispanic, Caucasian, and African-American mothers rated their children similarly with regard to this activity of daily living measure.

RESULTS FOR THE PUERTO RICAN FAMILIES

Comparisons among Three Ethnic Groups at the Albert Einstein College Site

We now present some IHDP results at the Albert Einstein College of Medicine site in the Bronx, New York City. This site had a relatively large number of Puerto Rican families (n = 55), as well as a number of African-American and Caucasian families (n = 63 and 20, respectively). The neonatal and familial characteristics of these three groups at the beginning of the study are shown in Table 2. Similar proportions of lighter and heavier low-birth-weight children are represented in the three groups, as would be expected given the randomization procedure. However, African-American infants are somewhat lighter in weight than the other two groups. Others have reported that African-American infants are lighter at birth than Caucasian infants.[72] The three groups did not differ on neonatal health (which controlled for birth weight). Mothers from the three groups were the same age. The Puerto Rican mothers were less likely to have a high school diploma than the other two groups, however, and the African-American mothers were less likely to have graduated from high school than the Caucasian mothers.

Table 3 shows means and standard deviations (SDs) for the primary outcome measures by ethnicity. The Puerto Rican and African-American children had lower cognitive test scores at age 3 than the Caucasian children, as has been found in other studies.

The Puerto Rican mothers reported that their children had more behavior problems than did the Caucasian mothers (with the African-American mothers intermediate). These findings parallel those for the total Hispanic sample reported earlier.

Mainland Puerto Rican children had twice the rate of serious illnesses of Caucasian children. In a further review of clinic records, this finding was primarily accounted for by serious lower respiratory infec-

Table 2 Initial Status Measures by Ethnicity, Bronx Site and All Sites

Measure		Bronx site: PR ($n = 55$)	Bronx site: Caucasian ($n = 20$)	Bronx site: African-American ($n = 63$)	IHDP Sample
Birthweight	Mean	1882	2007	1707	1795
	SD	420	328	424	458
			($p < 0.008$)		
BW group	% lighter	62%	55%	73%	63%
	% heavier	38%	45%	27%	37%
			(N.S.)		
Sex of child	% male	56%	30%	51%	49%
	% female	44%	70%	49%	51%
			(N.S.)		
Maternal age	Mean	25.5	26.8	24.8	24.8
	SD	6.9	7.1	5.6	6.0
			(N.S.)		
Maternal education	Mean	2.64	3.35	2.78	3.01
	SD	1.01	1.18	1.05	1.10
			($p < 0.036$)		
Neonatal Health Index	Mean	98.8	99.6	101.1	100.0
	SD	14.7	19.5	16.0	15.9
			(N.S.)		

tions, chronic asthma, and hospitalizations resulting from asthma. Differences were also found on the General Health Ratings Index, as the Puerto Rican mothers perceive their children to be more ill than the Caucasian or African-American mothers at the Einstein site.

Intervention Effects at the Bronx Site

Comparisons among the two treatment groups were made for all three ethnic groups at the Bronx site. Given the small sample size, these analyses are frankly exploratory. The IHDP was not designed to detect difference between treatment groups at the individual site level, let alone within subgroups at a site. Keeping this caveat in mind, we looked at the patterns of treatment effects for Puerto Rican, Caucasian, and African-American families. Table 4 presents simple mean values; the comparisons in Table 5, on which the *p*-values are based, have been adjusted for differences in variables defined at baseline (see the Table 5 footnote for the list of variables).

Table 3 Primary Outcome Measures by Ethnicity, Bronx Site and All Sites

		Bronx site			
Measure		Puerto Rican (n = 50)	Caucasian (n = 19)	African-American (n = 53)	IHDP Sample
Stanford-Binet scale, form L-M	Mean	74.6	96.3	74.9	88.0
	SD	14.9	25.9	11.5	20.1
			($p < 0.001$)		
Child behavior checklist for age 2–3 years	Mean	52.2	37.1	47.5	45.9
	SD	20.2	20.4	21.5	20.0
			($p < 0.030$)		
Mother's report: Morbidity index	Mean	6.7	6.4	5.9	7.2
	SD	2.7	3.8	2.6	3.2
			(N.S.)		
Mother's report: Serious morbidity index	Mean	1.31	0.63	0.96	1.20
	SD	0.94	0.76	0.86	0.97
			($p < 0.013$)		
Functional status II (R) scale	Mean	0.95	0.99	0.97	0.96
	SD	0.11	0.02	0.06	0.08
			($p < 0.08$)		
General health ratings index	Mean	25.3	28.6	28.5	27.2
	SD	4.7	5.2	4.2	5.2
			($p < 0.001$)		

Table 4 Effects of Treatment on Primary Outcome Measures by Ethnicity, Bronx Site and All Sites

Measure		Bronx site			
		PR	Caucasian	African-American	IHDP Sample
Stanford-Binet scale, form L-M	F Mean	71.0	87.0	73.7	84.5
	I Mean	81.6	107.9	77.4	93.5
	Difference	10.6	20.9	3.7	9.0
Child behavior checklist for age 2–3 years	F mean	49.1	41.2	46.9	47.2
	I mean	58.0	32.6	48.7	43.7
	Difference	8.9	−8.6	1.8	−3.5
Mother's report: Morbidity index	F mean	7.0	6.7	5.4	6.9
	I mean	6.2	6.2	7.1	7.6
	Difference	−0.8	−0.5	1.7	0.7
Mother's report: Serious morbidity index	F mean	1.31	0.70	0.74	1.20
	I mean	1.29	0.56	1.41	1.19
	Difference	−0.02	−0.14	0.67	−0.01
Functional status II (R) scale	F mean	0.96	0.99	0.97	0.96
	I mean	0.91	1.00	0.97	0.97
	Difference	−0.05	−0.01	0.00	0.01
General health ratings index	F mean	25.4	26.2	29.5	27.1
	I mean	25.1	31.3	26.4	27.5
	Difference	−0.3	5.1	−3.1	0.4

Cognitive Domain

The Puerto Rican and Caucasian children in the treatment group had higher cognitive scores at age 3 than those in the follow-up only group. These findings for the Puerto Rican and Caucasian children in the Bronx parallel those for the sample as a whole.

A treatment effect was not seen in the African-American children at the Einstein site, however, unlike the findings for the entire IHDP African-American sample. What might account for this difference? One possibility is that the sample is too small to detect treatment differences, as mentioned earlier; another is that the African-American families in the Bronx differ from the African-American families in other sites on dimensions other than maternal education and age.

Behavior Domain

No treatment effects were seen for behavior problems at the Einstein site. Given that the treatment effect for the entire IHDP sample was

Table 5 Adjusted Effect Size (ES) by Ethnicity, Bronx Site only

Measure		Bronx site				
		PR	Caucasian	African-American	Total	IHDP Sample
Stanford-Binet scale, form L-M	ES	9.54	20.61	4.84	10.29	9.42
	(p I vs F)	(0.046)	(0.006)	(0.165)	(0.001)	(0.001)
Child behavior checklist for	ES	10.21	−10.64	−0.86	1.20	−3.99
age 2–3 years	(p I vs F)	(0.138)	(0.105)	(0.900)	(0.773)	(0.003)
Mother's report: Morbidity	ES	−0.90	0.30	1.59	0.46	0.82
index	(p I vs F)	(0.289)	(0.795)	(0.056)	(0.406)	(0.001)
Mother's report: Serious	ES	0.04	−0.20	0.51	0.24	0.01
morbidity index	(p I vs F)	(0.878)	(0.576)	(0.038)	(0.144)	(0.846)
Functional status II (R) scale	ES	−0.045	0.008	0.011	−0.011	0.002
	(p I vs F)	(0.195)	(0.335)	(0.554)	(0.466)	(0.664)
General Health Ratings Index	ES	−0.06	5.81	−2.99	−0.30	0.40
	(p I vs F)	(0.965)	(0.019)	(0.026)	(0.728)	(0.261)

Estimates adjusted for birthweight, sex, maternal age, maternal education, Neonatal Health Index (and race for the total Bronx site; and site for entire IHDP group) using a multiple linear regression model.
(p I vs. F) = p value for intervention vs. follow-up group comparison.

very small (although statistically significant), the sample was probably too small to detect a difference (i.e., a difference of over 10 points for the Caucasian families in the Bronx did not reach significance, while the overall effect for the total sample was 3.99 points, which was significant at the $p < 0.005$ level).

At the same time, the patterns of intervention effects were very different for the three ethnic groups. The Caucasian mothers reported a 10-point reduction in behavior problem scores if their children were in the Intervention group. No such differences were seen for the African-American children. The Hispanic mothers reported more behavior problems if their children were in the treatment group. The Puerto Rican mothers reported more behavior problems overall, compared to the other two groups in the Bronx, as did the Hispanic mothers in the total sample.

Why might participation in an early intervention program result in the report of more, rather than less, behavior problems? Several possibilities exist: The Puerto Rican mothers might report more problems because the home visitors, in discussing their children's behavior, sensitized the mothers to such behavior (similar to such effects on health surveillance). On the other hand, participation in the intervention may have resulted in children becoming less compliant, more active, more exploratory, and more peer-oriented.[73,74] These behaviors may be seen as negative by the Puerto Rican mothers, if they value quiet and obedience. The fact that the Hispanic children in the sample as a whole were not rated by their teachers as having more behavior problems lends some support to this premise.[71] Finally, the center-based schooling might have altered the children's behavior, though it is difficult to see how it would alter Puerto Rican children negatively, Caucasian children positively, and African-American children not at all. For these reasons, we believe that these ethnic group patterns are due to cultural differences in what is deemed appropriate behavior by 3-year-olds.

Health Domain

The only health outcome that shows an intervention effect is the General Health Ratings Index. Caucasian mothers reported better health ratings for the children receiving the treatment, African-American mothers reported poorer health ratings for the children receiving the treatment, and Puerto Rican mothers reported no treatment differences.

CONCLUSIONS

The home-based and center-based early intervention services provided by the IHDP increased the cognitive functioning of the Hispanic children as well as the African-American and Caucasian 3-year-olds. The effects were most pronounced in those cognitive skills in which low-birth-weight children are likely to show deficits—verbal and visual–spatial skills. These effects were also seen in the Puerto Rican children in one of the IHDP sites. This site was located in New York City, where the majority of mainland Puerto Ricans live.[75]

These IHDP results are limited to those Hispanic families with at least limited English proficiency. At the time of the IHDP, the curriculum had not been used in any language except English (it is currently being used in Rumania). Unfortunately, funding constraints did not allow for a Spanish version to be developed and pretested. Whether this set of early intervention services would show similar effects for exclusively Spanish-speaking Hispanic families is not known.

Another possible limitation involves the testing of children in English. The decision to test in English was made based on the provision of the intervention in English. For children exposed to two languages in the home (as was the case for the majority of Puerto Rican families in the Einstein IHDP site), administration of the Stanford-Binet Test in English might have resulted in slightly lower scores than would administration in Spanish. Hispanic children tend to score slightly higher on cognitive tests, with better performance in nonverbal than verbal items.[76] Comparisons between verbal ability scores based on English and Spanish proficiency have been made using the Peabody Picture Vocabulary Test-Revised.[63] Using the English version of the PPVT-R, Caucasian children tend to score highest, followed by African-Americans, and Hispanics.[76] Our findings for the Follow-up group only, as illustrated in Figure 1, parallel these previous results, using the Stanford-Binet Test. Interestingly, at the Einstein site, the African-American and Puerto Rican children are less divergent (three points in the follow-up only group) than for the total sample of African-American and Hispanic children (seven points in the follow-up group only). These findings may be due to the fact that more Puerto Rican children in the Bronx site hear English spoken in their homes or the homes of relatives than the Mexican-American children in the Dallas site or the Cuban-American children in the Miami site. Alternatively, the African-American sample in the Bronx may be more disadvantaged than the

African-American samples in other sites, which results in their Stanford-Binet scores being an average lower than the total sample of African-Americans.

Testing on Spanish versions of the PPVT-R results in slightly lower (nonsignificant) scores for mainland Hispanic 3-year-olds compared to Puerto Rican and Mexican children. With age, the mainland children fall further behind the Puerto Rican and Mexican cohorts; presumably, the entrance into schools with classes in English depresses the mainland Hispanic children's knowledge of Spanish vocabulary.[77] Thus, mainland Hispanic children lag behind Caucasian children in English and Puerto Rican and Mexican children in Spanish vocabulary.

Low cognitive test scores may be more common in mainland Puerto Rican children compared to Mexican-American children.[78] School achievement is also depressed for the former group.[76] These differences are in part accounted for by the greater poverty of mainland Puerto Rican children, as discussed in this volume. Thus, the IHDP has the potential to alter the cognitive skills exhibited by mainland Puerto Rican children. Whether these effects continue into school is currently being evaluated.

The findings for behavior are particularly interesting, in that Hispanic mothers report that their children have more problems than do Caucasian or African-American mothers. Such differences are likely to be due to variations in child-rearing attitudes and practices across cultural groups.[79–81] As Wasserman points out (see chapter 9 this volume), such differences may be due to culture, poverty, and education (in that certain groups are more likely to be poor than others, as is the case for mainland Puerto Ricans), or an interaction between the two (e.g., mainland Puerto Ricans in New York City are likely to be not only poor but from rural and low education origins, which might influence childrearing attitudes). This type of interaction is elegantly illustrated by Sameroff and his colleagues. One study directly tested the premise that degree of acculturation would be associated with more differentiated concepts of development (using the Concepts of Development Questionnaire). Three groups of Mexican-American mothers were assessed: (1) those who immigrated in the last several years (Mexican in America); (2) those who had lived in the United States for a decade or more and were bilingual (Mexican-American); and (3) those who were born in the United States and were English-speaking (Chicano). A group of native-born Anglos were also included.[82,83] One-half of each group was high socioeconomic status and one-half low. Acculturation was associated with being able to take a perspectivisitic approach to child development, with these effects only being seen in the high socioeconomic women.

Cultural differences also may be influenced by the age of the parent.[60,84,85] For example, if teenage parenthood is accepted in one cultural group but not another, a mother in the former group will probably receive more social support for and be more comfortable with being a young parent, as Garcia Coll[60] has reported in her sample of island Puerto Ricans and mainland African-Americans and Caucasians.

Differences in child-rearing attitudes are probably also associated with degree of acculturation.[86,87] In the IHDP, we have no measures of acculturation—length of residence, generational continuity on the mainland, relatives (and visits to) Puerto Rico.

One possible methodological limitation of this finding is related to the cultural influences summarized above. The behavior problem scales used in the IHDP (as well as in most studies) were normed on primarily Caucasian samples, and this may result in some undetermined bias.[88,89]

In another study of New York City mainland Puerto Rican, Dominican, and African-American mothers,[80] Puerto Rican women had more negative child-rearing attitudes than did African-American women (although Dominican mothers, who were the most disadvantaged group, had even more negative child-rearing attitudes and parenting behavior than did the Puerto Rican mothers). These findings might be akin to our findings of Hispanic mothers' reports of more behavior problems.

The IHDP also has data on child-rearing attitudes (not reported in this chapter). When the low-birth-weight children were 1 year of age, mothers filled out the Knowledge of Infant Development Inventory[90,91] and the Concepts of Development Questionnaire.[82] Scores were calculated on the accuracy of mothers' knowledge about developmental milestones (KIDI), their categorical concepts of development (the mother tends to use a single simplistic explanation of behavior; for example, either genetic or environmental determinants influence child functioning, but not both; CODQ), and their perspectivistic concepts of development (the mother sees multiple influences operating; CODQ). Controlling for maternal education, income, age and number of children, as well as neonatal characteristics (gender, birth weight, and neonatal health), the Hispanic and African-American mothers had more categorical and less perspectivistic views of development than did Caucasian mothers.[92]

The Puerto Rican low-birth-weight infants as a group at the Einstein site had higher ratings on the Serious Morbidity Index. In a review of their hospital and clinical records, this was accounted for by higher levels of respiratory illnesses and by asthma requiring hospitalization or lengthy periods of convalescence at home. This finding mirrors those of other investigators. Newacheck,[93] using the National Health Interview Survey (1979–1981), found that the overall prevalence of activity-limiting chronic conditions among U.S. children younger than 17 years was 3.8%. A chronic medical condition was defined as an event that had limited activity for the prior three months. Trevino and Moss,[94] also examining the National Health Interview Survey (1978–1980), determined the prevalence of limitation due to chronic conditions among Mexican-American (3.0%), mainland Puerto Rican (6.2%), Cuban-American (3.5%), African-American (3.7%), and Caucasian (4.0%) children. The overall prevalence of chronic medical conditions in Mexican-American and Cuban-American children is similar to that in non-Hispanic children of the United States. The prevalence of chronic medical conditions for mainland Puerto Ricans was significantly higher than for the other two Hispanic subgroups and appeared to be higher than the national average. Newacheck's findings were due primarily to the high prevalence of asthma reported for mainland Puerto Rican children.

Mainland Puerto Rican children have a distribution of conditions that were highly skewed with a high prevalence of respiratory disorders. In a study reported by Mendoza,[78] 62% (50/81) of mainland Puerto Rican children with a chronic medical condition had a respiratory disorder and of these 98% (49/50) were classified as asthmatics. The prevalence of asthma among mainland Puerto Rican children appears to have the worst health status among the major Hispanic groups, although access to health care is the highest.[78] The findings of the Puerto Rican children enrolled in the IHDP study in the New York City area clearly support previous reports of increased rates in asthma and serious morbidity ratings. The higher rate of respiratory illness among Puerto Rican children may be due in part to the fact that Puerto Rican families tend to be poorer than other Hispanic groups or white groups. Hispanics families are less likely to have health insurance or continuity of care.[95] This pattern is more pronounced in Puerto Rican than Cuban-American or Mexican-American families.[95] Thus, it is not surprising that mainland Puerto Rican children have the worst health status of the three major Hispanic groups.[96]

The higher rate of poverty make it likely that mainland Puerto

Rican children have inadequate preschool and school experiences. Since poor children generally are ill-prepared for school, lower quality education sets many children on a trajectory for failure. Early educational intervention programs, like IHDP, are designed in order to improve the life chances of poor children. Beginning with Head Start and a number of small, educationally-oriented programs in the 1960s, early education has become one of the major programs to serve the poor (the others being more health oriented—WIC, EPDST, Education for All Handicapped Children). Cognitive and school performance improvements have been found in disadvantaged children from early educational services.[97] Perhaps the most widely cited study is the evaluation of eleven separate (mostly preschool) programs, which were summarized by Lazar and colleagues.[98] When compared to controls, children who had attended the preschool intervention programs demonstrated higher intelligence scores at ages five and six, were less likely to have been held back a grade or to be in special classes by third grade, and were more likely to have high math achievement scores in the early grades.[99–103]

A limitation of these program evaluations is that most included primarily African-American children, making it impossible to determine whether early intervention services are effective for other ethnic groups. One exception is the Parent Child Development Center evaluation, which provided services to poor families in the first three years of a child's life. Significant effects were seen on IQ tests at ages three and four in all three centers, and one of the centers which had a substantial number of Hispanic families.[104–105]

One limitation of the IHDP vis-a-vis Hispanic group is that it was based on interventions developed for other ethnic groups. As such, the IHDP might not have been particularly sensitive to the cultural needs of Hispanic families (or more accurately, the subgroups of Hispanic families, given the cultural diversity among Hispanic groups). The approach used by IHDP was to take an intervention used for poor children of normal birth weight and modify it for use with premature children of low birth weight across the socioeconomic spectrum. We suspect that if this intervention were to be targeted for Hispanic children specifically, further modifications might be necessary. However, two strategies for the development of interventions are possible. One takes existing interventions and alters them for a particular ethnic or cultural group; while the other takes as a starting point the values and behaviors of a particular cultural group and designs an intervention around them.[106–109] Both are legitimate avenues of inquiry and implementation.

Thus, the IHDP is one of the few randomized clinical trial programs for young children that includes Hispanic families. This chapter presents exploratory analyses of the results of the IHDP for the Hispanic children in general and mainland Puerto Rican children in particular. Our results suggest interventions such as the IHDP could be implemented on a large scale for Hispanic families.

ACKNOWLEDGMENT. Supported by grant MCJ-360593, Maternal and Child Health Bureau, HRSA, DHHS.

REFERENCES

1. Brooks-Gunn J: Promoting healthy development in young children: What educational interventions work? in Rogers DE, Ginzberg E (eds): *Improving the life chances of children at risk*. Boulder, CO, Westview Press, 1990, pp 125–145
2. Werner EE, Smith RS: *Vulnerable but Invincible: A Longitudinal Study of Resilient Children and Youth*. New York, McGraw-Hill, 1982
3. Garmezy N, Rutter M (eds): *Stress, Coping and Development in Children*. Baltimore, MD: Johns Hopkins University Press, 1988
4. Sameroff AJ, Chandler MJ: Reproductive risk and the continuum of caretaking casualty, in Horowitz FD, Hetherington M, Scarr-Salapatek S, Siegal G (eds): *Rev. Child Develop. Res*. 4:187–244, 1975
5. Brown G, Bhrolchain M, Harris T: Social class and psychiatric disturbance among women in an urban population. *Sociology* 9:225–254, 1975
6. Sandler I, Miller P, Short J, Wolchik S: Social support as a protective for children in stress, in Belle D (ed): *Children's Social Networks and Social Supports*. New York: Wiley, 1989, pp 277–307
7. Lee KS, Paneth N, Gartner LM, Pearlman MA, Gross L: *Neonatal Mortality: An Analysis of the Recent Improvement in the United States*. ASPH. Vol. 70, No. 1. Washington, DC: National Center for Health Statistics, 1980
8. McCormick MC: Long-term follow-up of infants discharged from neonatal intensive care units. *JAMA* 261:1767–1772, 1989
9. McCormick MC: The contribution of low birth weight to infant mortality and childhood morbidity. *N. Eng. J. Med*. 321:82–90, 1985
10. Institute of Medicine: *Preventing Low Birthweight*. Washington, DC, National Academy Press, 1985
11. Garcia Coll CT: Developmental outcome of minority infants: A process-oriented look into our beginnings. *Child Develop* 61:270–289, 1990
12. Drillien CM: *The Growth and Development of the Prematurely Born Infant*. Edinburgh, Livingstone, 1964
13. Kopp CB: Risk factors in development, in Campos JJ, Haith M (eds): *Handbook of Child Psychology*, Vol 2. New York, John Wiley, 1983, pp 1081–1088
14. Klein NK, Hack M, Gallagher, J, Fanaroff AA: Preschool performance of children with normal intelligence who were very low-birthweight infants. *Pediatrics* 75:531–537, 1985
15. McCormick MC, Brooks-Gunn J, Workman-Daniels K, Turner J, Peckham G: The infant health and development status of very low birth weight children at school age. *JAMA* 267:2204–2208, 1992

16. Meisels SJ, Plunkett JW: Developmental consequences of preterm birth: Are there long-term effects? In Baltes PB, Featherman DL, Lerner RM (eds): *Life-span Development and Behavior*. Hillsdale, NJ, Lawrence Erlbaum, 1988, pp 87–128
17. Friedman SL, Sigman MD (eds): *The Psychological Development of Low Birth Weight Children: Advances in Applied Developmental Psychology*. Norwood, NJ, Ablex Publishing Co, 1991
18. Petersen PE, Jencks C (eds): *Urban Underclass*. Washington, DC, Brookings Institute, 1991
19. Tienda M: Puerto Ricans and the underclass debate. *Ann. Amer. Acad. Pol. & Soc. Sci.* 501:105–119, 1989
20. US Bureau of the Census: *The Hispanic Population in the United States: March, 1986 and 1987* (Advance Report). Washington, DC, US Government Printing Office, 1987, No. 416; series P-20
21. McCormick MC, Brooks-Gunn J: Health care for children and adolescents, in Freeman H, Levine S (eds): *Handbook of Medical Sociology*. Englewood Cliffs, NJ, Prentice Hall, 1989, pp 347–380
22. Chase-Lansdale PL, Brooks-Gunn J (eds): *Escape From Poverty: What Makes a Difference for Poor Children?* New York, Cambridge University Press, in press
23. Liaw FR, Brooks-Gunn J: Patterns of low birth weight children's cognitive development and their determinants. *Develop. Psychol.*, 1992
24. Sameroff AJ, Seifer R, Zax M, Greenspan S: Intelligence quotient scores of 4-year-old children: Social environmental risk factors. *Pediatrics* 79:343–350, 1987
25. Bronfenbrenner U: Contexts of child rearing: Problems and prospects. *Amer. Psychologist* 34:844–850, 1979
26. Huston A (ed): *Children in Poverty: Child Development and Public Policy*. New York, Cambridge University Press, 1991
27. Duncan GJ, Klebanov PK, Brooks-Gunn J: Economic deprivation and early childhood development. *Child Develop.*, in press
28. Parker S, Greer S, Zuckerman B: Double jeopardy: The impact of poverty on early childhood development. *Pediatr. Clin. N. Amer.* 35:1227–1240, 1988
29. Egbuonu L, Starfield B: Child health and social status. *Pediatrics* 69:550–557, 1982
30. Benasich AA, Brooks-Gunn J, Clewell BC: How do mothers benefit from early intervention programs? *J. Appl. Develop. Psychol.* 13:311–362, 1992
31. Brooks-Gunn J, Hearn P: Early intervention and developmental dysfunction: Implications for pediatrics. *Av. Pediatr.* 29:497–527, 1982
32. Ramey CT, Bryant DM, Suarez TM: Preschool compensatory education and the modifiability of intelligence: A critical review, in Detterman D (ed): *Current Topics in Human Intelligence*. Norwood, NJ, Ablex Publishing, 1983, pp 247–296
33. Bennett FC: The effectiveness of early intervention for infants at increased biologic risk, in Guralnick M, Bennett FC (eds): *The Effectiveness of Early Intervention For At-Risk and Handicapped Children*. New York, Academic Press, 1983, pp 79–112
34. Field TM: Interventions for premature infants. *J. Pediatrics.* 109:183–191, 1986
35. Olds DL: Can home visitation improve the health of women and children at risk? in Rogers DL, Ginsberg E (eds): *Improving the Life Chances of Children at Risk*. Boulder, CO, Westview Press, 1990, pp 79–103
36. Patteson DM, Barnard KE: Parenting of low birth weight infants: A review of issues and interventions. *Inf. Ment. Health J.* 11:37–56, 1990
37. Infant Health and Development Program Staff: Enhancing the outcomes of low birthweight, premature infants: A multisite randomized trial. *JAMA* 263:3035–3042, 1990
38. McCormick MC, Brooks-Gunn J, Shapiro S, Benasich A: Health care use among young children in day care. Results in a randomized trial of early intervention. *JAMA* 265:2212–2217, 1991

39. Scott DT, Bauer CR, Kraemer HC, Tyson J: A neonatal health index for preterm infants. *Pediatr. Res.* 25:263A, 1989
40. Bayley N: *Manual for the Bayley Scales of Infant Development*. New York, Psychological Corporation, 1969
41. Terman LM, Merrill MA: *Stanford Binet Intelligence Scale: Manual for the Third Revision, Form L-M*, Boston, Houghton Mifflin Co, 1973
42. Brooks-Gunn J, Klebanov PK, Liaw F, Spiker D: Enhancing the development of low birth weight, premature infants: Changes in cognition and behavior over the first three years. *Child Develop.* 64:815–829, 1993
43. Brooks-Gunn J, Liaw F, Klebanov PK: Effects of early intervention on low birth weight preterm infants: What aspects of cognitive functioning are enhanced? *J. Pediatrics* 120:350–359, 1992
44. Brooks-Gunn J, Klebanov P, Duncan GJ: The impact of neighborhood poverty on three-year-old black children's IQ and home environment. Presented to the Symposium on Effects of Neighborhood Poverty on the Development of Children and Adolescents, at the meeting of the Society for Research in Child Development, Seattle, 1991
45. Bornstein MH, Sigman MD: Continuity in mental development from infancy. *Child Develop.* 57:251–274, 1986
46. Lewis M, McGurk H: Evaluation of infant intelligence: Infant intelligence scores—true or false? *Science* 178:1174–1177, 1972
47. Lewis M: *Origins of Intelligence: Infancy and Early Childhood*, ed 2. New York, Plenum Press, 1983
48. McCall RB, Hogarty PS, Hurlburt N: Transitions in infant sensorimotor development and the prediction of childhood IQ. *Amer. Psychologist* 27:728–743, 1972
49. Brooks-Gunn J, Gross RT, Kraemer HC, Spiker D, Shapiro S: Enhancing the cognitive outcomes of low-birth-weight, premature infants: For whom is the intervention most effective? *Pediatrics* 89:1209–1215, 1992
50. McLoyd VC, Spencer MB (eds): Special issue on minority children. *Child Develop.* 61, 1990
51. Dunn LM, Dunn LM: *Peabody Picture Vocabulary Test-Revised*. American Guidance Service, 1981
52. Billings AG, Moos RH: The role of coping response and social resources in attenuating the stress of life events. *Journal of Behavioral Medicine* 4, 139–157, 1981
53. McLoyd VC: The impact of economic hardship on Black families and development. *Child Development* 61:311–346, 1990
54. Orvaschel H, Weissman M, Kidd KK: The children of depressed parents: The childhood of depressed patients. *Journal of Affective Disorders* 2:1–16, 1980
55. Goldberg S: Prematurity: Effects of parent-infant interaction. *Journal of Pediatric Psychology* 3:137–144, 1978
56. Cohen JB, Lazarus RS: *Social Support Questionnaire*. Berkeley, CA, University of California, 1977
57. McCormick MC, Brooks-Gunn J, Shorter T, Wallace CY, Holmes JH, Heagarty MC: The planning of pregnancy among low-income women in central Harlem. *American Journal of Obstetrics and Gynecology*, 156:145–149, 1987
58. McCormick MC, Brooks-Gunn J: The health of children and adolescents, in Freeman HE, Levine S (eds), *Handbook of medical sociology*, Englewood Cliffs, NJ, Prentice Hall, 1989, pp 347–379
59. Liaw FR, Brooks-Gunn J: Cumulative familial risks and low-birth-weight children's cognitive and behavioral development. *J. Clin. Child. Psych.*, in press
60. Garcia Coll CT: The consequences of teenage childbearing in traditional Puerto Rican culture. In Nugent JK, Lester BM, Brazelton TB (eds), *The cultural context of infancy* Vol 1. Norwood, NJ, Ablex, 1988, pp 111–132

61. Garcia Coll CT, Hoffman J, Vohr W: The social ecology and early parenting of Caucasian adolescent mothers. *Child Development* 58:955–963, 1987
62. Oppel W, Roystom A: Teenage births: Some social, psychological, and physical sequelae. *American Journal of Public Health*, 61:751–756
63. Roosa MW, Fitzgerald HE, Carlson NA: A comparison of teenage and older mothers: A systems analysis. *Journal of Marriage and Family* 32:367–377.
64. Sameroff AJ, Feil LA: Parental concepts of development, in Sigel IE (ed), *Parental Belief Systems*. Hillsdale, NJ: Erlbaum, 1985, pp 85–105
65. Klein NK, Hack M, Breslau N: Children who were very low birthweight: Development and academic achievement at nine years of age. *Dev. Behav. Pediatr.* 10:32–37, 1989
66. Vohr BR, Garcia Coll CT: Neurodevelopmental and school performance of very low-birth-weight infants: A seven year longitudinal study. *Pediatrics* 76:345–350, 1985
67. Brooks-Gunn J, Lewis M: The prediction of mental functioning in young handicapped children. In: Vietze P, Vaughan HG Jr. (eds): *Early Identification of Infants with Developmental Disabilities*, Philadelphia, Grune & Stratton, 1988
68. Richman N, Graham PJ: A behavioral screening questionnaire for use with three-year-old children: Preliminary findings. *J. Child Psychol. & Psychiatry* 12:5–33, 1971
69. Richman N, Stevenson J, Graham PJ: Prevalence of behavior problems in three-year-old children: An epidemiological study in a London Borough. *J. Child Psychol. & Psychiatry* 16:277–288, 1975
70. Achenbach TM, Edelbrock CS, Howell CT: *Empirically Based Assessment of the Behavioral/Emotional Problems of 2- and 3-Year-Old Children*. Monographs of the Society for Research in Child Development 46 (1, Serial No. 188), 1987
71. Spiker D, Ferguson J, Brooks-Gunn J: Enhancing maternal interactive behavior and child social competence in low-birth-weight, premature infants. *Child Develop.* 64:754–768, 1983
72. Brenner WE, Edelman DA, Hendricks CH: A standard of fetal growth for the United States of America. *Amer. J. Obstet. & Gynec.* 126:555–564, 1976
73. Feagans L, Haskins R: Neighborhood dialogues of Black and White 5-year-olds. *J. Appl. Develop. Psychol.* 7:181–200, 1986
74. Kagan J, Kearsley RB, Zelazo PR: The emergence of initial apprehension to unfamiliar peers in Lewis M, Rosenblum LA (eds): *Friendship and Peer Relations* Vol 4. New York, John Wiley & Sons, 1975, pp 187–206
75. Lash T, Sigal II, Dudzinski D: *Children and Families in New York City: An Analysis of the 1976 Survey of Income and Education*. New York, Foundation for Child Development, 1979
76. Dunn LM: *Bilingual Hispanic Children on the U.S. Mainland: A Review of Research on their Cognitive, Linguistic, and Scholastic Development*. Circle Pines, MN, American Guidance Services, 1986
77. Dunn LM, Dunn LM: *Peabody Picture Vocabulary Test—Revised*. Circle Pines, MN, American Guidance Service, 1981
78. Mendoza FS, Takata: *Measures of Health Status and Health Care Access* for Mainland Puerto Rican Children: Results from the Hispanic Health and Nutrition Examination Survey.
79. Durrett ME, O'Bryant S, Pennebaker JW: Childbearing reports of White, Black and Mexican-American families. *Develop. Psychol.* 11:871, 1975
80. Wasserman GA, Rauh VA, Brunelli SA, Garcia-Castro M, Necos B: Psychosocial attributes and life experiences of minority mothers: Age and ethnic variations. *Child Develop.* 61:566–580, 1990
81. Ramos-McKay JM, Comas-Diaz L, Rivera LA: Puerto Ricans. In: Comas-Diaz L, Griffith EEH (eds). *Clinical guidelines in cross-cultural mental health*. New York, John Wiley, 1988, pp 204–232

82. Sameroff AJ, Feil LA: Parental concepts of development. In: Sigel IE (ed). *Parental Belief Systems*. Hillsdale, NJ, Erlbaum, 1985
83. Armendariz JB, Sameroff AJ, Karrer B: Effects of Mexican-American acculturation on parents' concepts of development. Unpublished manuscript, 1983.
84. Furstenberg FF, Brooks-Gunn J: Teenage childbearing: Causes consequences and remedies. In: Aiken L, Mechanic D (eds). *Applications of Social Science to Clinical Medicine and Health Policy*. New Brunswick, NJ, Rutgers University Press, 1986, pp 307–334
85. Furstenberg FF, Brooks-Gunn J, Morgan SP: *Adolescent Mothers in Later Life*. New York, Cambridge University Press, 1987
86. Padilla AM: The role of cultural awareness and ethnic loyalty in acculturation. In: Padilla AM (ed), *Acculturation*. Boulder, CO: Westview, 1980, pp 85–110
87. Rogler L, Cortes D, Malgady R: Acculturation and mental health status among Hispanics: Convergence and new directions for research. *American Psychologist* 46:585–597, 1991
88. Clarke-Stewart KA, Apfel N: Evaluating parental effects on child development. In: Shulman LS (ed): *Review of Educational Research*, Vol 6. New York, Academic Press, 47–119, 1978
89. Spencer MB, Markstrom-Adams C: Identity processes among racial and ethnic minority children. *Amer. Child Develop.* 61:290–310, 1990
90. MacPhee D: Manual: Knowledge of Infant Development Inventory. Unpublished manuscript: University of North Carolina, 1981
91. MacPhee D: The nature of parents' experiences with knowledge about infant development. Presented at the Meeting of the Society for Research in Child Development, Detroit, 1983
92. Benasich AA, Brooks-Gunn J, Spiker D, Kreitman W, Black GW: Maternal attitudes and knowledge about child development: Concurrent and predictive effects on child outcome and home environment, in: Gross RT, Spiker D (eds). The Infant Health and Development Program For Low Birth Weight Premature Infants. Palo Alto, CA, Stanford University Press (in press)
93. Newacheck PW, Budetti PD, Halfon N: Trends in activity-limiting chronic conditions among children. *American Journal of Public Health* 76:178–184, 1986
94. Trevino F, Moss J: Health indicators for Hispanic, black, and white Americans. *Vital Health Stat.* 10:50–51, 1984
95. Hispanic Health and Nutrition Examination Survey, 1982–84: Findings on Health Status and Health Care Needs. *American Journal of Public Health* 80:1–72 (Supplement), 1990
96. Mendoza FS, Takata GS: *Measures of Health Status and Health Care Access for Mainland Puerto Rican Children: Results from the Hispanic Health and Nutrition Examination Survey*, 1991
97. Shonkoff J, Meisels S: Early childhood intervention: The evolution of a concept, in Meisels S, Shonkoff J (eds), *Handbook of early childhood intervention*. New York, Cambridge University Press, 1990
98. Lazar I, Darlington RB, Murray H, Royce J, Snipper A: Lasting effects of early education: A report from the Consortium for Longitudinal Studies. Monographs of the Society for Research in Child Development, 47 (No. 2–3, Serial No. 195), 1982
99. Benasich AA, Brooks-Gunn J, Clewell BC: How do mothers benefit from early intervention programs? *Journal of Applied Developmental Psychology* 13:311–362, 1992
100. Haskins R: Beyond metaphor: Efficacy of early childhood education. *American Psychologist* 44:274–282, 1989
101. Zigler EF: Early childhood intervention: A promising preventative for juvenile delinquency. *American Psychologist* 47:997–1006, 1992
102. Clarke-Stewart KA, Fein GG: Early childhood programs. In Mussen PH (eds),

Handbook of Child Psychology, 4th ed, Vol 4. New York, John Wiley & Sons, 1983, pp 918–999

103. Ramey CT, Bryant DM, Suarez TM: Preschool compensatory education and the modifiability of intelligence: A critical review, in Detterman D (ed), *Current topics in human intelligence*. Norwood, NJ, Ablex Publishing, 1983, pp 247–293
104. Bridgeman B, Blumenthal JB, Andrews SR: Parent Child Development Center: Final Evaluation Report. Department of Health and Human Services, Office of Human Development Services, Washington, DC, April, 1981
105. Lee KS, Brooks-Gunn J, Schnur E: Does Head-Start work? A one-year follow-up comparison of disadvantaged children attending head start, no preschool, and other preschool programs. *Developmental Psychology* 24:210–222, 1988
106. Betancourt H, Lopez SR: The study of culture, ethnicity, and race in American psychology. *American Psychologist* 48:629–637, 1993
107. Hammel EA: A theory of culture for democracy. *Population and Development Review* 16:455–485, 1990
108. Rugler LH: The meaning of culturally sensitive research in mental health. *American Journal of Psychiatry* 146:296–303, 1989
109. Wilkinson DY, King G: Conceptual and methodological issues in the use of race as a variable: Policy implications. *Milbank Quarterly* 65:56–71, 1987

11

Distinguishing among Proficiency, Choice, and Attitudes in Questions about Language For Bilinguals

KENJI HAKUTA

INTRODUCTION

The issue of language has played a particularly prominent role in defining Puerto Rican culture and identity. This has to do, in part, with the history of attempts at the imposition of English through government and schools.[1,2] This legacy continues to seep into current political debates about the status of English and Spanish, a controversy that is inseparable from the issue of the political status of the island vis-à-vis the United States.

As a measure of acculturation to mainstream U.S. mainland cul-

KENJI HAKUTA • School of Education, Stanford University, Stanford, California 94305.

Puerto Rican Women and Children: Issues in Health, Growth, and Development, edited by Gontran Lamberty and Cynthia Garcia Coll. Plenum Press, New York, 1994.

ture, language variables take on particular importance. The purpose of this paper is to dissect, from the perspective of a language specialist, the various dimensions of bilingualism. In particular, I argue for the importance of considering separately three aspects: language proficiency (a primarily cognitive psychological or psycholinguistic dimension); language choice (a sociolinguistic dimension having to do with the particulars of conversational settings and interlocutors); and language attitudes (a social psychological dimension).

Sociologists who study bilingual communities have long noted that stable and balanced bilingualism over generations is rarely observed.[3] The bilingualism of language minority communities including Puerto Ricans on the U.S. mainland is no exception. It is generally characterized by a rapid shift into monolingual usage of English within two to three generations,[3,4] even in the case of Spanish.[5] Indeed, Veltman[5] concludes the following with respect to the status of Spanish on the mainland:

> Given the age structure of the immigrant population, more than three-fourths of any given group of immigrants will come to speak English on a regular basis after approximately 15 years of residence on the U.S. mainland. Even more important, approximately 70 percent of the youngest immigrants and 40 percent of those aged 10–14 at time of arrival will make English their usual, personal language. As a result, they will give birth to children of English, not Spanish, mother tongue [p. 45].

Variability in this shift from minority language to mainstream language is assumed to be correlated with acculturation, the extent of the correlation depending upon the theory of the relationship between language and culture to which one subscribes. The phenomenon of language shift needs close scrutiny not only because it increases our understanding of language, communication, and acculturation of Puerto Rican families, but also because of the measurement issues involved. In analyses of the Hispanic Health and Nutrition Examination Survey (HHANES), for example, the language and acculturation variables have proven to be significant predictors of health preventive behavior,[6], alcohol use,[7] marijuana and cocaine use,[8] and even use of *curanderos*.[9] A closer look at the questions asked in the acculturation scale in light of our conceptualization of language shift may help sharpen our future inquiry.

This chapter presents data on language shift obtained in the course of research conducted in a Puerto Rican bilingual education program in New Haven, Connecticut. I will also make reference to data collected in Watsonville, California from students of Mexican background. The value of these data lie in the fact that they contain actual measures of English and Spanish proficiency, whereas most of the quantitative research on language shift, such as the pioneering works of Joshua Fishman and Calvin Veltman, use self-reported language data collected by the Census Bureau and the High School and Beyond survey gathered by the National Opinion Research Center. Naturally, the latter data sets are infinitely superior with respect to sampling and generating population estimates, but they are possibly subject to distortion in self-report.

METHODOLOGICAL ISSUES IN THE MEASUREMENT OF LANGUAGE SHIFT

Language shift has at least three components that should be measured separately: (1) an individual's actual proficiency in the two languages; (2) an individual's choice to use differential amounts of the languages (in different discourse settings) given threshold proficiency in the languages; and (3) an individual's personal identification with the cultures associated with the languages. These components are in principle separable (i.e., there may be an individual with high proficiency in both English and Spanish who chooses to use mostly English, but maintains an identity that is primarily Puerto Rican); in reality, they are probably related. For example, Veltman focuses on language choice over language proficiency, not just because the census bureau questions have tended to ask the question on usual language practice (e.g., "What language does [this person] usually speak?" in the Survey of Income and Education, 1976),[10] but also because he considers it a logical outcome that if a language is not usually spoken in the home, the children will not develop proficiency in it.

In addition to distinguishing between these components of language shift, it is important to ask whether the data are based on self-report or on direct observation. For example, the High School and Beyond survey asked: "How well do you speak *that* language?" with response choices varying from "very well," "pretty well," "not very well," and "not at all." How accurate would this self-report be when compared with direct observation of proficiency in the language? Obviously, self-reported data are the easiest to obtain, but they sacrifice objectivity; however, in some cases, direct observation may be extremely difficult or impractical, such as in the case of language identification.

The rough measurement model in the study of language shift, then, can be thought of as a 2 × 3 table as follows:

	Type of Data	
Aspect of Bilingualism	Self-Report	Observation
Language Proficiency	1	2
Language Choice	3	4
Language Identification	5	6

In an ideal situation, one would look at the correlations between 2, 4, and 6 based on actual observations; however, we are often dependent on self-report and other indirect means of inference.

PUERTO RICAN CHILDREN, NEW HAVEN, CONNECTICUT

The data on Puerto Rican children were collected from a bilingual education program in New Haven in the fall of 1980. The program uses a transitional rather than a maintenance model of bilingual education. Students are placed in the program on the basis of the home language reported by the parents, and exited to English-only classes on the basis of their English proficiency as determined by a standardized language test and teacher assessment (see Hakuta, Ferdman, Diaz,[11] for more information on bilingualism in the New Haven Puerto Rican community). The primary purpose of the study was to test the hypothesis that degree of bilingualism would be related positively to performance on various measures of cognitive flexibility.[12,13] Because the study was not originally designed to investigate language shift, the data have severe limitations. They are nevertheless informative because language proficiency and language choice measures were obtained.

The subjects included in this analysis were a total of 226 children in Kindergarten (n = 54, Mean Age = 5.23, SD = .43); Grade 1 (n = 60, Mean Age = 6.55, SD = .55); Grade 4 (n = 63, Mean Age = 10.02, SD = .78); and Grade 5 (n = 49, Mean Age = 10.76, SD = .65). In order to obtain background information on the subjects, a brief questionnaire was distributed to the parents, on which the following questions were asked:

- What language does your child use with you and the other adults in the household? (Only Spanish, Mostly Spanish, Both English and Spanish, Mostly English, Only English) [¿Qué idioma usa su hijo/a con usted y con otras personas adultas en la casa? (español solamente, mayormente español, igual español que inglés, mayormente inglés, inglés solamente)]
- What language does your child use with his or her brothers and sisters? [¿Qué idioma usa su hijo/a con sus hermanos y hermanas?]
- What language do the adults in your household use with each other? [¿Qué idioma usan las personas adultas en la casa?]

In addition, parents were asked to indicate the number of years that the family had lived on the mainland (we did not ask for the entire history of migration, although clearly such data would be highly relevant).

In order to assess the relative bilingual proficiency of the child, the Peabody Picture Vocabulary Test (PPVT) was administered in both languages by separate testers.[14,15] The PPVT measures receptive vocabulary; uncertainty about the validity of standardized norms in either language led us to use the raw scores as estimates of language proficiency.

With reference to the measurement model described above, we have parental report of language used (Cell 3; in this case as reported by the parents, and actual observations of language proficiency in English and Spanish (Cell 2). We also have some background information, including years of residence on the mainland.

Figure 1 displays Spanish and English proficiency as a function of years of residence on the mainland, reported separately by grade level (K,1,4,5). The smoothing function fitted on the data in this and all other figures used in this paper applies a locally weighted regression method,[16] available on SYGRAPH.[17] The first notable feature of these figures is the fact that there is a clear subtractive relationship between English and Spanish proficiency. Years of residence on the mainland is associated with higher English proficiency and lower Spanish proficiency. The second notable feature is that there is a sharp break at about 10 years of residence. The relationship between years of residence and proficiency is evident in those who have been on the mainland for about 10 years or less. If one considers only those whose families have been here for over 10 years (i.e., in the case of this sample, this would mean

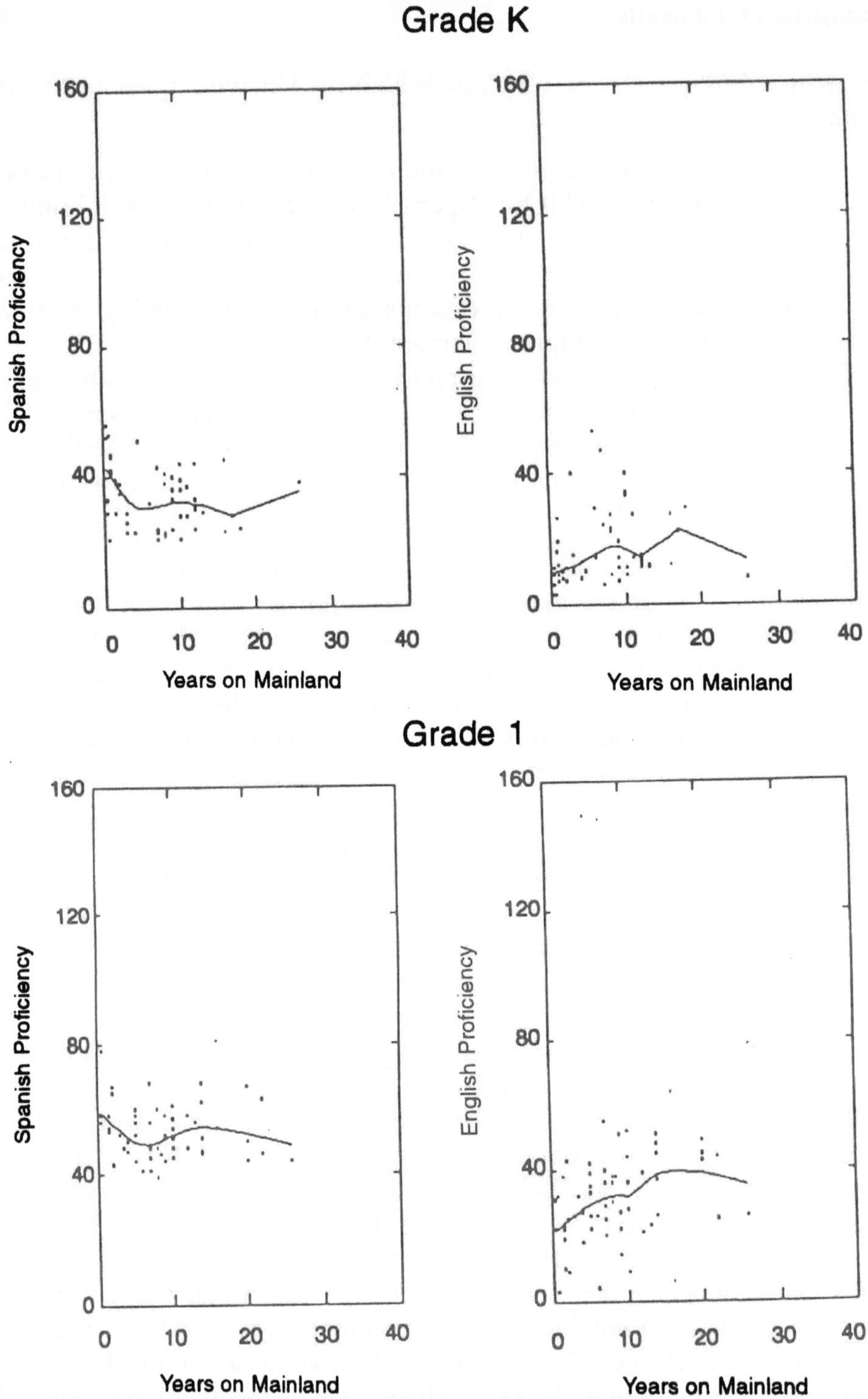

Figure 1. Spanish and English proficiency (as measured by raw scores on receptive vocabulary tests, Dunn, 1965 for English, Wiener, Simmonds & Weiss, 1978 for Spanish) as a function of years of residence on the mainland, separately by grade level. A locally

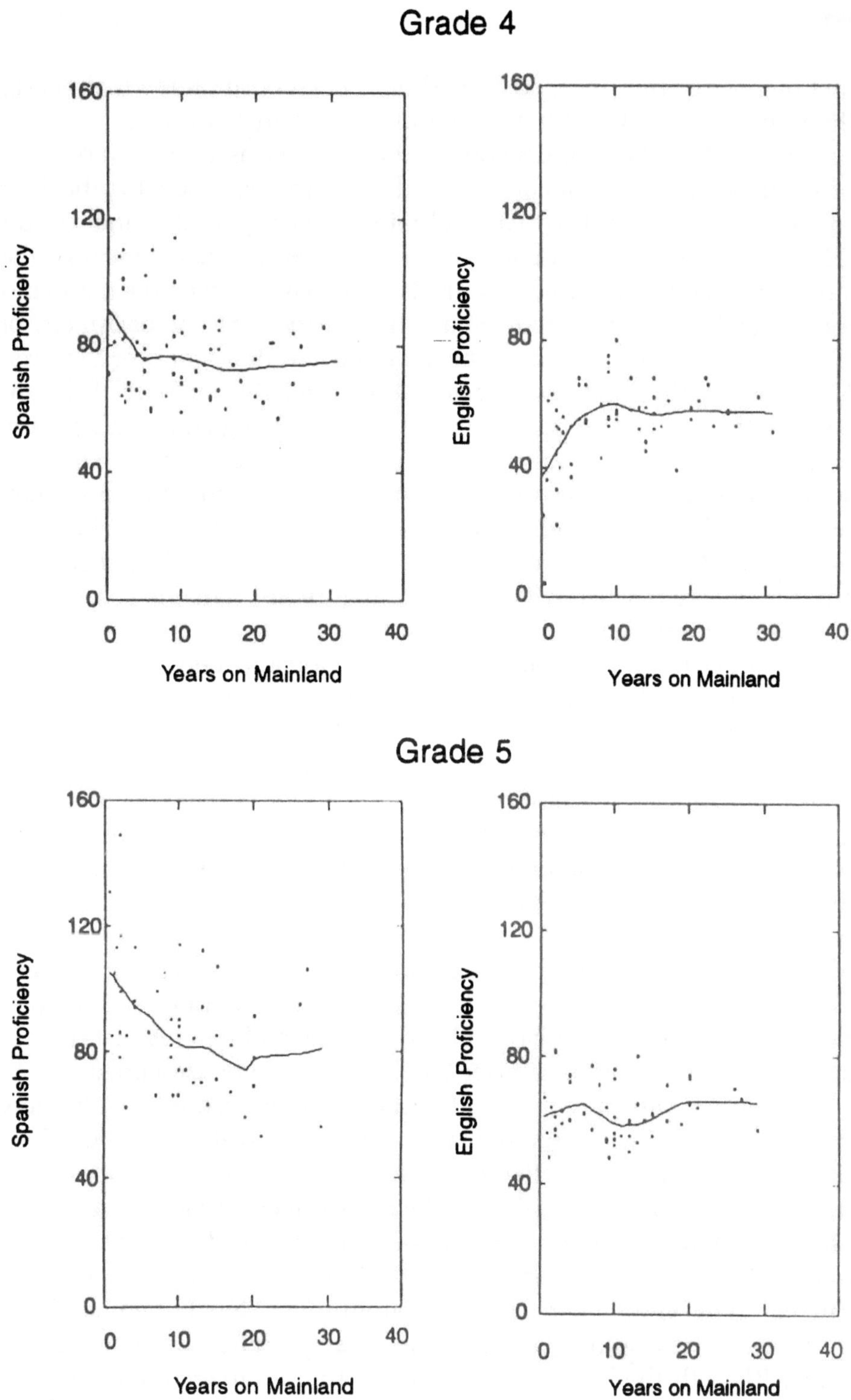

weighted regression was applied to summarize the data trend (Wilkinson, 1987). *Ss* were Puerto Rican children enrolled in a bilingual education program in New Haven, Connecticut.

that on average most of them would have been born on the mainland), the trends in both English and Spanish proficiency are flat.

Figure 2 displays the data on language choice as a function of years of residence on the mainland. The data were combined for the four cohort groups since they were obtained from parents, and cohort differences were not evident. Several features are notable. First, the language used by the adults (Figure 2a) who have been on the mainland for under 15 years is mostly Spanish, but there is encroachment of English among those who have been on the mainland for over 15 years. Nevertheless, there are few values that use "mostly" or "only" English. Second, the language reportedly used among siblings (Figure 2c) shifts much earlier (within 10 years of residence) to a value of approximately somewhere between "mostly Spanish" and "both equally," and then remains at about that level. Among the siblings, there are considerably more individuals who reportedly use "mostly" or "only" English. The adult language practice with children (Figure 2b) remains somewhere between these two.

In order to understand better the relationship between language proficiency and language choice (reported by parents), a measure combining the proficiency scores of English and Spanish was constructed, by subtracting Spanish from English. Recall that the choice scales run from 1 = only Spanish to 3 = both equally, to 5 = only English. Thus, to the extent that proficiency and choice are related, the correlation between the English minus Spanish scale and the choice measures should be a positive one. Figure 3a displays the data for the *S*s from Grades K–1, and Figure 3b for the *S*s from Grades 4–5. The magnitude of the linear correlations are $r = .32$ and $r = .23$ respectively. We must consider this to be both good news and bad news. The good news is that they are positively related, but the bad news is that there is a large amount of variance (over 90%) still left to be explained.

There are probably at least two factors that account for this low correlation. The first is that the language choice scale is very crude—one question that uses a five-point scale. More questions would undoubtedly increase the reliability. The second fact is that this sample of bilingual children is quite selective, i.e., they are students who are in a bilingual education program, and by definition, they are dominant in English. If the entire Puerto Rican community in New Haven had been included, there would have been considerably higher variances associated with both the language proficiency and language choice scores. These factors are controllable by sharpening the instruments and the sampling procedures.

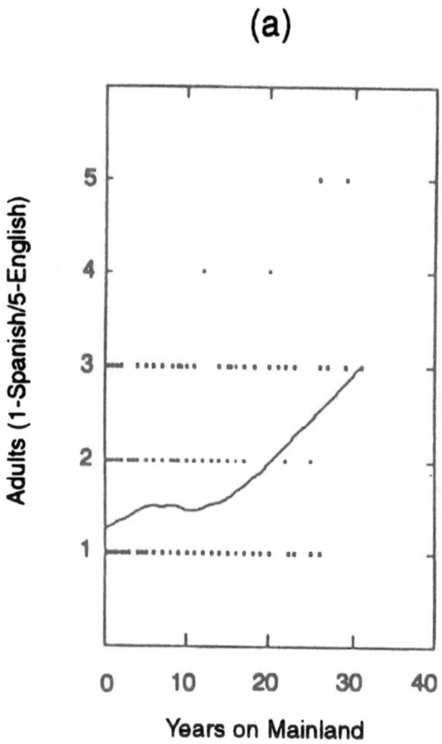

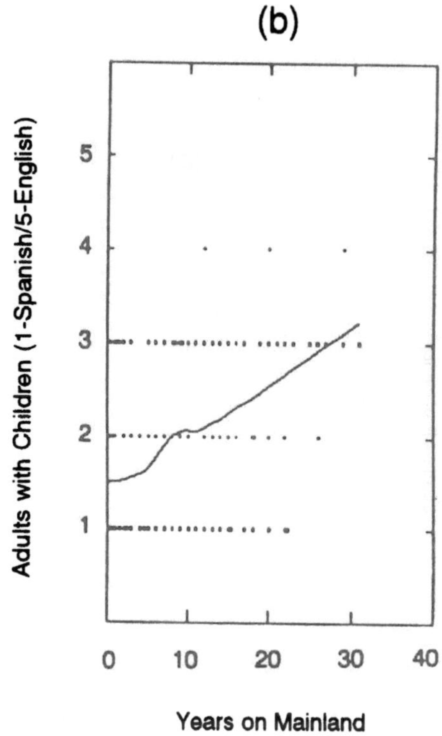

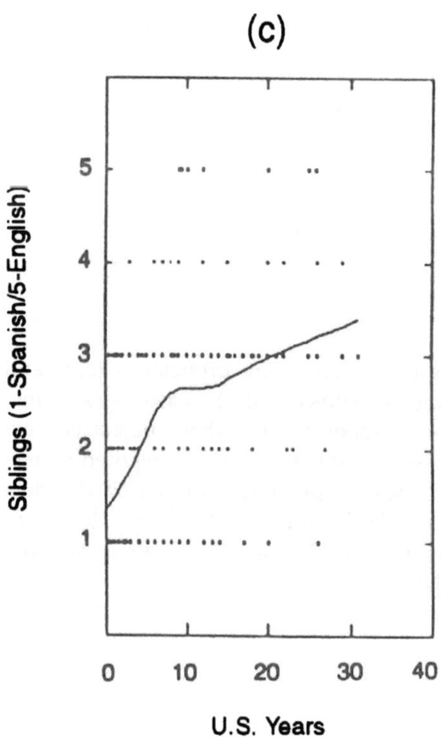

Figure 2. Language choice (as reported by parents, 1 = only Spanish, 2 = mostly Spanish, 3 = both English and Spanish, 4 = mostly English, 5 = only English) as a function of years of residence on mainland. A locally weighted regression was applied to summarize the data trend (Wilkinson, 1987). The three panels are for (a) language among adults, (b) language between children and adults, and (c) language among siblings. Respondents were parents of Puerto Rican children enrolled in a bilingual education program in New Haven, Connecticut.

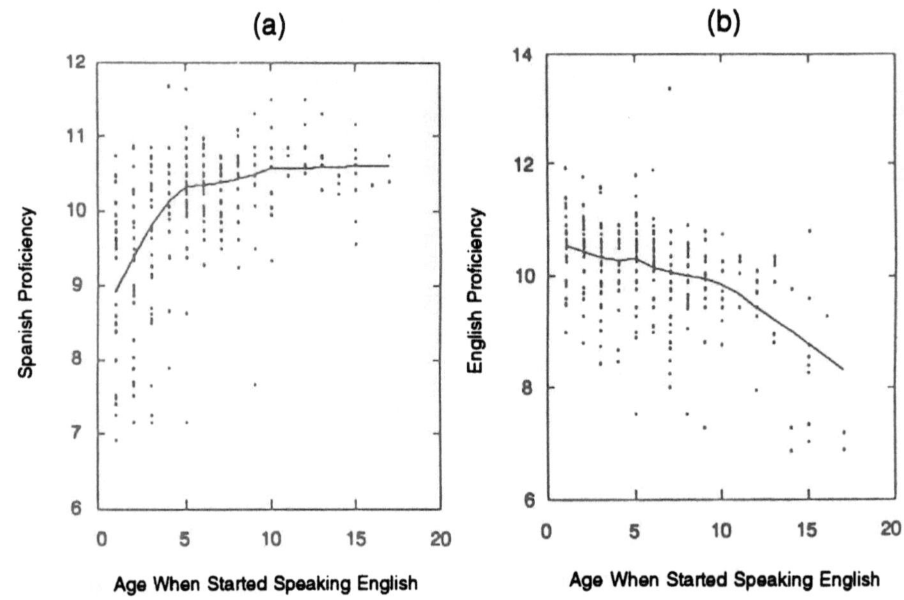

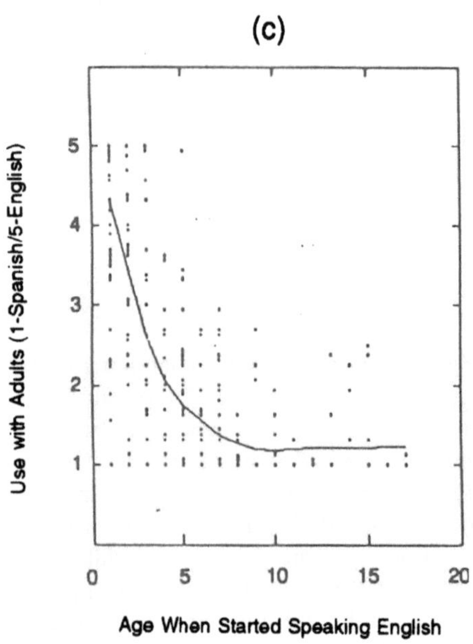

Figure 3. Language proficiency (a,b) and language choice (c,d,e) measures as a function of reported age when subject was exposed to English. A locally weighted regression was applied to summarize the data trend (Wilkinson, 1987). *Ss* were Mexican-American high school students in Watsonville, California.

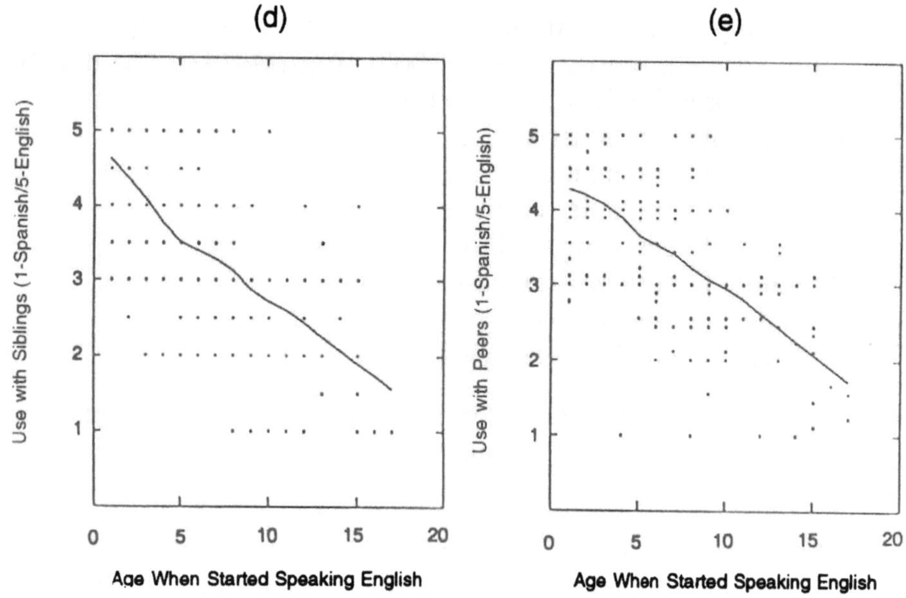

Figure 3. *(continued)*

MEXICAN-AMERICAN HIGH SCHOOL STUDENTS, WATSONVILLE, CALIFORNIA

In our Watsonville data,[18] we examined the language proficiency, choice, and identification of over 300 high school students of Mexican descent from different generational backgrounds. With reference to the measurement model above, we directly assessed English and Spanish proficiency by one of three measures (vocabulary, grammatical knowledge, and a measure of whole language knowledge called "cloze"), i.e., Cell 2. In addition to study the validity of self-reported ability in the languages, we asked them to rate their own ability in reading, writing, and speaking the two languages (Cell 1) through the following questions:

- How well do you speak and understand English/Spanish? (not at all, hardly at all, not so good, so-so, good, well, but not perfect, perfect)
- How well do you read in English/Spanish?
- How well do you write in English/Spanish?

To assess language choice, we asked for a self-report (Cell 3) of what language they used with various parties including adults at home, their siblings, and their peers at school, using the following questions:

- The adults in my home usually speak with each other in . . . (only Spanish, mostly Spanish, both languages equally, mostly English, only English, not applicable)
- I speak with my father in ____
- I speak with my mother in ____
- I speak with my older brothers and sisters in ____
- I speak with my younger brothers and sisters in ____
- At school I speak with my friends in ____
- Outside of school I speak with my friends in ____
- My friends usually speak with me in ____

Finally, we obtained their attitudes toward maintenance of bilingualism and Mexican culture by Likert scale responses to the following questions:

- Knowing how to speak Spanish is important to understand a person's family history. (strongly disagree/strongly agree)
- How important is it for you to know Spanish well? (not at all/very much)
- A person who knows Spanish, in addition to English, has more chances to express his or her feelings. (strongly disagree/strongly agree)
- How important is it for you to know both English and Spanish well? (not at all/very much)
- Using Spanish allows a person to feel good about him or herself. (strongly disagree/strongly agree)
- People who know Spanish should use it daily, especially at home. (strongly disagree/strongly agree)
- A person often needs to use Spanish for daily communication. (strongly disagree/strongly agree)
- It's okay if a person grows up speaking Spanish, and later forgets it. (strongly agree/strongly disagree)

These attitude questions are clearly an aspect of identification, and are probably best classified as self-report on this aspect of bilingualism (Cell 5).

The first major finding with respect to generational background was that Spanish proficiency appeared to be maintained through the second generation (the group who were born in the United States, but whose parents were born in Mexico, but drops sharply for the third generation. This dip in proficiency was associated with the reported home language choice of the adults, very much along the lines predicted by Veltman.[5] Language shift, as defined by a drop in Spanish proficiency, appears discontinuous. On the other hand, when we looked at language choice across the different generational backgrounds, the shift appeared incremental and synchronous to the acquisition of English proficiency in both languages and by language attitude; however, neither proficiency in Spanish nor English was predicted by language attitude. Thus, we concluded that language choice is a socially mediated variable having to do with ethnic identification, but it is constrained by the limits of proficiency in the two languages (i.e., if one does not have proficiency in either language, the choices are not even available).

Some of the interesting properties of the time course of shift in language proficiency and choice can be observed in Figure 3 (not reported in Hakuta, D'Andrea,[18] which plots these variables as a function of the age at which the individual started learning English. (We obtained an estimate of this age from the subjects.) A quick look at the figures shows that age of exposure to English is a powerful predictor for all of the variables, although with differently shaped functions.

Early exposure to English before the age of 5 shows a negative relationship with Spanish proficiency (Figure 3a). It is likely that those who were exposed before age 5 never fully acquired proficiency, especially in light of the reported language choice in favor of English of the adults at home (Figure 3b). The English slope (Figure 3b) requires a more careful interpretation, because those with exposure after age 10 are still in the process of second language acquisition.

Figure 4c shows the pattern for adult language choice, and suggests that the low Spanish proficiency in the early exposure group is most likely due to the adult language practice. Indeed, as can be seen in Figure 5, when English and Spanish proficiency are plotted as a function of the language choice of adults in the home (selecting only those subjects who were exposed to English before age 6), it is evident that adult language practice maps directly onto Spanish proficiency in their children. Equally interesting from the viewpoint of the debate about the role of home language practice in accelerating the children's English proficiency, is the fact that adult language practice evidently has no effect on English proficiency.

Returning to Figure 3, the data on language choice for siblings and peers (Figure 3d, e) suggest a linear trend toward English with earlier exposure. Notable (though predictable) is the discrepancy in language

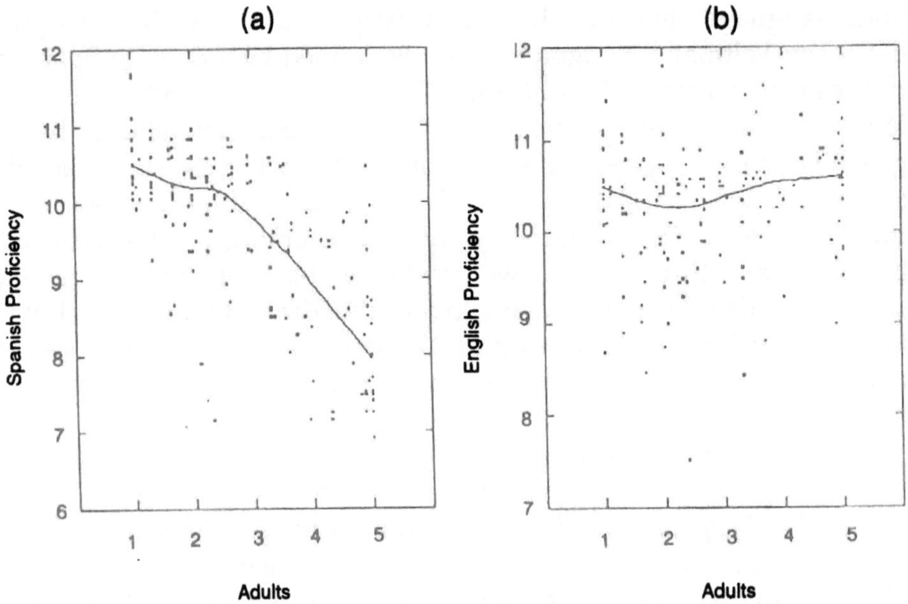

Figure 4. Spanish and English proficiency as a function of reported language choice with adults at home (1 = only Spanish, 5 = only English, selecting only *S*s who were exposed to English before age 6). A locally weighted regression was applied to summarize the data trend (Wilkinson, 1987).

choice with that for the adults (Figure 3c), with a stronger gravitation toward English when choosing language with siblings and peers. This finding underscores the importance of specifying the interlocutors in asking questions about language choice.

To parallel the analysis of the relationship between reported language choice and observed language proficiency that was reported for the Puerto Rican sample, Spanish proficiency scores were subtracted from English proficiency scores, and used to predict self-reported language choice with siblings. The results can be found in Figure 5, which also incorporates some data collected from seventh and eighth grade students (n = 95) from two feeder schools in the course of a pilot work (the language proficiency measure was a test of productive vocabulary, and questions were also asked about language use with siblings and friends). The linear correlations are $r = .39$ for the Grades 7 to 8 sample, and $r = .62$ for the Grades 9 to 12 sample. In the discussion of the results from the Puerto Rican sample, I speculated that the low correlation might be due to the coarseness of measurement as well as

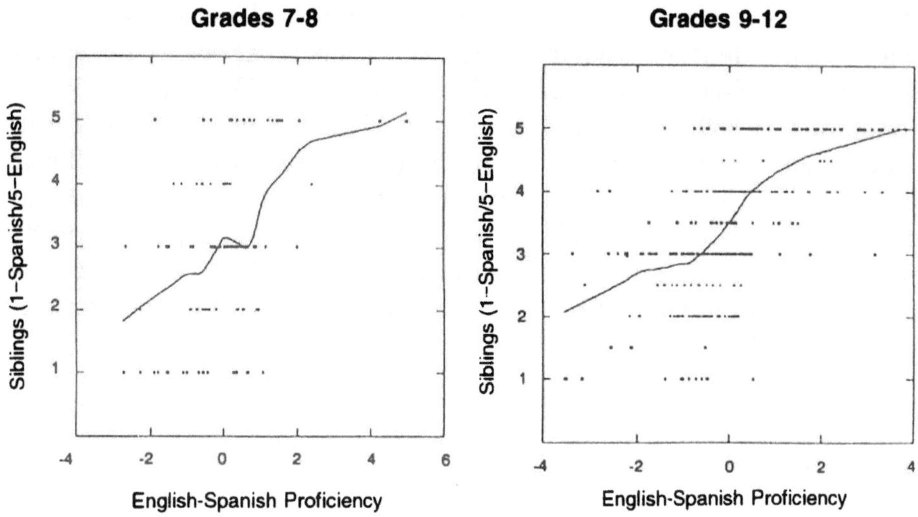

Figure 5. Correlation between reported language choice among siblings and proficiency difference between English and Spanish (English raw vocabulary score minus Spanish raw vocabulary score). A locally weighted regression was applied to summarize the data trend (Wilkinson, 1987). Data for Grades 7–8 were obtained from feeder schools to the high school in Watsonville, California. Linear correlation coefficient for Grades 7–8 was $r = .39$, and for Grades 9–12, $r = .62$.

restriction of range. The Watsonville sample is reasonably representative of the Latino population in the community (see Hakuta, D'Andrea[18] for discussion), and in the case of the high school study, two questions were asked about language choice with siblings. Thus, both factors may have been at work, in explaining the differences in the magnitude of the language choice with siblings. Thus, both factors may have been at work in explaining the differences in the magnitude of the correlative, although there are other significant differences between the samples.

Finally, the study revealed an important methodological finding about the relationship between self-reported and observed language proficiency (the relationship between Cells 1 and 2 in the measurement model above). Regression analyses were conducted using the following model with simultaneous entry of the predictors:

Self-reported Spanish (or English) proficiency = Constant + Spanish (or English) Proficiency + Maintenance Attitude + Subtractive Attitude + Pragmatic Attitude

(the latter two attitudinal orientations were also extracted from the attitude questionnaire using factor analytic techniques).

The results indicated a significant contribution of the attitudinal variables independent of actual measured proficiency, especially for Spanish. Thus, for Spanish self-reported proficiency, the *b*'s were as follows: Constant (−1.889), Spanish Proficiency (.53), Maintenance Attitude (.407), Subtractive Attitude (−.135), Pragmatic Attitude (.007). All but the last predictor were significant, and it is indeed notable that the attitudinal variables were about as predictive of self-reported proficiency as actual measured proficiency itself. Thus, we concluded that Cell 1 is contaminated by Cell 5, and as such, it is an imperfect approximation of Cell 2.

DISCUSSION

The New Haven Puerto Rican and the Watsonville Mexican-American data both support the claims of demographers that there is considerable on-going language shift from Spanish to English in the United States. This shift is evident both in language choice and language proficiency measures. The time course of shift in these two measures, however, appears to be different. In the Watsonville high school data, for example, the shifts in both language use with siblings and with peers were quite linear and gradual (Figure 4d, 4e), whereas the shift in Spanish proficiency was characterized by a relatively sharp break at age of exposure to English of 5 years (Figure 4a). Likewise, the Puerto Rican sample showed discontinuities in English and Spanish proficiencies at about 10 years on the mainland (Figure 1), whereas the shift in choice was more gradual (Figure 2). It remains for future researchers to sort out the finer differences between these two aspects of language. I would speculate that a main source of difference might lie in the fact that language proficiency is more cognitive in nature, and thus it is bounded by maturational factors associated with first and second language acquisition. On the other language, language choice is primarily social in nature, and may exhibit more of a dosage relationship with experience.

Finally, we are in a position to examine the language and acculturation questions used by the HHANES survey. According to Delgado, Johnson, Roy, and Treviño,[19] the following questions comprise the acculturation scale:

1. What language do you speak?
2. What language do you prefer?

3. Can you read Spanish? Can you read English? Which do you read better?
4. Can you write Spanish? Can you write English? Which do you write better?
5. What ethnic identification do you use?
6. What ethnic identification does/did your mother use?
7. What ethnic identification does/did your father use?
8. Where was the birthplace of yourself, your mother, your father?

Perhaps the most informative and instructive findings to emerge from analyses of the HHANES dataset to this point is the work by Solis, Marks, Garcia, and Shelton.[6] These investigators factor analyzed these questions, and found three groups: language preferred and spoken (Items 1 and 2); language written and read (Items 3 and 4), and ethnic identification (Items 5–8). They compared the relative contributions of these factors in predicting preventive health behavior in the Mexican-American sample, and found spoken language to be better than reading and writing ability, and they also found that acculturation was not a significant factor.

In the terminology that we have been using in this paper, the first two questions on spoken and preferred language are the closest to questions about language choice, whereas questions 3 and 4 are most closely associated with proficiency. The last four questions on identification would most likely be related to language attitude, but probably only indirectly so. Indeed, based on the Watsonville study, we might argue that the questions on language choice are related to both language attitude *and* language proficiency, and that the question about language proficiency, because it is based on self-report, probably also picks up on language attitude. It is then not altogether surprising that language choice emerges as the most powerful of Solis et al.'s three groups.

The power of the language variable is attested to further by the findings of Marks et al.[6] who were able to use the full scale for the Mexican-American sample in predicting alcohol use, but were only able to use the language items for the Cuban-Americans and the Puerto Ricans due to highly restricted variance on the identification items. Nevertheless, the magnitude of prediction was similar across the three groups, suggesting that the identification items (5–8) added little predictive power for the Mexican-American sample.

In conclusion, there is considerable evidence for language shift among various Hispanic communities in the United States, and this shift is influenced by a combination of processes related to proficiency, choice, and attitudes. These components of language shift may have different developmental time courses, and therefore should be measured separately. Further, self-report of the proficiency variable is likely to contain a substantial attitudinal component, and therefore should be measured through observation to obtain valid proficiency estimates. It is to be hoped that a better understanding of the community and psychological processes involved in language shift will contribute to a better understanding of the acculturation process of how to measure in studies of health and development in language minority populations.

ACKNOWLEDGMENT. Preparation of this paper was supported in part by a grant from the Spencer Foundation.

REFERENCES

1. Morales Carrion A: *Puerto Rico: A Political and Cultural History*. New York, W. W. Norton, 1983
2. Negron de Montilla A: *The Americanization of Puerto Rico and the Public-School System: 1900/1930*. 2nd ed. San Juan, University of Puerto Rico Press, 1975
3. Fishman J: *Language Loyalty in the United States*. The Hague, Mouton, 1966
4. Veltman C: *Language Shift in the United States*. Berlin, New York, and Amsterdam, Mouton, 1983
5. Veltman C: *The Future of the Spanish Language in the United States*. Hispanic Policy Development Project, New York City and Washington, D.C., 1988
6. Solis J, Marks G, Garcia M, Shelton D: Acculturation, access to care, and use of preventive services by Hispanics: Findings from HHANES 1982–84. *Amer. J. Pub. Health* 80:11–19, 1990
7. Marks G, Garcia M, Solis J: Health risk behaviors of Hispanics in the United States: Findings from HHANES, 1982–1984. *Amer. J. Pub. Health* 80(Suppl):20–26, 1990
8. Amaro H, Whitaker R, Coffman G, Heeren T: Acculturation and marijuana and cocaine use: Findings from HHANES 1982–84. *Amer. J. Pub. Health* 80(Suppl):54–60, 1990
9. Higginbotham J, Treviño F, Ray L: Utilization of curanderos by Mexican Americans: Prevalence and predictors: Findings from HHANES 1982–84. *Amer. J. Pub. Health* 80(Suppl):32–35, 1990
10. US Bureau of the Census: Survey of Income and Education. Washington, Bureau of the Census, US Dept of Commerce, 1976
11. Hakuta K, Ferdman BM, Diaz RM: Bilingualism and cognitive development: Three perspectives. In: Rosenberg S (ed). *Advances in Applied Psycholinguistics*. Vol. 2. *Reading, Writing and Language Learning*. Cambridge, U.K., Cambridge University Press, 1987, pp 284–319
12. Hakuta K, Diaz R: The relationship between degree of bilingualism and cognitive ability: A critical discussion and some new longitudinal data. In: Nelson KE (ed). *Children's Language*. Vol. 5. Hillsdale, N.J., Lawrence Erlbaum Associates, 1985, pp 319–344

13. Hakuta K: Degree of bilingualism and cognitive ability in mainland Puerto Rican children. *Child Develop.* 58:1372–1388, 1987
14. Dunn L: *Peabody Picture Vocabulary Test*. Circle Pines, MN, American Guidance Service, 1965
15. Wiener FD, Simmond AJ, Weiss FL: *Spanish Picture Vocabulary Test*. New York, Marymount Manhattan College
16. Cleveland WS: LOWESS: A program for smoothing scatterplots by robust locally weighted regression. *Amer. Statist.* 35:54, 1981
17. Wilkinson L: *SYGRAPH*. Evanston, Ill., SYSTAT, 1987
18. Hakuta K, D'Andrea D: Some properties of bilingual maintenance and loss in Mexican background high school students. *Appl. Linguist.* 13:72–99, 1992
19. Delgado J, Johnson C, Roy I, Treviño F: Hispanic Health and Nutrition Examination Survey: Methodological considerations. *Amer. J. Pub. Health* 80(Suppl):6–10, 1990

12

Health Status and Health Care Access for Mainland Puerto Rican Children: Results from the Hispanic Health and Nutrition Examination Survey

FERNANDO S. MENDOZA, GLENN S. TAKATA,
AND REYNALDO MARTORELL

INTRODUCTION

Although the Hispanic population has grown more rapidly than any other on the U.S. mainland over the past decade, the health status of

FERNANDO S. MENDOZA • Department of Pediatrics, Lucile Salter Packard Children's Hospital at Stanford University, Stanford, California 94305. GLENN S. TAKATA • Division of General Pediatrics, Children's Hospital of Los Angeles, Los Angeles, California 90027. REYNALDO MARTORELL • Center for International Health, Emory University School of Public Health, Altanta, Georgia 30329.

Puerto Rican Women and Children: Issues in Health, Growth, and Development, edited by Gontran Lamberty and Cynthia Garcia Coll. Plenum Press, New York, 1994.

Hispanic children has been poorly documented. This dearth of information can be partially attributed to the failure of health surveys, prior to 1975, to differentiate Hispanic from non-Hispanic children, and the inability of these surveys to sample Hispanic children adequately. The problems in obtaining basic information on the health status of Hispanic children has resulted in a limited understanding of the major health issues facing them, and uncertainty as to whether the current system is able to meet their health care needs.

Hispanic children tend to live in impoverished households two to three times more frequently than non-Hispanic children.[1] Their families are usually larger and more likely to be headed by a single parent than non-Hispanic Caucasian families. In families in which these latter two factors exist together, it is economically and socially more tenuous for children. These social and economic conditions are not equally distributed across the three major Hispanic subgroups: Mexican-Americans, mainland Puerto Ricans, and Cuban-Americans. One cannot assume that if two subgroups have similar poverty rates that their health status will be similar. For example, although Mexican-Americans have a rate of poverty similar to that of mainland Puerto Ricans, their rate of babies with low birth weight is half as prevalent.[2] Furthermore, Mexican-Americans have a poverty rate twice that of Cuban-Americans, yet they have similar rates of babies with low birth weight.[2] Therefore, other factors may contribute to the variability among Hispanic subgroups, including demographic variables such as the proportion of families headed by single parents, the degree of urbanization, the percentage of parents that are U.S. citizens, and thereby eligible for government assistance, and other socioeconomic and historical–cultural factors.

For example, all Puerto Ricans, whether born in Puerto Rico or on the mainland, are U.S. citizens as a result of Puerto Rico's commonwealth status to the United States. In contrast, all other Hispanics, unless they were born in the United States, have to apply for citizenship. Therefore, although Puerto Rican children are U.S. citizens, some children from other Hispanic subgroups are not. This produces differential access to health care among Hispanic children.

To insure that appropriate health policies are formulated for Hispanic children, basic health status measures must be assessed for each subgroup. Studies using only the generic grouping "Hispanic" without reference to subgroup differences, will not provide the accurate data needed for appropriate and effective health and social policies directed at Hispanic children. This review describes the health status and health care access of one of these subgroups: mainland Puerto Rican children.

BACKGROUND

Using data from the Hispanic Health and Nutrition Examination Survey (HHANES), 1982–1984, and another large-scale governmental health survey, National Health Interview Surveys (NHIS)[3], this review describes the medical needs and characteristics of mainland Puerto Rican children. (Prior to the HHANES the NHIS was the only other large-scale source of health information on mainland Puerto Rican children.)[4] The National Center for Health Statistics conducted both the HHANES and NHIS. However, the NHIS contains only household interview data while the HHANES also contains physical examination and biochemical data. Moreover, the HHANES was specifically designed to assess the health status of mainland Puerto Ricans, and did so by sampling mainland Puerto Ricans in the New York City area. This sampling technique obtained health information on 53% of all mainland Puerto Ricans living in the United States in 1980, thereby making the HHANES the most comprehensive health survey of mainland Puerto Ricans to date. The HHANES sample contained 1,289 mainland Puerto Rican, 3,622 Mexican-American, and 387 Cuban-American children ages 6 months to 18 years. The mainland Puerto Rican sample represents 487,168 children living in the New York City area. In contrast, the NHIS is a national probability study that does not oversample for mainland Puerto Ricans, and therefore provides useful but somewhat limited information on these children, due to small sample size.

Information from NHIS on health indicators for Hispanics, non-Hispanic Caucasians, and African-Americans has been previously published by Trevino and Moss from the National Center for Health Statistics.[5] Information from this report included the number of physician visits and hospitalizations per year, the prevalence of acute and chronic medical conditions, and the days of restrictive activity for non-Hispanic Caucasian, non-Hispanic African-American, Mexican-American, mainland Puerto Rican, and Cuban-American children surveyed during the period 1978 to 1980. In all of these categories, mainland Puerto Rican children had the highest prevalence rates for these health indicators. They reported the greatest number of acute conditions (489 per 100 children), the highest percentage of children with limitations due to chronic medical conditions (6.2%), and the most days of restricted activity per child per year (18.0 days per child per year). In conjunction with their high health needs, mainland Puerto Rican children also reported the highest health care utilization rates of any group studied. They averaged six physician visits per year, and 7% reported a short-stay hospitalization. Only Cuban-American children reported higher physician visits per year (6.2 visits per year), but these children had a lower rate of hospitalization (5.7%).

In general, these data show that mainland Puerto Rican children reported 50 to 100% greater prevalence of acute conditions, limitations due to chronic medical conditions, and restrictive activity compared to non-Hispanic Caucasian and African-American children as well as Mexican-American and Cuban-American children. While African-American and Mexican-American children have similar levels of poverty as mainland Puerto Rican children, they describe lower levels of health care problems. The NHIS data, however, are not supported with physical examination data as in the HHANES. Therefore, these differences in reported health concerns may not reflect the true health status difference between these groups.

METHODS

The data used to measure the health status of mainland Puerto Rican children in HHANES were obtained from questionnaire information, biochemical assessments, and physical examination data. These data sources were used to assess a variety of health status parameters for mainland Puerto Rican children, including (1) prevalence and types of chronic medical conditions; (2) maternal reported medical conditions and their state of treatment; (3) subjective rating of the children's heath status by surveying physicians, children, and their mothers; (4) prevalence of iron deficiency anemia; (5) prevalence of high lead levels; and (6) access to health care services. Since HHANES did not have a non-Hispanic Caucasian sample to act as a control group, the Mexican-American group was used as a comparison Hispanic group when possible, or alternatively, reported literature values were used for national comparisons.

Chronic Medical Conditions among Mainland Puerto Rican Children

Children in the HHANES were labeled as having chronic medical conditions if these conditions had caused functional impairment for the prior three months. These assessments were made by survey physicians after reviewing findings from the patient's standardized health questionnaires and physical examinations. The HHANES data showed that mainland Puerto Rican children's prevalence of chronic medical condition was 6.24%.[2] This prevalence was significantly higher than that for Mexican-American or Cuban-American children, 3.93 and 2.49% respectively. The reported prevalence of chronic medical conditions for U.S. children in general is approximately 4%.[6] The definition of a chronic medical condition is variable, however, and the prevalence may range from 3 to 6%. Therefore, mainland Puerto Rican children seem to have a prevalence of chronic medical conditions that may be slightly higher than the national average.

Although there were no significant differences in the severity of chronic medical conditions among the three groups or in the survey physicians' confidence in diagnosing these conditions, there was a significant difference in the primary method of determining the presence of a chronic medical condition for each group.[2] In particular, mainland Puerto Ricans were most likely to have chronic medical conditions determined by history alone. This could indicate that the parent may be more aware of the child's condition because of greater contact with the health care system, or that the condition, although causing chronic impairment, is not always physically present, but instead is episodic (i.e., asthma). It is also interesting to note that the prevalence of chronic medical conditions was not affected by the children's sex, age, poverty status, or language usage (a proxy measure of acculturation).[2]

Chronic medical conditions identified among mainland Puerto Rican children in HHANES were classified according to the international categories of diseases, ninth revision.[7] The distribution of categories of chronic medical conditions among mainland Puerto Rican children was skewed and different from the Mexican-American sample.[2] Sixty-two percent (50/81) of mainland Puerto Rican children with chronic medical conditions had respiratory diseases, and 98% of these children (49/50) were asthmatics, resulting in a prevalence rate of chronic asthma of 3.4%. This rate is high when compared to a prevalence of 0.3% for chronic asthma among Mexican-American children. In a recent report by Gergen et al., however, the national prevalence of asthma reported to be diagnosed by physicians and currently active was 3.6%.[8] The severity of the asthma was not taken into account in Gergen's study, therefore the comparisons of prevalence from one study to another is problematic. Certainly, a clear difference exists between mainland Puerto Rican and Mexican-American children in the prevalence of asthma. To what degree differences in geographic distributions of the samples (i.e., the New York City area vs. the Southwest) affect the prevalence for each subgroup needs further investigation. Without the higher prevalence of asthma, mainland Puerto Ricans would have a prevalence of chronic medical conditions similar to or lower than the Mexican-American sample. Other chronic conditions occurred too infrequently to provide useful information for comparative purposes.

Reported Medical Conditions and Their Treatment Status

The HHANES also contains information reported by mothers about whether their children's medical conditions were mild, moderate, severe, or chronic. Tables 1 to 4 show the prevalence of these conditions reported for mainland Puerto Rican children from 6 months to 4 years, and 5 to 11 years of age.* The prevalence of each condition is shown by whether the child has ever had the condition, whether he or she has it now, and if the child is currently being treated for the condition or has been in the past.

Asthma is the most frequently reported currently active condition, comprising approximately 11% for both age groups (it is interesting to note that about one in five have had at least one attack of asthma). This estimate includes both mild, moderate, and severe asthma. The rates are higher than the 2 to 3% prevalence reported by Mexican-American mothers for their children. Gergen et al. reported that approximately 9.5% of children in the new national sample have had at least one attack of wheezing or asthma.[8] The prevalence of a wheezing episode was higher for African-American (13.1%) than Caucasian (8.9%) children. Therefore, we can conclude from both the prevalence of chronic medical conditions and maternal reported conditions that asthma is a significant medical problem for mainland Puerto Rican children.

Anemia was the next most common condition reported by mothers. Approximately 7% of the 6-month- to 4-year-olds, and almost 3% of the 5- to 11-year-olds had this condition at the time of the survey. In comparison, Mexican-American children were reported to have 1 and 2% prevalence of anemia for the younger and older age groups, respec-

*The prevalence less than 5% are not reliable population estimates because of small samples. However, they do provide an indication of the percent of sampled children with the specific condition.

Table 1 Reported Medical Conditions of Mainland Puerto Rican Children Ages 6 Months to 4 Years from HHANES[a]

	Percent with condition		Percent of children	
Type	Ever	Now	Treatment	Treated
Anemia	19.7	7.3	89	100
Asthma	17.8	11.4	97	100
Other lung conditions	2.4	0.3	100	100
Rheumatic fever	0.3	0.3	100	—
Heart conditions	3.4	1.5	72	100
Urinary tract infections	1.3	0.5	100	100
Convulsions	3.3	1.1	100	100
Poisons	0.9	0	0	100

[a]Percentages less than 5% are not reliable.

tively. Nationally, the prevalence of iron deficiency anemia, the major cause of anemia in children, is 3%.[9] The higher prevalence of anemia among mainland Puerto Rican children could reflect their poor nutritional intake of iron-rich foods. However, other causes of anemia should be considered for these children, such as lead, which can mimic iron deficiency anemia, and is a major health problem in older urban areas like New York City.[10]

Among the other medical conditions reported for mainland Puerto Rican children, only heart conditions and convulsions were above 1% prevalence. Those children with heart conditions most likely had benign heart murmur, since only seven children were found to have a chronic medical condition which was cardiovascular (0.5%). Further

Table 2 Reported Medical Conditions of Mainland Puerto Rican Children Ages 6 Months to 4 Years from HHANES[a]

	Percent with condition		Percent of children	
Type	Ever	Now	Treatment	Treated
Coordination problems	0.8	0.6	53	100
Weakness/paralysis	0.3	0.3	100	—
Psychologic/behavioral problems	1.0	1.0	24	—
Speech problems	1.3	1.3	80	—
Mental retardation	0.2	0.2	100	—

[a]Percentages less than 5% are not reliable.

Table 3 Reported Medical Conditions of Mainland Puerto Rican Children Ages 5 to 11 Years from HHANES[a]

	Percent with condition		Percent of children	
Type	Ever	Now	Treatment	Treated
Anemia	16.0	2.7	92	96
Asthma	22.0	11.5	100	98
Other lung conditions	3.0	1.0	100	98
Rheumatic fever	0.7	0.2	100	100
Heart conditions	7.3	5.0	51	100
Urinary tract infections	3.2	0.6	100	100
Convulsions	5.3	1.3	85	96
Poisons	1.9	0	100	0

[a]Percentages less than 5% are not reliable.

more, mainland Puerto Rican children did not have high prevalence rates of elevated blood pressure, either by report or measurement.[11] On an average, about 5% of all children will experience at least one convulsion. Since febrile convulsions should not occur beyond 5 years of age, those children 5 to 11 years old with convulsions most likely include children with true epilepsy. A 1% occurrence of epilepsy would, therefore, be similar to the national average.[12]

Although maternal reported prevalence of neurodevelopmental conditions (coordination problems, weakness/paralysis, psychological and behavioral problems, speech problems, and mental retardation) were lower than those reported for medical conditions (asthma, anemia, heart conditions, etc.), the neurodevelopmental conditions were

Table 4 Reported Medical Conditions of Mainland Puerto Rican Children Ages 5 to 11 Years from HHANES[a]

	Percent with condition		Percent of children	
Type	Ever	Now	Treatment	Treated
Coordination problems	2.3	1.5	74	100
Weakness/paralysis	1.7	1.3	82	100
Psychological/behavioral problems	5.9	5.7	74	100
Speech problems	8.6	6.7	70	81
Mental retardation	3.1	3.1	88	—

[a]Percentages less than 5% are not reliable.

more likely to be ongoing in comparison to the medical conditions. This is particularly evident in school-age children: 6.7% were reported to have speech problems and 5.7% psychological and behavioral problems. Depending upon whether these two conditions occur in the same child or not, these rates suggest that 30,000 to 60,000 mainland Puerto Rican children in the New York City area are in need of either speech therapy or psychological and behavioral services. In comparison, Mexican-American mothers reported their school-age children to have speech and psychological/behavioral problems at a rate of 3.5 and 1.3% respectively. Similarly, mental retardation was reported to have higher prevalence rate of 3.1% among mainland Puerto Rican children 5 to 11 years old, compared to a rate of 0.5% for Mexican-American children. The general prevalence of mental retardation is estimated to be 3%.[12]

Although these data suggest significant differences in neurodevelopmental conditions between mainland Puerto Rican and Mexican-American children, these prevalence rates should be viewed cautiously since the mainland Puerto Rican sample is small, and comparable national data do not always exist to know whether Mexican-Americans are lower than the national average in these areas or mainland Puerto Ricans are higher. Moreover, more frequent recognition of neurodevelopmental problems in Puerto Rican children may be a result of better case findings which, in a more geographically confined area be easier and more consistent. In contrast, Mexican-American children were sampled from five different states, thereby creating much greater variability in case-finding.

In addition to reporting whether children had a specific medical condition, mothers also specified whether the condition had been treated or was being treated at the time. This information is also shown in Tables 1–4. Medical conditions tended to be treated more often than those conditions which were neurodevelopmental. Only heart conditions were reported to have a lower level of treatment. This may be secondary to the limited and benign nature of many of the conditions in this category. This suggests that conditions which traditionally have been treated with medical interventions are more likely to receive those therapies than are neurodevelopmental problems which may require nonmedical, long-term therapies. Therefore, although neurodevelopmental conditions may be less prevalent, children with these conditions may be at a greater risk for not receiving appropriate care. For children in poverty who already face obstacles in achieving their full developmental potential, this may prove an additional burden.

SUBJECTIVE HEALTH STATUS RATINGS OF MAINLAND PUERTO RICAN CHILDREN

Another assessment of children's health status used in HHANES was a subjective measure completed by surveying the physicians, mothers, and the children themselves. This assessment provided a global measure of health status, rating the child's health as excellent, very good, good, fair, or poor. This type of health status assessment is usually affected by the rater's view of the child's physical, mental, and developmental health. The rater's perspective of the definition of "health" can also have a major influence on the assessment.

The prevalence of mainland Puerto Rican children rated to be in poor health (fair and poor percentages) by the survey physicians in HHANES was less than 1%.[13] The prevalence of poor health ratings for children with chronic medical conditions was 6.4%.[13] This implies that most children who had a chronic medical condition were not rated to be in poor health by survey physicians. This finding, along with the seemingly low percentage of mainland Puerto Rican children in HHANES who were determined by survey physicians to need medical referral within one month (less than 6%),[13] suggests that physicians' appraisal of these children's health is generally good. These ratings by survey physicians were similar for Mexican-American children in HHANES; however, a greater proportion of Mexican-American children with chronic medical conditions were found to be in poor health (11.6%).

When mothers were asked to rate their children's health, their ratings of poor health were significantly higher than those of survey physicians. Approximately 20% of mainland Puerto Rican mothers rated their children in poor health.[13] Similarly, 15.2% and 17.0% of mainland Puerto Rican children and adolescents, respectively, rated themselves in poor health. Compared to mothers of Mexican-American and Cuban-American children, mothers of mainland Puerto Rican children were more likely to rate their children in poor health.[13] This rate is also higher than that of the U.S. parents in general who rate 6% of their children in poor health.[14]

The influence of maternal demographic variables on mothers' ratings of their children's health status for children less than 12 years showed that older children (23.3 vs. 15.7%) and those living in poverty (22.5 vs. 14.7%) were significantly more likely to be rated in poor health.[13] Those children who lived in a household in which Spanish was spoken, either as the sole language or in combination with English, were also more likely to be rated in poor health by their mothers (Spanish: 27.1%; bilingual: 20.3%; English: 15.2%).[13] This latter finding suggests that the process of acculturation may affect the maternal perception of the child's health, or at least the concept of health. This finding may be confounded by maternal education and socioeconomic status, since these variables are linked with the home language spoken. Lastly, the presence of a chronic medical condition in the child significantly increased the likelihood of a poor health rating by the mother (40.6% vs. 18.3%).

The findings among mainland Puerto Rican mothers and children concerning the subjective assessment of health status suggest that they differ significantly when compared to physicians' evaluations. Although a variety of factors may affect this measure, including environmental and psychosocial factors, as well as medical conditions, it is clear that a high proportion of mainland Puerto Rican mothers consider their children to be in poor health. What actions are taken as a result of this perception and what factors can significantly influence it besides the ones noted above need further investigation.

BIOCHEMICAL HEALTH STATUS: IRON STATUS AND LEAD LEVELS

In addition to data from health questionnaires and physician examinations, HHANES also obtained biochemical measures, including iron and lead levels, which helped provide an additional estimate of mainland Puerto Rican children's health status. Iron levels reflect a child's nutritional status. Poor intake of iron is the most common reason for a low level of this nutrient, and its resultant, anemia. As noted above, mothers reported that 7.3% of children 6 months to 4 years, and 2.7% of children 5 to 11 years were anemic, which is presumed to be the result of iron deficiency anemia. In contrast, the iron levels for mainland Puerto Rican children suggest that less than 2% of the children in these age groups have actual iron deficiency anemia as documented by biochemical measures.[15] In comparison to the national average of 2%, mainland Puerto Rican children have adequate iron levels suggesting that their intake of this nutrient is similar to that of other U.S. children.[16] This provides additional evidence that in general American children suffer less often from iron deficiency anemia than in the previous decade, when 10% of children had this nutritional problem.

The presence of lead, in contrast, leads to significant central nervous system disorders, including behavioral and developmental problems.[16] Significant impairment of learning can occur even at seemingly low levels. The Centers for Disease Control have defined an elevated lead level to be 25 μg per dl or greater.[17] Using this definition, Carter-Pokras et al. examined the HHANES to determine lead levels for mainland Puerto Rican and Mexican-American children ages 4 to 11 years.[18] Sixty-nine percent of Mexican-Americans (n = 1390) and 60% of mainland Puerto Rican (n = 397) children sampled had values available for analysis. Among children in this age group, 3.9% of mainland Puerto Rican children had elevated lead levels, compared to 1.2% of Mexican-American children. This distribution, however, was not equal for all ages. Children 4 to 5 years of age, toward the end of the pica period (age at which children eat nonfood items), had the highest proportion of elevated lead levels: 10.6% for mainland Puerto Ricans and 4.9% for Mexican-Americans. Lead levels decreased for mainland Puerto Rican children 6 to 8 years old (1.1% elevated), but increased in late childhood (9 to 11 years old) to 4.0%. This study noted no significant difference between mainland Puerto Rican children born in Puerto Rico and those born in the United States. This study estimated that 8,000 mainland Puerto Rican children in the New York City area had elevated lead levels. These findings from HHANES for mainland Puerto Rican children are higher than comparable national data from 1976 to 1978, showing 3.5% of non-Hispanic Caucasian children having elevated lead levels, but lower than that for non-Hispanic African-American children who had a 20% prevalence.[19]

Recently, learning difficulties have been associated with lower lead levels, between 15 and 25 μg per dl.[16] If a cutoff of 15 μg per dl was used to determine risk, then 20% or 41 000 mainland Puerto Rican children would be at risk in the New York City area,[18] and this figure may correlate with the large percentage of mothers expressing concern about their children's development. A more recent study by Daniel et al. in New York City found an elevated lead level rate (25–34 μg per dl) of 0.3 per 100 children screened; 27% of children with an elevated level were Hispanic.[10] Of the 796 cases of childhood lead poisoning, 59% were African-American and 27% were Hispanic; the majority were presumably mainland Puerto Rican (New York City also has other Hispanic groups). Although this is a lower rate than that in HHANES, the authors believe that this is an underestimation of the prevalence. In either situation, lead poisoning is a clear public health problem for mainland Puerto Rican children living in the New York City area.

HEALTH CARE UTILIZATION BY MAINLAND PUERTO RICAN CHILDREN

In order to appraise health care utilization, health care needs must be evaluated. In addition to chronic and reported medical conditions, subjective health ratings, and biochemical assessments, it was also possible to determine functional impairment from questionnaire data that were obtained in the HHANES. This provided an additional assessment of health needs, and indicated that one-third of all sampled children had some functional impairment due to a health problem or injury in the past year.

Once health needs are assessed, it is possible to determine if the subjects in need were able to access services at a health care facility. Among mainland Puerto Rican children, only 2.4% reported having no regular source of health care.[20] Nonetheless, 18% of parents of mainland Puerto Rican children also reported that they had encountered a barrier—frequently financial—to obtaining care for their child.[20]

The utilization of health care services by mainland Puerto Ricans is shown in Table 5. Twelve percent of mainland Puerto Rican children had neither a routine nor sick care visit in the past year.[20] About half of the children reporting a routine or sick care visit indicated that these were made to a public sector health care facility.[20] This was significantly higher than the percentage for Mexican-Americans or Cuban-Americans.

A comparison of utilization patterns from HHANES to the 1984 National Health Interview Survey, and the 1986 National Access Survey (Table 5) shows that mainland Puerto Rican children have the lowest rate of no regular source of health care and no visits in the past year.[20] However, they have a higher rate of uninsured children, as reported by parents (18.1%), compared to the national average of 10.7%. Compared to Mexican-American children who have an uninsured rate of 34.0%, mainland Puerto Rican children have better health coverage and concurrently better utilization.[20] These findings support those found previously by Trevino and Moss in the National Health Interview Survey.[5]

In addition, compared to the National Access Survey 1986, where 2.2% of mothers were not satisfied with their children's last health care

Table 5 Comparison of the Hispanic Health and Nutrition Examination Survey to National Surveys[a]

	HIS (1984)		NAS (1986)	HHANES (1982–1984)		
Access measure	Caucasian	African-American	Total	MEXAM	PRAM	CUBAM
No regular source	—	—	9.9	3.3	2.4	8.4
No health coverage	—	—	10.7	34.0	18.1	30.7
Fair or poor health	2.8	5.4	6.0	15.6	19.1	5.4
No visit in past 12 months	19.6	24.8	26.8	26.2	12.0	18.4
Not at all satisfied with visit	—	—	2.2	4.3	4.5	3.4

[a]Comparison of the pediatric Hispanic Health and Nutrition Examination Survey (H-HANES) subjects to Caucasian and African-American children in the National Health Interview Survey (NHIS) of 1984 and to the general pediatric population in the National Access Survey (NAS) of 1986 demonstrated differences in self-report of health status and the proportion with health care coverage and a medical visit in the past year.

visit, 4.5% of mainland Puerto Rican mothers were not satisfied with their children's last health care visit, a higher proportion than either Mexican-American or Cuban-American children.[20]

DISCUSSION

Mainland Puerto Rican children may have a somewhat higher rate of chronic medical conditions than Mexican-American, Cuban-American, or other U.S. children due to the higher frequency of asthma. The high prevalence of asthma or respiratory problems raises some concern that geographic factors (e.g., living in an inner city) may affect the prevalence of this condition. There are clinical reports of a high prevalence of asthma on the island of Puerto Rico, however, suggesting a possible genetic predisposition. The other health measures of concern, specifically higher lead levels and the greater maternal concern about children's health, may also be related to or result from living in an inner city. Since HHANES data are derived only from a sample of mainland Puerto Rican children living in an inner city, the New York City area, there may be an inherent bias in this study which, when compared to other samples (i.e., Mexican-Americans and non-Hispanic Caucasians), may result in an overly negative health profile. We should ask: what is the health status of mainland Puerto Rican children who do not live in inner city ghettos? Is there health status similar to that of Mexican-American children who live in the Southwest?

Some of the health status measures reported in HHANES indicate a mixed picture for mainland Puerto Rican children. Reported medical conditions do not appear to be higher than the national averages although comparisons are difficult. While medical health problems are somewhat more prevalent than neurodevelopmental conditions, the latter are less often treated. This should be of concern since poverty rates in the mainland Puerto Rican community are second only to the African-American community. If children from these communities are going to pull themselves out of poverty, then their ability to succeed educationally will be a cornerstone in that process. Therefore, children's neurodevelopmental problems should be as much a concern as other physical health problems such as asthma.

Overall, physicians' assessment of mainland Puerto Rican children is quite favorable. Nevertheless, this perspective is not shared by the mainland Puerto Rican family, mothers or children. Why this difference exists between physicians' assessments and those made by mothers and children, needs further intensive investigation. It is important to understand not only the causes of this difference in perspective between physicians and mothers and children, but also the effect that this greater concern about the child's health has on the mother–child relationship and the child's development.

Mainland Puerto Rican children appear to be utilizing the health care system more frequently than Mexican-Americans and Cuban-Americans. Whether this is enough to meet their total health care need, and is effectively resolving the children's health care problems is not known. The data from HHANES are now a decade old, and changes in the U.S. economy may have worsened the situation for Hispanic children, particularly for Puerto Rican children. The prior limitation of data on Hispanic children hampered efforts to address the health care needs of this population of children during most of the 1980s. A similar scenario can occur if continued monitoring of each subpopulation of Hispanic children (Mexican-Americans, mainland Puerto Ricans, Cuban-Americans, and now also Central Americans and Dominicans) is not undertaken.

In conclusion, mainland Puerto Rican children appear to have the worst health status among the three major Hispanic groups on the U.S. mainland, even though their access to health care appears to be the highest. This finding may be partly related to the higher poverty rate among mainland Puerto Ricans in comparison to the other groups. Yet poverty, as synthesized by demographers or epidemiologists, may not be a homogenous experience for all families. Differences in the life experience of poverty may be affected by geographic location, historical perspectives, cultural identity, social stability, and environmental factors. A deficit model, therefore, shows only the final common pathway to poor health outcomes. What it fails to show are the facets of poverty which contribute to poor health status, and the strengths of the individual, family, and community which attempt to buffer them. A better understanding of these factors is needed in order to improve the health status of U.S. mainland Puerto Rican children.

ACKNOWLEDGMENT. Supported by grant MCJ-060-518, Maternal and Child Health Bureau, HRSA, DHHS.

REFERENCES

1. The Hispanic Population in the United States: Current Population Reports, Population Characteristics, series p-20, no. 444, March, 1989
2. Mendoza F, Ventura S, Valdez R: Selected measures of health status for Mexican-American, mainland Puerto Rican, and Cuban-American children. *Journal of the American Medical Association* 265:227–232, 1991
3. Plan and Operation of the Hispanic Health and Nutrition Examination Survey 1982–84: Hyattsville, MD, National Center for Health Statistics, Vital and Health Statistics Program and Collection Procedure Series 1, No. 19; Department of Health and Human Services Publication No. (PHS) 85–1321
4. Data Systems of the National Center for Health Statistics: Programs and Collection Procedures Series 1, No. 16. Department of Health and Human Services Publication No. (PHS) 82–1318
5. Trevino F, Moss J: Health indicators for Hispanic, black, and white Americans. *Vital Health Statistics* 10:50–51, 1984
6. Newacheck PW, Budetti PD, Halfong N: Trends in activity-limiting chronic conditions among children. *American Journal of Public Health* 86:178–184
7. World Health Organization: *International Classification of Diseases, Ninth Revision.* Geneva, Switzerland, 1977
8. Gerngen PJ, Mullally DI, Evans R: National survey of prevalence of asthma among children in the United States, 1976 to 1980. *Pediatrics* 81:1–6, 1988
9. Filer L: Iron needs during rapid growth and mental development. *Journal of Pediatrics* 117:S143–146, 1990
10. Daniel K, Sedlis M, Polk L: *Childhood Lead Poisoning, New York City, 1988*. Bureau of

Lead Poisoning Control, New York City Department of Health, MMWR CDC surveillance summary, 39:1–7, 1990

11. Saldivar L, Mendoza F, Martorell R: Blood pressure in Hispanic children. *Clinical Research* 38:214A, 1990
12. Behrman R and Vaughn V: *Nelson Textbook of Pediatrics, Thirteenth Edition*. W.B. Saunders Company, Philadelphia, PA, 1987
13. Mendoza F, Ventura S, Valdez R: Health status of U.S. Hispanic children, in Furino A: *Health Policy and the Hispanic*. Boulder, CO, Westview Press (in press)
14. National Center for Health Statistics: Current Estimates from the National Health Interview Survey, United States 1985, Series 10, No. 160 Vital and Health Statistics, Hyattsville, Maryland, 1985
15. Castillo R, Garcia M, Pawson I: Iron status of U.S. Hispanic children. *Clinical Research* 38:1, 1990
16. Needleman H, Schell A, Bellinger D: The long-term effects of exposure to lead in childhood: An 11-year follow-up report. *New England Journal of Medicine* 322:83–88, 1990
17. Centers for Disease Control: *Preventing Lead Poisoning in Young Children*. Atlanta, GA, January 1985
18. Carter-Porkas O, Pirkle J, Chavez G: Blood lead levels of 4–11-year-old Mexican American, Puerto Rican, and Cuban Children. *Public Health Reports* 105:388–393, 1990
19. Annest J and Mahaffey K: Blood lead levels for persons age 6 months–74 years, United States 1976–80. Vital Health Statistics No. 233. Department Health and Human Services Publication No. (PHS) 84–1683. National Center for Health Statistics. Hyattsville, MD, 1984
20. Takata G: *Differential Access to Health Care of Latino Children in the Hispanic Health and Nutrition Examination Survey*. Masters thesis, Stanford University, 1991

13

Effect of Comprehensive Pediatric Care on the Health of Poor High-Risk Puerto Rican and American Black Children in New York City

JACK ELINSON AND PENNY LIBERATOS

INTRODUCTION

The present report is based on data generated by a larger study that was designed to evaluate the impact of a model of comprehensive pediatric care on the health of poor, high-risk children living in areas of the City of New York characterized by the worst health and economic statistical indicators. These New York City areas are almost entirely inhabited by

JACK ELINSON • Division of Sociomedical Sciences, Columbia University School of Public Health, New York, New York 10032, and Medical and Health Research Association of New York City, Inc., New York, New York 10013. PENNY LIBERATOS • Medical and Health Research Association of New York City, Inc., New York, New York, 10013.

Puerto Rican Women and Children: Issues in Health, Growth, and Development, edited by Gontran Lamberty and Cynthia Garcia Coll. Plenum Press, New York, 1994.

Hispanics and American Blacks.* Of the Hispanics, the largest group are Puerto Rican. This chapter will focus on comparisons of Puerto Rican and American Black children participating in the study.

The pediatric care model being evaluated was designed to provide high-quality, comprehensive health services to high-risk population groups. The model had been applied earlier by the Children and Youth programs legislated in the 1960s, now defunct in New York City. A decade ago, the Select Panel for the Promotion of Child Health[2] specifically called for an expansion of this type of service delivery model. Significant features of the model include: availability, accessibility, continuity, comprehensiveness, and coordination. Key elements of the model continue to be advocated, by the pediatric community.[3–5]

Under mandated cutbacks in funding in recent years, however, it has proved difficult for policy and decision makers to point to solid evidence that such models are indeed effective. The overall aim of this study is to evaluate the effectiveness of a model of comprehensive pediatric care for poor children at relatively high risk of preventable morbidity.

Measures were developed to assess quantitatively certain essential components of the model.[6] The effectiveness of implementing the model was assessed by its impact on important outcomes for poor, high-risk children. The model studied was that implemented at seven Pediatric Resource Centers (PRC) situated in four counties of New York City.

STUDY DESIGN AND SAMPLE

The essential design of the evaluation research is a quasi-experimental study of equivalent groups: children enrolled as patients in PRC's (PRC group); and children equally eligible for enrollment in the PRC's, but who were not enrolled, and who received care from more generally available community sources (Comparison group).

Among the children served by the PRC's, two high-risk groups were selected for inclusion in the evaluation study: low birth weight children and children of adolescent parents. Pediatric Resource Center

*Although the term "African-American" is consistently used throughout this volume, this study differentiated between those individuals born in the United States and those born in the Caribbean or Africa; thus the term "American Black" will be used in this chapter.

study children also had family incomes less than 185% of the federal poverty level, resided in areas with the worst health and social indicators, and were new patients to the PRC at the time of enrollment into the study. Comparison children, matching the PRC group in essential characteristics (i.e., poverty status, risk category, area of residence), were drawn from birth certificate registries, child health clinics operated by the local health department, hospital nurseries, friends of participants, and late registrants (i.e., PRC registrants who had been eligible to enroll for at least a year, but had not done so). Comparison children had never attended a PRC and the child was at least 10 months of age at the time of enrollment in the study.

For analysis purposes, a subgroup of the PRC children (n = 323) who had made all their nonemergent visits to the PRC exclusively (to be referred to as PRC "pure") was compared to the Comparison group (n = 472).

The study population was diverse in its racial/ethnic background. Included were Hispanics (from Puerto Rico, the Dominican Republic, and other Hispanic American countries), American Black, Haitian and other Caribbean Blacks (non-Hispanic). A substantial number of Study children were identified as Puerto Rican (n = 124).* The remaining Hispanic children number 77 and came from all parts of the Caribbean and Central and South America. Among those of African ancestry, most children were designated by the respondent as American Black (n = 477) and the rest as Other Black (n = 40). The remaining children were designated as Other (of neither Hispanic nor African descent) (n = 77). This chapter compares the Puerto Rican children with their African-American counterparts for a total of 601 children.

METHODS

Data were collected by means of structured interviews and medical examinations. Interviews were usually conducted with the child's

*Early in the study, it became apparent that the designation of someone as "Puerto Rican" was neither simple nor clear-cut.[7] An operational definition for study purposes had to be developed. Respondents were asked to identify the child's and the respondent's race/ethnicity. In addition, respondents were offered the option of an "Other" category. In those cases where the respondent reported the "Other" category for the child, the child was allocated the same race/ethnicity as the mother.

mother, but occasionally with a grandmother or guardian. Interviews were conducted by specially trained bilingual (English and Spanish) interviewers. Medical examinations were conducted by on-site pediatricians who completed a data collection form specifically designed for the study. Data were collected at two points, approximately one year apart, for the PRC group; and for one point for the Comparison group, matching the second point for the PRC children.

Almost 200 variables were utilized to assess outcomes in a variety of areas. These variables can be grouped under the following seven categories: physical health, psychosocial health, functional health, preventive health behaviors, health knowledge and practices, utilization of health services and unmet needs for care. Information for some variables (e.g., physical and psychosocial well-being, symptoms) were collected by both sociomedical interviews and by pediatric examinations, which provided a validity check. For the most part, variables were assessed using measures derived for, and used, in prior studies.

The analytic method used to assess the impact of the PRC model was logistic regression. Each outcome variable was dichotomized at a logical cutpoint to simplify analysis. The regression equation included any demographic characteristics identified as significantly different between groups (see next section). This analysis was performed separately for Puerto Rican and for American Black children in order to examine the impact of the model on each group.

COMPARABILITY OF STUDY GROUPS

The two analytic groups (PRC "pure" and Comparison) comprising the focus of this analysis, were assessed on several characteristics for comparability. The two racial/ethnic groups (Puerto Rican and American Black) were also examined as to comparability on these same characteristics. Those characteristics that were found to differ significantly ($p < .05$) between the analytic or racial/ethnic groups were used as covariates in all analyses.

Assessment of the comparability of the study groups utilizes demographic, antecedent (prenatal and intrapartum experience with the index child), and environmental variables (residential crowding and mobility, problems in the home and neighborhood, and economic constraints). None of these variables are expected to be affected by the PRC program.

Demographic Variables (Table 1)

The ages of both the children and the respondent were significantly different between the PRC and Comparison groups. The PRC children were younger (91 vs. 32% under age 2). Their corresponding respondents (usually the mother) were also younger (41 vs. 26% under age 20).

In comparing the Puerto Rican with the American Black families, more Puerto Rican respondents had not completed high school (61 vs. 46%), a larger proportion of the Puerto Rican households were smaller (59 vs. 44% with <5 persons), and the mother was the respondent more often for the Puerto Rican children (94 vs. 86%). There were no other differences between the two groups on the remaining nine variables in this area.

Antecedent Variables (Table 2)

The PRC group did differ from the Comparison group on several variables that occurred prior to entry in the PRCs. The Comparison group was more likely to have sought prenatal care during the first trimester (for the pregnancy with the index child) (67 vs. 51%) and was less likely to have consumed alcoholic beverages during the pregnancy (4 vs. 9%). The children of the Comparison group were more likely to have been born full term (65 vs. 51%), and spent less time in the hospital (71 vs. 59% spent one week or less). Although not significant, there was also a tendency ($p < .10$) for the Comparison group to have been born at a higher birth weight (53 vs. 47% weighed more than 2500 grams) and for the mothers to have had fewer problems during the pregnancy (3 vs. 5%).

All these differences favor the Comparison group. These children appear to have begun life with fewer problems and their mothers practiced better preventive health behaviors. Thus, these preexisting differences between the two groups should operate counter to the study hypotheses.

There were two significant differences between the Puerto Rican and American Black families in the area of antecedent conditions. Puerto Rican mothers were more likely to have sought prenatal care during the first trimester of pregnancy (with the index child) (67 vs. 54%) and the Puerto Rican child was more likely to have spent one week or less in the hospital after birth (80 vs. 67%). Both of these differences

Table 1 Demographic Characteristics PRC "Pure" and "Comparison"

Variables	PRC Pure (n = 323) n (%)	Comparison (n = 472) n (%)	Puerto Rican (n = 124) n (%)	American Black (n = 477) n (%)
Risk category				
Low birthweight	166 (52)	236 (48)	48 (39)	230 (49)
Child of adolescent	140 (43)	237 (48)	69 (56)	224 (47)
Low birthweight child of adolescent	17 (5)	19 (4)	7 (5)	20 (4)
Birthweight (grams)				
≤2500	174 (54)	246 (46)	52 (42)	241 (51)
2501+	150 (46)	253 (54)	72 (58)	236 (49)
Child's age (months)				
<24	296 (91)	153 (32)	72 (59)	267 (56)
24+	28 (9)	326 (68)[a***]	51 (41)	208 (44)
Respondent's age (years)				
<20	129 (41)	119 (26)	49 (41)	147 (33)
20+	182 (59)	336 (74)[a***]	70 (59)	303 (67)
Respondent's education (years)				
0–11	148 (47)	220 (47)	73 (61)	214 (46)
12+	164 (53)	249 (53)	46 (39)	256 (56)[b**]
Household size				
<5	149 (46)	243 (51)	73 (59)	210 (44)
5+	174 (54)	230 (49)	51 (41)	263 (56)[b**]
Poverty level				
<100%	181 (61)	277 (63)	77 (66)	268 (63)
100–185%	115 (39)	160 (37)	40 (34)	159 (37)
Respondent's relationship to child				
Mother	288 (89)	425 (89)	115 (94)	406 (86)
Other	35 (11)	53 (11)	8 (6)	67 (14)[b*]
Child's sex				
Male	162 (50)	219 (46)	61 (50)	226 (48)
Female	161 (50)	257 (54)	62 (50)	246 (52)

[a] = PRC Pure significantly different from Comparison, chi-square.
[b] = Puerto Rican significantly different from American Black, chi-square.
* = $p < .05$ ** = $p < .01$ *** = $p < .001$

imply that the Puerto Rican children began life a little healthier and their mothers practiced better preventive health behavior.

Environmental Variables (Table 3)

The Comparison group reported more neighborhood problems (45 vs. 35% with 3+ problems). Although the two groups did not differ in

Table 2 Antecedent Variables PRC Pure and Comparison Children

Variables	PRC Pure (n = 323) n (%)	Comparison (n = 472) n (%)	Puerto Rican (n = 124) n (%)	American Black (n = 477) n (%)
Trimester saw M.D.				
First	158 (51)	292 (67)	79 (67)	240 (54)
Second/Third	154 (49)	144 (35)[a***]	39 (33)	201 (46)[b*]
Health habit talk during pregnancy				
No	18 (6)	33 (8)	6 (5)	27 (6)
Yes	283 (94)	381 (92)	109 (95)	392 (94)
Smoked during pregnancy				
No	253 (80)	336 (77)	92 (79)	322 (72)
Yes	63 (20)	98 (23)	24 (21)	124 (28)
Drank alcohol during pregnancy				
No	288 (91)	414 (96)	111 (97)	401 (92)
Yes	27 (9)	19 (4)[a*]	3 (3)	37 (8)
Prematurity				
Normal term	155 (51)	285 (65)	75 (65)	271 (62)
Premature	148 (49)	151 (35)[a***]	41 (35)	165 (38)
Birthweight (grams)				
<2000	89 (27)	95 (20)	19 (15)	114 (23)
2000–2499	86 (26)	131 (28)	31 (25)	128 (26)
⩾2500	154 (47)	250 (53)	73 (59)	245 (50)
Hospitalization during pregnancy				
Nonpregnancy problems				
No	298 (95)	430 (97)	116 (98)	427 (95)
Yes	17 (5)	12 (3)	3 (2)	22 (5)
Pregnancy complications				
No	291 (92)	398 (90)	107 (90)	417 (93)
Yes	24 (8)	44 (10)	12 (10)	32 (7)
Problems with baby at birth				
No	228 (72)	322 (74)	85 (73)	332 (74)
Yes	89 (28)	113 (26)	31 (27)	120 (26)
Child's length of hospital stay at birth				
⩽1 week	185 (59)	313 (71)	95 (80)	298 (67)
>1 week	130 (41)	126 (29)[a***]	24 (20)	148 (33)[b**]
Ever breast-fed				
No	215 (67)	327 (73)	82 (70)	361 (78)
Yes	104 (33)	122 (27)	35 (30)	104 (22)

[a] = PRC Pure significantly different from Comparison, chi-square.
[b] = Puerto Rican significantly different from American Black, chi-square.
* = $p < .05$ ** = $p < .01$ *** = $p < .001$

Table 3 Environmental Variables PRC Pure and Comparison Children

Variables	PRC Pure (n = 323) n (%)	Comparison (n = 472) n (%)	Puerto Rican (n = 124) n (%)	American Black (n = 477) n (%)
Housing type				
House/apartment	317 (99+)	448 (98)	118 (99)	452 (99)
Hotel/shelter/group home	1 (<1)	8 (2)	1 (1)	6 (1)
Crowding (persons/room)				
<2	225 (71)	335 (72)	80 (66)	349 (74)
2+	92 (29)	131 (28)	42 (34)	125 (26)
Bathroom crowding (persons/bathroom)				
<5	178 (56)	280 (60)	80 (66)	261 (55)
5+	142 (44)	185 (40)	42 (34)	211 (45)[b*]
Housing satisfaction				
Satisfied	176 (54)	264 (56)	73 (59)	251 (53)
Somewhat/not satisfied	147 (46)	208 (44)	50 (41)	226 (47)
House problems				
0–2	251 (78)	367 (78)	92 (76)	384 (81)
3+	69 (22)	105 (22)	29 (24)	89 (19)
Neighborhood problems				
0–2	205 (65)	259 (55)	80 (66)	258 (55)
3+	111 (35)	213 (45)[a**]	41 (34)	212 (45)[b*]
Mobility (last year)				
Moved once +	50 (16)	82 (17)	24 (20)	72 (15)
Didn't move	272 (84)	390 (83)	99 (81)	404 (85)
Adequacy of money for				
Food				
All/most of the time	277 (87)	386 (82)	100 (83)	397 (84)
Some/little/none of the time	42 (13)	86 (18)	21 (17)	76 (16)
Clothes				
All/most of the time	239 (75)	292 (62)	77 (64)	332 (70)
Some/little/none of the time	80 (25)	180 (38)[a***]	44 (36)	141 (30)
Medical care				
All/most of the time	292 (92)	388 (82)	106 (88)	421 (89)
Some/little/none of the time	27 (8)	83 (18)[a***]	15 (12)	52 (11)

[a] = PRC Pure significantly different from Comparison, chi-square.
[b] = Puerto Rican significantly different from American Black, chi-square.
* = $p < .05$ ** = $p < .01$ *** = $p < .001$

terms of family income, their perceptions of their economic circumstances did differ. The PRC group was more likely to report that they had adequate money all the time for food (87% vs. 82%), clothes (75 vs. 62%), and for the child's medical care (92 vs. 82%).

A smaller proportion of Puerto Rican families reported bathroom crowding (34 vs. 45%; with 5+ persons per bathroom) and neighborhood problems (34 vs. 45% with 3+ problems).

SUMMARY

A total of five demographic variables (i.e., child's age, household size, and respondent's age, education, and relationship to child) were significantly different either between the PRC and Comparison groups or between the Puerto Rican and American Black children. All of these variables were used as covariates in the analyses.

There were 12 other variables (out of a possible 42) in the antecedent and environmental areas which were also significantly different between groups. Preliminary analyses showed that inclusion of these variables in the analytic equation had no effect on the outcome, therefore they were not used as covariates.

PROGRAM IMPACT

These analyses were done to evaluate the efforts of participation in the PRC on the outcome measures as compared to a group who did not participate for each of the two racial/ethnic groups. As noted in the comparability section above, five variables were found to be possible confounders and were therefore used as covariates in logistic regression analyses examining the relationship between each health outcome and the PRC and Comparison groups.

Physical Health Variables

General Health Perception and Health Problems

There were no differences between the groups in the respondent's perception of the child's health (as excellent, very good, good, fair, or poor). Among the Puerto Rican children, the Comparison group reported more health problems (33 vs. 15%, $p < .01$) and health problems of greater severity (25 vs. 13%, $p < .01$) than the PRC group. There were no differences in the number or severity of health problems reported for American Black children.

Physical Symptoms

Table 4 shows the physical health variables for Puerto Rican and American Black PRC and Comparison children. Among the Puerto Rican children, the Comparison group reported a higher frequency of occurrence during the previous three months for sore throat (32 vs. 15%, $p < .01$) and coughs with fever (23 vs. 6%, $p < .05$). However, the two groups did not differ on the overall number of symptoms experienced.

For the American Black children, the Comparison group reported a greater frequency of occurrence of high (>102°) fevers (27 vs. 21%, $p < .05$) but no difference in the remaining 17 symptoms or on the total number of symptoms reported.

Judgment of Completeness of Prior Care and Well-Being

When physicians were asked to judge the completeness of prior care and well-being in three areas (physical, mental/emotional, and social), they rated the PRC and Comparison groups about the same in all areas for both racial/ethnic groups.

Judgment of Development and Weight

Physicians' judgment of development in the areas of gross motor, fine motor, language, and personal/social (see Table 5) was similar for both groups, but the PRC group was more likely to be judged as having delays in the fine motor area among American Black children (7 vs. 1%, $p < .05$). There were no differences in weight assessments.

Physical Health Screening

Among American Black children, the PRC group was more likely to be anemic (14 vs. 4%, $p < .05$) the groups were similar for all other physical health screening variables (blood lead and blood pressure).

Table 4 Physical Health Variables Physical Symptoms for PRC and Comparison Children

Variables	Puerto Rican			American Black		
	PRC Pure (n = 52) n (%)	Comparison (n = 72) n (%)	Total (n = 124) n (%)	PRC Pure (n = 197) n (%)	Comparison (n = 280) n (%)	Total (n = 477) n (%)
Physical symptoms (last 3 mos.)						
Accidental poisoning	1 (2)	1 (1)	2 (2)	4 (2)	4 (1)	8 (2)
Constipation	7 (14)	10 (14)	17 (14)	31 (15)	41 (15)	72 (15)
Cough	29 (56)	41 (58)	70 (57)	118 (59)	168 (60)	286 (60)
with fever 3 days	3 (6)	16 (23)	19 (15)[a*]	27 (13)	47 (17)	74 (15)
Cranky	13 (25)	14 (20)	27 (22)	35 (17)	51 (18)	86 (18)
Diarrhea	14 (27)	16 (23)	30 (24)	50 (25)	64 (23)	114 (24)
for 3 days	5 (10)	10 (14)	15 (12)	26 (13)	27 (10)	53 (11)
Ear infection	20 (39)	32 (45)	52 (42)	59 (29)	84 (30)	143 (30)
with fever	13 (25)	25 (35)	38 (31)	41 (20)	57 (21)	98 (21)
Fever	33 (64)	43 (61)	76 (62)	113 (56)	146 (53)	259 (54)
+102 or >2 days	16 (31)	21 (30)	37 (30)	42 (21)	74 (27)	116 (24)[b*]
Poor appetite	13 (25)	24 (34)	37 (30)	40 (20)	73 (26)	113 (24)
Sore throat	8 (15)	23 (32)	31 (25)[a**]	20 (10)	27 (10)	47 (10)
with fever for 3 days	4 (8)	11 (16)	15 (12)	11 (6)	18 (7)	29 (6)
Unexplained weight loss	4 (8)	10 (14)	14 (11)	17 (9)	16 (6)	33 (7)
Vomiting	9 (17)	17 (24)	26 (21)	52 (26)	62 (22)	114 (24)
for 2 days	3 (6)	9 (13)	12 (10)	10 (5)	22 (8)	32 (7)
Other	3 (6)	6 (9)	9 (7)	5 (3)	22 (8)	27 (6)
Total symptoms						
0–2	22 (42)	24 (34)	46 (37)	90 (45)	116 (42)	206 (43)
3+	30 (58)	47 (66)	77 (63)	110 (55)	161 (58)	271 (57)

[a] = PRC Pure significantly different from Comparison for Puerto Rican children, logistic regression.
[b] = Puerto Rican significantly different from Comparison for American Black children, logistic regression.
* = $p < .05$ ** = $p < .01$ *** = $p < .001$

Table 5 Physical Health Variables, M.D. Judgments: Judgment of Development and Weight for PRC and Comparison Children

	Puerto Rican			American Black		
Variables	PRC Pure (n = 52) n (%)	Comparison (n = 72) n (%)	Total (n = 124) n (%)	PRC Pure (n = 197) n (%)	Comparison (n = 280) n (%)	Total (n = 477) n (%)
Judgment of development						
Gross motor						
Advanced/average	39 (98)	41 (100)	80 (99)	130 (93)	156 (97)	286 (95)
Delayed	1 (2)	0 (0)	1 (1)	10 (7)	5 (3)	15 (5)
Fine Motor						
Advanced/average	38 (97)	41 (100)	79 (99)	130 (93)	155 (99)	285 (96)
Delayed	1 (3)	0 (0)	1 (1)	10 (7)	2 (1)	12 (4)[a]**
Language						
Advanced/average	36 (92)	39 (98)	75 (95)	126 (90)	146 (92)	272 (91)
Delayed	3 (8)	1 (3)	4 (5)	14 (10)	13 (8)	27 (9)
Personal/social						
Advanced/average	37 (95)	41 (100)	78 (98)	130 (94)	152 (97)	282 (96)
Delayed	2 (5)	0 (0)	2 (2)	8 (6)	5 (3)	13 (4)
Assessment of weight						
Failure to thrive/ underweight/average	35 (92)	32 (80)	67 (86)	126 (94)	140 (90)	266 (92)
Overweight/obese	3 (8)	8 (20)	11 (14)	8 (6)	15 (10)	23 (8)

[a] = PRC Pure significantly different from Comparison for American Black children, logistic regression.
* = $p < .05$ ** = $p < .01$ *** = $p < .001$

Chronic Conditions

Children in the PRC and Comparison groups were reported by the physicians to have a similar number of chronic conditions with a similar severity distribution.

Psychosocial Health Variables

There were no differences between the two groups for the three variables examined in this area (general psychosocial health, family relationships, and friendships).

Functional Health Variables

Restricted Activity/Bed Disability

There were no differences between the groups in the reporting of restricted activity and bed disability days.

Eating and Sleeping Patterns

Among American Black children, the PRC group was more likely to eat lunch (93 vs. 83%, $p < .05$) everyday. There was no difference between the groups in any other eating or sleeping patterns.

Preventive Health Behavior Variables

There were no differences between the groups for testing for any of the six screening variables (lead, TB, blood pressure, vision, hearing, dental).

Nutrition

There were no differences between the groups for types of foods eaten (number of high fat, sugar, empty calories, high fiber, poor diet foods consumed).

Immunizations (Table 6)

American Black children from the Comparison group were more likely to be delayed in receiving DPT (36 vs. 26%, $p < .05$) and OPV (76

Table 6 Preventive Health Behavior Variables: Immunizations for PRC and Comparison Children

	Puerto Rican			American Black		
Variables	PRC Pure (n = 52) n (%)	Comparison (n = 72) n (%)	Total (n = 124) n (%)	PRC Pure (n = 197) n (%)	Comparison (n = 280) n (%)	Total (n = 477) n (%)
DPT						
Delayed	12 (27)	22 (39)	34 (33)	47 (26)	78 (36)	125 (32)
Not delayed	33 (73)	35 (61)	68 (67)	131 (74)	140 (64)	271 (68)[a]*
OPV						
Delayed	25 (54)	41 (72)	66 (64)	77 (44)	162 (76)	239 (61)
Not delayed	21 (46)	16 (28)	37 (36)	100 (56)	52 (24)	152 (39)[a]***
MMR[b]						
Delayed	5 (17)	11 (17)	16 (17)	22 (16)	39 (16)	61 (16)
Not delayed	24 (83)	53 (83)	77 (83)	116 (84)	206 (84)	322 (84)
HIB[b]						
Delayed	12 (63)	24 (42)	36 (47)	70 (69)	76 (36)	146 (47)
Not delayed	7 (37)	33 (58)	50 (53)	31 (31)	136 (64)	167 (53)[a]**
All immunizations						
Delayed	31 (65)	53 (82)	84 (74)	117 (62)	201 (78)	318 (72)
Not delayed	17 (35)	12 (18)	29 (26)	71 (38)	56 (22)	127 (28)[a]**

[a] = PRC Pure significantly different from Comparison for American Black children, logistic regression.
[b] = Applies to children 15 months and older since that is when the immunization is due.
* = $p < .05$ ** = $p < .01$ *** = $p < .001$

vs. 44%, $p < .001$) immunizations and in having a delay in at least one immunization (78 vs. 62%, $p < .01$). The PRC group was more delayed for the HIB immunization (69 vs. 36%, $p < .01$). There was no difference in timeliness of the MMR immunization. Although not significant, there was a tendency ($p < .10$) for Puerto Rican children's DPT immunizations from the comparison group (39 vs. 27%) to be delayed, and in there being a delay in at least one immunization (82 vs. 65%).

Health Knowledge and Practice Variables (Table 7)

All but one of the differences in this area favor the PRC group. For American Black children, the PRC group was more likely to make sure that all medicines have child-proof caps (85 vs. 77%, $p < .01$); check toys for safety (63 vs. 49%, $p < .05$); to have less pica (19 vs. 26%, $p < .05$); and to have fewer injuries/bruises (30 vs. 43%, $p < .05$). In contrast, the Comparison group was less likely to drink cereal from a bottle (9 vs. 22%, $p < .01$). Among Puerto Rican children, the PRC respondents were more likely to possess a fever thermometer (92 vs. 78%, $p < .05$) and reported having discussed more health education topics with their provider (76 vs. 56%, $p < .05$). There were no other differences for Puerto Rican children in this area.

Utilization of Health Services Variables (Table 8)

Puerto Rican PRC children were reported to have had fewer episodic visits (11 vs. 15%, $p < .01$) and fewer preventive visits (28 vs. 48%, $p < .01$) than the Comparison group during the previous three months. American Black PRC children were also reported to have had fewer preventive visits (25 vs. 48%, $p < .001$) during the three months prior to the study interview. There were no differences, however, for either racial/ethnic group for episodic and preventive visits for the previous 12-month period. There were no differences between the groups for ER visits and hospitalizations (both number and severity of conditions).

Unmet Needs for Care Variables (Table 9)

There were no differences for unmet health needs variables between the two groups. In the social service needs area, American Black PRC children were more likely to have WIC services (69 vs. 52%, $p < .05$) and to be more likely to report needing help with housing (43 vs. 26%, $p < .01$).

Table 7 Health Knowledge and Practices Variables for PRC and Comparison Children

Variables	Puerto Rican			American Black		
	PRC Pure (n = 52) n (%)	Comparison (n = 72) n (%)	Total (n = 124) n (%)	PRC Pure (n = 197) n (%)	Comparison (n = 280) n (%)	Total (n = 477) n (%)
Has window guards						
No	6 (16)	2 (4)	8 (9)	15 (10)	10 (5)	25 (7)
Yes	32 (84)	50 (96)	82 (91)	132 (90)	185 (95)	317 (93)
Has smoke detector						
No	12 (23)	11 (16)	23 (19)	29 (15)	41 (15)	70 (15)
Yes	40 (77)	56 (84)	96 (81)	169 (85)	232 (85)	401 (85)
Response in case of fire						
Use elevator	0 (0)	1 (2)	1 (1)	5 (3)	3 (1)	8 (2)
Use stairs/other	52 (100)	67 (98)	119 (99)	195 (97)	270 (99)	465 (98)
Has peeling paint[c]						
Yes	0 (0)	6 (37)	6 (24)	13 (33)	14 (19)	27 (24)
No	9 (100)	10 (63)	19 (76)	26 (67)	58 (81)	84 (76)
Electrical outlets covered						
No	9 (17)	15 (22)	24 (20)	32 (16)	58 (21)	90 (19)
Yes	43 (83)	53 (78)	96 (80)	168 (84)	214 (79)	382 (81)
Poisons kept out of reach						
None/few/some/most	7 (13)	18 (26)	25 (21)	28 (14)	65 (24)	93 (20)
All	45 (87)	50 (74)	95 (79)	173 (86)	201 (76)	374 (80)
Medicines have child-proof caps						
None/few/some/most	15 (29)	18 (26)	33 (28)	30 (15)	64 (23)	94 (20)
All	36 (71)	50 (74)	86 (72)	171 (85)	209 (77)	380 (80)[b**]
Action if poison swallowed						
Correct action	19 (37)	32 (47)	51 (43)	84 (42)	133 (49)	217 (46)
Other action	33 (63)	36 (53)	69 (57)	116 (58)	139 (51)	255 (54)

Ever heard of ipecac						
No	46 (89)	59 (89)	105 (89)	183 (93)	246 (91)	429 (92)
Yes	6 (11)	7 (11)	13 (11)	14 (7)	25 (9)	39 (8)
Has ipecac[d]						
No	2 (33)	5 (71)	7 (54)	7 (50)	16 (64)	23 (59)
Yes	4 (67)	2 (29)	6 (46)	7 (50)	9 (36)	16 (41)
Ever heard of poison control center						
No	16 (31)	31 (47)	47 (40)	65 (33)	95 (35)	160 (34)
Yes	36 (89)	35 (53)	71 (60)	135 (67)	178 (65)	313 (66)
Method of contacting poison control center[d]						
Correct response	31 (94)	32 (94)	63 (94)	125 (93)	164 (93)	289 (93)
Other response	2 (6)	2 (6)	4 (6)	9 (7)	13 (7)	22 (7)
Has fever thermometer						
No	4 (8)	15 (22)	19 (16)	24 (12)	56 (21)	80 (17)
Yes	48 (92)	53 (78)	101 (84)[a*]	175 (88)	215 (79)	390 (83)
How often use thermometer when child is sick						
None/little/some	6 (13)	10 (19)	16 (16)	35 (22)	33 (16)	68 (19)
Most/always	41 (87)	42 (81)	83 (84)	128 (78)	171 (84)	299 (81)
Toy safety						
Very safe	42 (81)	48 (71)	90 (75)	167 (84)	206 (76)	373 (79)
Not too/somewhat/mostly safe	10 (19)	20 (29)	30 (25)	32 (16)	67 (24)	99 (21)
Checks toys for safety						
All the time	36 (69)	36 (54)	72 (61)	126 (63)	133 (49)	259 (55)
None/little/some/most of the time	16 (31)	31 (46)	47 (39)	74 (37)	140 (51)	214 (45)[b*]
Car safety[e]						
Always in car seat	12 (39)	9 (21)	21 (28)	37 (30)	45 (24)	82 (26)
Sometimes in car seat	19 (61)	34 (79)	53 (72)	86 (70)	143 (76)	229 (74)
Drinks cereal from bottle						
No	32 (71)	12 (55)	44 (66)	129 (78)	82 (91)	211 (83)
Yes	13 (29)	10 (45)	23 (34)	36 (22)	8 (9)	44 (17)[b**]

(Continued)

Table 7 *(Continued)*

Variables	Puerto Rican			American Black		
	PRC Pure (n = 52) n (%)	Comparison (n = 72) n (%)	Total (n = 124) n (%)	PRC Pure (n = 197) n (%)	Comparison (n = 280) n (%)	Total (n = 477) n (%)
Number of injuries/bruises						
None	36 (69)	37 (54)	73 (61)	141 (70)	155 (57)	296 (62)
1+	16 (31)	31 (46)	47 (39)	60 (30)	118 (43)	178 (38)[b*]
Ever eaten nonfood substances						
No	43 (83)	52 (77)	95 (79)	162 (81)	201 (74)	363 (77)
Yes	9 (17)	16 (23)	25 (21)	39 (19)	72 (26)	111 (23)[b*]
Number of health education topics discussed by provider						
0–4	12 (24)	30 (44)	42 (35)	79 (40)	113 (42)	192 (41)
5+	39 (76)	38 (56)	77 (65)[a*]	119 (60)	159 (58)	278 (59)
Kept follow-up appointments[f]						
Always/usually	8 (89)	14 (78)	22 (82)	26 (72)	40 (77)	66 (75)
Half the time/sometimes/never	1 (11)	4 (22)	5 (18)	10 (28)	12 (23)	22 (25)
Number of missed appointments[f]						
None	20 (41)	33 (53)	53 (48)	77 (40)	93 (36)	170 (38)
1+	29 (59)	29 (47)	58 (52)	118 (60)	163 (64)	281 (62)

How soon usually fill prescriptions[f]						
Same day	46 (96)	55 (93)	101 (94)	183 (96)	232 (94)	415 (95)
Next day +	2 (4)	4 (7)	6 (6)	7 (4)	15 (6)	22 (5)
Number of medicines used (last 3 mos.)						
None	8 (15)	11 (16)	19 (15)	27 (13)	41 (15)	68 (14)
1+	44 (85)	60 (84)	104 (85)	173 (87)	236 (85)	409 (86)
Number of medicines recommended by doctor						
None	13 (25)	20 (28)	33 (27)	42 (21)	76 (27)	118 (25)
1+	39 (75)	51 (72)	90 (73)	158 (79)	201 (73)	359 (75)
Total number of medicines used	104 —	184 —	288 —	450 —	597 —	1,047 —
Total number of medicines recommended by M.D.	86 (83)	136 (74)	222 (77)	398 (88)	500 (84)	898 (86)
Total number used not recommended by doctor	18 (17)	48 (26)	66 (23)	52 (12)	97 (16)	149 (14)
Mean number medicines used per child using medicines	2.4 —	3.1 —	2.8 —	2.6 —	2.5 —	2.6 —

[a] = PRC Pure significantly different from Comparison for Puerto Rican children, logistic regression.
[b] = PCR Pure significantly different from Comparison for American Black children, logistic regression
[c] = Asked only if child has pica.
[d] = Asked only if respondent had ever heard of ipecac/poison control center.
[e] = Asked only if child rides regularly in a car.
[f] = Asked only if child ever had: follow-up appointment/appointment/prescription.
* = $p < .05$ ** = $p < .01$ *** = $p < .001$

Table 8 Utilization of Health Services Variables for PRC and Comparison Children

	Puerto Rican			American Black		
Variables	PRC Pure (n = 52) n (%)	Comparison (n = 72) n (%)	Total (n = 124) n (%)	PRC Pure (n = 197) n (%)	Comparison (n = 280) n (%)	Total (n = 477) n (%)
Number of episodic visits						
Last 12 months						
0–4	32 (62)	44 (62)	76 (62)	161 (81)	212 (77)	373 (78)
5+	20 (38)	27 (38)	47 (38)	39 (19)	65 (23)	104 (22)
Last 3 months						
0–2	46 (89)	60 (85)	106 (86)	186 (93)	263 (95)	449 (94)
3+	6 (11)	11 (15)	17 (14)[a]**	14 (7)	14 (5)	28 (6)
Number of preventive visits						
Last 12 months						
0–4	22 (42)	33 (47)	55 (45)	60 (30)	118 (42)	178 (37)
5+	30 (58)	38 (53)	68 (55)	140 (70)	159 (58)	299 (63)
Last 3 months						
0–2	36 (72)	34 (52)	70 (61)	146 (75)	134 (52)	280 (62)
3+	14 (28)	31 (48)	45 (39)[a]**	49 (25)	124 (48)	173 (38)[b]***
Number of emergency room visits						
Last 12 months						
0–1	25 (48)	41 (58)	66 (54)	134 (67)	180 (65)	314 (66)
2+	27 (52)	30 (42)	57 (46)	66 (33)	97 (35)	163 (34)

Last 3 months						
None	35 (67)	53 (75)	88 (72)	142 (71)	212 (77)	354 (74)
1+	17 (33)	18 (25)	35 (28)	58 (29)	65 (23)	123 (26)
Number of lifetime hospitalizations						
Child[c]						
None	40 (77)	54 (76)	94 (76)	157 (79)	221 (80)	378 (79)
1+	12 (23)	17 (24)	29 (24)	43 (21)	56 (20)	99 (21)
Mother[d]						
None	44 (85)	59 (83)	103 (84)	155 (78)	231 (84)	386 (81)
1+	8 (15)	12 (17)	20 (16)	45 (22)	46 (16)	91 (19)
Hospitalizations—severity of conditions[e]						
Child[f]						
None/minor	43 (83)	60 (85)	103 (84)	169 (86)	236 (85)	405 (86)
Potentially serious/serious	9 (17)	11 (15)	20 (16)	27 (14)	41 (15)	68 (14)
Mother[g]						
None/minor	45 (87)	62 (87)	107 (87)	159 (81)	243 (88)	402 (85)
Potentially serious/serious	7 (13)	9 (13)	16 (13)	37 (19)	34 (12)	71 (15)

[a] = PRC Pure significantly different from Comparison for Puerto Rican Children, logistic regression.
[b] = PRC Pure significantly different from Comparison for American Black children, logistic regression.
[c] = Not including birth.
[d] = Not including birth of index child.
[e] = Problems classified based on most serious problem reported.
[f] = Includes hospitalizations for tests and unspecified conditions.
[g] = Includes hospitalizations for birth-related and reproductive conditions.
* = $p < .05$ ** = $p < .01$ *** = $p < .001$

Table 9 Unmet Needs for Care Variables for PRC and Comparison Children

	Puerto Rican			American Black		
Variables	PRC Pure (n = 52) n (%)	Comparison (n = 72) n (%)	Total (n = 124) n (%)	PRC Pure (n = 197) n (%)	Comparison (n = 280) n (%)	Total (n = 477) n (%)
Child takes medicine recommended by doctor[b]						
No	4 (19)	4 (18)	8 (19)	12 (21)	17 (21)	29 (21)
Yes	17 (81)	18 (82)	35 (81)	45 (79)	64 (79)	109 (79)
Takes medicine that mother feels child needs[b]						
No	2 (22)	5 (39)	7 (32)	12 (32)	21 (38)	33 (36)
Yes	7 (78)	8 (61)	15 (68)	25 (68)	34 (62)	59 (64)
Needs help with housing[c]						
No	38 (73)	43 (61)	81 (66)	114 (57)	202 (74)	316 (66)
Yes	14 (27)	28 (39)	42 (34)	87 (43)	73 (26)	160 (34)[a**]
Has health education question not answered by provider						
No	45 (88)	62 (91)	107 (90)	181 (91)	239 (88)	420 (89)
Yes	6 (12)	6 (9)	12 (10)	18 (9)	33 (12)	51 (11)

Health insurance						
Child						
Medicaid/other	45 (87)	59 (83)	104 (85)	160 (80)	239 (86)	399 (84)
None	7 (13)	12 (17)	19 (15)	40 (20)	38 (14)	78 (16)
Mother						
Medicaid/other	43 (83)	56 (79)	99 (81)	156 (78)	224 (81)	380 (80)
None	9 (17)	15 (21)	24 (19)	44 (22)	53 (19)	97 (20)
Social services						
WIC						
No	16 (31)	27 (38)	43 (35)	62 (31)	132 (48)	194 (41)
Yes	36 (69)	44 (62)	80 (65)	138 (69)	145 (52)	283 (59)[a]*
Food stamps						
No	28 (54)	22 (31)	50 (41)	102 (51)	132 (48)	234 (49)
Yes	24 (46)	49 (69)	73 (59)	98 (49)	145 (52)	243 (51)
Welfare						
No	25 (48)	19 (27)	44 (36)	87 (44)	111 (40)	198 (42)
Yes	27 (52)	52 (73)	79 (64)	113 (56)	165 (60)	278 (58)

[a] = PRC Pure significantly different from Comparison for American Black children, logistic regression.
[b] = Asked only if child needs medicine.
[c] = Asked only if less than satisfied with current housing.
* = $p < .05$ ** = $p < .01$ *** = $p < .001$

SUMMARY

Among the 124 variables used in this analysis, 6 (or 5%) are expected to be significant by chance. The results adjusted for the five covariates showed 18 to be significant for American Black children and 8 for Puerto Rican children, with more than two-thirds favoring the PRC group. For Puerto Rican PRC children, mothers reported fewer and less serious health problems and fewer occurrences of some physical symptoms, although both groups reported the same number of symptoms overall. The PRC group had better health knowledge and practices in general. In addition, the PRC group had fewer episodic visits and preventive visits during the previous 3 months but not the previous 12 months.

Among American Black children in the PRC group, mothers and physicians reported fewer occurrences of some physical symptoms, although both groups reported the same number of symptoms overall. The Comparison group was found to have better fine motor development and the PRC group was more anemic. The PRC group had more regular eating habits, was less likely to be delayed in receiving DPT and OPV immunizations, was more likely to receive WIC services, and their mothers had better health knowledge and practices in general. In addition, the PRC group had fewer preventive visits in the previous 3 months (although not during the previous 12 months) and were more likely to need help with housing. The Comparison group was more likely to be up to date on the HIB immunization.

Overall, it appears that the PRC model may have had a greater impact on the health of its American Black participants as compared to their Puerto Rican counterparts, although the benefits are not seen in all areas. This may, however, be due to the fact that the Puerto Rican children may have been slightly healthier at birth (shorter hospital stay at birth, tendency toward higher birth weight) and their mothers practiced better preventive health by seeking prenatal care earlier. A more detailed analysis examining the possible differences in initial health status could help to clarify this issue.

Although not specifically designed to address racial/ethnic difference, this study was able to draw on the Puerto Rican and American Black children within its study sample. Future studies should be specifically addressed to assessing the health of Puerto Rican children and that of other racial/ethnic groups for comparison.

ACKNOWLEDGMENTS. This Study was supported by Grant MCJ-360539 from the Maternal and Child Health Program (Title V, Social Security Act), Health Resources and Services Administration, U.S. Department of Health and Human Services; Maternal and Child Health Block Grant from the New York State Health Department through the New York City Health Department; and the W.T. Grant Foundation.

REFERENCES

1. Elinson J, Liberatos P, and Haddow S: *Outcome Evaluation of a Pediatric Health Care Model: Final Report*. Final Report to Maternal and Child Health Research Program, HRSA, DHHS. New York, Medical and Health Research Association of New York City, September 1993.
2. Select Panel for the Promotion of Child Health, *Better Health for Our Children: A National Strategy, Vol 1*. DHHS (PHS) Pub. No. 79–55071, Washington DC: Government Printing Office, 1981
3. Starfield B: Primary care in the United States. *Internat. J. Health Serv.* 16:179–197, 1986
4. Schiff D: *The Medical Home*. Paper presented at the United Hospital Fund Child Health Policy Retreat, Tuxedo, New York, September 1989
5. Mayor's Commission on the Future of Child Health, Robert Haggerty, Chair: *The Future of Child Health in New York City*. New York, New York City Department of Health, August 1989
6. Rosenbluth L, Morehead MA, Grossi M, Theroux Oliver C, Uccellani C, Robinson P: A model for evaluating the delivery of pediatric primary care services. *Qual. Assur. Util. Rev.* 6:2–7, 1990
7. Root MP: *Racially-Mixed People in America*. Newbury Park, CA, Sage, 1992

Conclusion: Expanding on What Is Known about the Health and Development of Puerto Rican Mothers and Children

GONTRAN LAMBERTY
AND CYNTHIA GARCIA COLL

INTRODUCTION

For a racial or ethnic group to score last or next to last in an array of social, economic, health, and child development indicators is a double-edged sword. On the one hand, these low ranks document that problems exist and, that solutions need to be found. On the other hand,

GONTRAN LAMBERTY • Maternal and Child Health Bureau, HRSA, Public Health Service, U.S. Department of Health and Human Services, Rockville, Maryland 20857. CYNTHIA GARCIA COLL • Department of Pediatrics, Brown University School of Medicine, Women and Infants Hospital of Rhode Island, Providence, Rhode Island 02905 and The Stone Center, Wellesley College, Wellesley, Massachusetts 02181-8268.

Puerto Rican Women and Children: Issues in Health, Growth, and Development, edited by Gontran Lamberty and Cynthia Garcia Coll. Plenum Press, New York, 1994.

consistent poor performance can be interpreted as an inherent flaw. This interpretation can lead to negative stereotypes and support the argument that the situation cannot be changed.

In ethnic and racial group politics, low performances not only elicit attributions of inferiority from the majority camp, but from the minority side as well. Thus, non-Caribbean Hispanics argue that the high rate of low birth weight of Puerto Rican infants relates to their African genes. Two facts are claimed to validate this contention: (1) African-Americans consistently have the highest rate of low-birth-weight infants in the United States, and (2) other Hispanic groups, Mexican-Americans in particular, show rates equal or lower than non-Hispanic Caucasians, despite having socioeconomic and obstetrical risk profiles equal to worse than Puerto Ricans. Fact two inferentially argues that not having African genes explains the far better performance of non-Caribbean Hispanics. Residents on the East Coast of the United States have made a similar racially tinted assertion. They have claimed that the high infant mortality rate of African-Americans in their cities results from classifying the infant deaths of Puerto Ricans as African-American. Some Puerto Ricans share with African-Americans visible Negroid features and hospital personnel use these features to assign the race of the deceased infant in the death certificate.

The two assertions referred to above are important for several reasons. First, they show that groups who are targets of racism also practice it. Second, it underscores the universality of racism. Third, and most important, they are examples of untested assertions about Puerto Ricans that are currently in circulation. These assertions influence negatively the definition and interpretation of problems for this population group and the possible remedies offered to alleviate them. Testing the validity of these and other assertions made about Puerto Ricans through research and routine data collection would define what the true situation is and give proper direction to efforts to improve it.

Three generalizations are supported by what was presented in the preceding chapters: (1) the amount of information available on Puerto Rican mothers and children residing on the mainland is meager: (2) what little is available is primarily outcome oriented and disregards the processes that mediate between persons and outcomes; and (3) in what information is available, Puerto Ricans do not do as well as other Hispanic groups. All three generalizations support the need to increase the analysis and amount of data routinely collected on Puerto Ricans by government agencies and to expand research about Puerto Ricans.

Expansion in routinely collected data and research are needed in five areas: (1) migration from Puerto Rico to the mainland and vice versa; (2) life in established and emerging Puerto Rican settlements on the mainland; (3) health status and health services use; (4) normative health, growth, and development in children, including issues of identity, racism, bilingualism, and biculturalism; and (5) contexts and processes that promote resiliency and exceptional achievements in Puerto Rican children despite overwhelming odds for failure. All of these areas are interrelated and constitute a minimum of what is needed to develop and mount empirically informed and culturally sensitive interventions. While it may be argued that successful interventions can be developed and mounted for Puerto Ricans based on the culturally undifferentiated knowledge base, proper solutions of the problems Puerto Ricans face on the mainland in the long run will be dependent on how well we understand the complex forces that impinge on their lives and create the problems.

The remainder of this chapter will expand on the issues introduced above and will provide a series of recommendations on what areas of information and research should be expanded. The chapter will conclude with a discussion of policy. It should be noted that the areas of information and research identified for expansion are not mutually exclusive and that a large part of the information and scientific knowledge sought is not specific to either reproductive health or child development.

MIGRATION

The migration of Puerto Ricans to the mainland has been described in the preceding chapters from a historical point of view and with respect to the psychological demands it imposes on families and individuals. There are suggestions in these chapters that the effects of migration are all-pervasive and that they extend beyond the generation of the migrant and her or his progeny. Whether the effects are multigenerationally enduring or in the aggregate more positive than negative are conjectured to depend on the characteristics of the individual who migrates, the community of origin of the migrant, the push and pull factors that prompted the migration, the migration pathway taken, and the mainland community selected as the new place of residence. The combinations and permutations deriving from these theorized causes are many and disentangling them requires multiple research and routine data collection approaches.

Within migration, several subsets of information seem essential for an informed understanding of the process and its consequences. First, we need a detailed characterization of the migration patterns between Puerto Rico and the mainland as they unfold over time. This is best pursued through an ongoing system of routine data collection under the auspices of government agencies. The characterization should inform yearly who migrates, to what destinations, and under the impetus of what push and pull factors. It should also distinguish between an individual and a family move, and differentiate whether the move was or was not part of a "revolving" episode. In addition, the characterization should allow for relating the collected information to social, economic, and political events taking place in the island and on the U.S. mainland, quarterly or biannual publication of core information, and multivariate analyses of trends. A possible byproduct of such a system could be the creation of hypotheses-driven studies that seek to amplify on the casual conjectures that have evolved from the routinely collected data. Questions that could be answered through the routine characterization are:

- What is the sociodemographic (i.e., gender, age, education, marital status, etc.) composition of Puerto Ricans migrating for the first to the mainland? Does the composition vary across time? What are the push and pull factors responsible for first-time moves? Do the factors vary across time, educational, and occupational groupings? Are the destinations changing?
- What proportion of the first-time moves represents individual versus family unit moves, and what differentiates between the two?
- What is the sociodemographic (i.e., gender, age, education, marital status, etc.) composition of Puerto Ricans returning from the mainland to resettle in Puerto Rico? Does the composition vary across time? Can the returning migrants be further differentiated into "permanent" and "revolving" returnees?
- What proportion of the "permanent" and "revolving" moves represent individual versus family unit moves, and what differentiates between them?
- To what extent is migration from Puerto Rico to the mainland, and from the mainland to Puerto Rico, a function of economic and market forces? Personal and family problems? Do family and personal problems, economic and market forces differentially affect first-time and return moves?

"Circular" or "revolving door" migration is the second subset of information that needs to be addressed, particularly from a family, maternal, and child perspective. Today, no formal conceptual definition of the revolving door phenomenon exists. It is generally defined as frequent moves, of varying duration, back and forth to Puerto Rico. Even though the concept has fared prominently in after-the-fact interpretations of routinely collected outcome data, very few studies based on the concept have ever been done. Despite the scarcity of theoretical and empirical work on the subject, however, the consensus is present in island and U.S. mainland professional circles that circular migration is a contributor to school dropouts, maladaptive states in children, adolescents, and adults, and that it is a conduit for the one-way transmission of fads, fashions, and negative life-styles from the mainland to Puerto Rico. Clinical insights also suggest that circular migration might be an obstacle to the early initiation of prenatal care, the management of chronic conditions in children, and that it interferes with sick and well-child health supervision.

Not all the consequences of circular migration are conjectured to be negative. Circular migration has been hypothesized to strengthen kinship and family ties and to foster developmental resiliency, biculturality, and bilingualism. Recent research along the U.S.–Mexico border and in New York City and Miami suggests that a new pattern of biculturality and dual national identity is evolving made possible by relatively cheap rail, bus, and airline travel. This new pattern allows for maintaining strong identification and ties to the mother culture without compromising allegiance and full participation in the adopted country. Examples of research questions on revolving door migration that beg elucidation include:

- To what extent do circular migration moves represent lack of marketable skills, failures in acculturation, patterns of personal and/or family instability, or a combination of these and other factors? Are skin color and visible Negroid features determinants of in- and out-flow?
- Does circular migration have qualitatively different consequences when the move is to Puerto Rico as compared to the mainland? What ages are most affected and how?
- What are the adaptive demands that revolving door migration places on children and how do these demands influence identity formation and the attainment of social, emotional, and cognitive competencies?

- What are the effects of revolving door migration on the physical and mental health of parents and children? What specific demands do these revolving door moves place on the educational, social welfare, and public health care systems of Puerto Rico and mainland communities?
- What mechanisms are currently in place to assure continuity of care for existing conditions in children and adults who migrate back and forth from Puerto Rico to the mainland?

A third subset of information about the process of migration that needs scrutiny is the selective exchanges taking place between Puerto Rican and non-Puerto Rican communities on the mainland and between Puerto Rico and Puerto Rican communities on the mainland. These exchanges have been conjectured to result in talent and leadership drain for mainland Puerto Rican communities as well as in changes in the sociodemographic compositions of these communities. If these exchanges are taking place then one could expect that a "steady state" condition may be operative in some communities with respect to social and demographic characteristics and levels of health. Such a situation could, over time, mask within group gains. This could possibly artificially raise mortality and morbidity rates depending on how many enter or exit specific communities and who goes out and comes in. Questions that need to be addressed in selective migration are:

- How much selective migration is going on in mainland Puerto Rican communities? What is the nature of the selectivity? Is outflow skewed toward families and individuals of middle and high socioeconomic status, and inflow to low socioeconomic status? Is outflow considerably less than inflow? Is there selectivity on skin color and Negroid features between in- and outflow?
- How does selective migration impact on natality, morbidity, and mortality indicators?
- Is talent and leadership in Puerto Rican U.S. mainland communities home grown or developed, or is it imported from Puerto Rico and/or other U.S. mainland Puerto Rican communities?
- What are the processes that promote or deter the development and retention of home grown talent and leadership in U.S. mainland Puerto Rican communities? Are skin color and Negroid features influencers of retention?
- Are there gender differences in out- and inflow?

Both circular and selective migration processes merit independent study. They are more appropriately studied, however, as part of more inclusive community studies. All three migration areas can be informed in varying degrees by analyses of vital statistics and decennial census data.

COMMUNITY STUDIES

Migration from Puerto Rico to the mainland has concentrated on East Coast destinations. Within the East Coast, the tendency has been for Puerto Rican migrants to settle in large industrial cities that have high rates of unemployment, extreme concentrations of poverty, high percentages of racial and ethnic minorities, intractable patterns of discrimination in housing and employment, and power relationships constantly in flux as a result of political challenges along racial and ethnic lines. In many respects, the communities where Puerto Ricans have settled and continue to settle on the mainland are not the most hospitable ecologies in which to live and grow up.

Studies of Puerto Rican communities on the mainland are needed that seek to document life in all of its complexities. The specific investigations in mind would need to go beyond the typical ethnographic field studies. They would need to be longitudinal in study design, theoretically driven, and planned to systematically collect data in multiple domains and through different methods (i.e., ethnographic field work, psychological testing, health examination, blood chemistry analyses, laboratory testing of soil, water, and air samples, etc.). The studies would need to relate multivariately the data collected to health and developmental outcomes and be able to track individuals and families in and out of the communities through imaginative forms of tracking. What is proposed is a series of large-scale investigations, in themselves composed of smaller ethnographic, community epidemiology, health, and development examination studies, which are ecologically based and guided by social stratification considerations.

Within the many research questions that could be addressed by the studies just described, some would be more critical than others. Regardless of what is selected, the studies would profit immensely by focusing on families and children as they are affected by and as they affect the communities in which they live. Answering the questions stated below appear to be critical:

- What are the nature and quality of the physical environments that are part of and surround Puerto Rican enclaves? How do these environments influence health and development in mothers and children?
- How residentially segregated are Puerto Rican communities from the larger context? Do these communities operate as self-contained enclaves? How open or closed are the lives of Puerto Rican families and children to what proximally and distally surrounds their communities? What institutions link the Puerto Rican enclaves to the rest of the community and to the larger society?
- What are the predominant child-rearing practices in Puerto Rican communities and what goals do they address? What values do these practices emphasize and how much do these values differ or resemble that of Puerto Rico and the larger mainland communities in which Puerto Ricans reside? What family processes promote community bridging of socialization patterns and outcomes?
- How much of a prominent role does the imputed African racial identity of Puerto Ricans play in the socialization of mainland Puerto Rican children? Are children prepared early to deal with racism and its derivatives—residential segregation, prejudice, and discrimination? How are they prepared?
- How much contact is there between the Puerto Rican communities on the mainland and the sending communities in Puerto Rico? What situations and practices are conducive to revolving door migration? What is the frequency of revolving door moves? In the aggregate, what specific patterns do the moves follow?

HEALTH SERVICES USE AND HEALTH STATUS

Puerto Ricans residing on the mainland have extremely high rates of unemployment and levels of poverty. They also have considerably higher than average incidence and prevalence of acute and chronic diseases, and one of the lowest proportions of medically insured heads of households in the United States. This is in part reflected in: (1) the high rates of late or no prenatal care; (2) the elevated rates of untreated neurological and behavioral conditions in children; (3) the high use of hospital emergency units by women and children; (4) the above average hospital stays when women and children are hospitalized; and (5) the high use of publicly supported health clinics. In short, Puerto Ricans on the mainland have a medical care problem of sizable proportions. Ironically, most Puerto Ricans on the mainland reside in cities containing the highest concentration of modern health care facilities and premier medical research centers in the world. These cities traditionally have been at the forefront of the social welfare and public health movements. The serious medical care problem of mainland Puerto Ricans then, is to a large extent, a problem of access and equity that is being compounded apparently by public and private apathy.

Good information on the health status of Puerto Rican women and children residing on the mainland and their use of medical care services is not available. An excellent beginning was made by the special National Hispanic Health and Nutrition Examination Survey (HHANES) conducted by NCHS between 1982 and 1983. This extremely valuable source of information is no longer available as NCHHS decided not to repeat the HHANES. Instead they opted for combining the objectives of the HHANES with the regular national health examination and interview survey (HHANES). The new "regular" approach will oversample African-Americans and Mexican-Americans but not mainland Puerto Ricans. Cost is the reason given by NCHS for excluding mainland Puerto Ricans from the new "regular" survey.

Several of the health and development problems of Puerto Ricans residing on the mainland described in this volume derive in part from the consequences of early childbearing. They also stem from maladaptive patterns of gender functioning. These patterns are not unique to mainland Puerto Ricans but part and parcel of life struggles characteristic of low income, urban populations everywhere in the United States. Fueling these patterns for Puerto Ricans are also historical antecedents, value orientations, and socialization patterns unique to the culture of Puerto Rico that might have been adaptive in other historical periods. These forces dictate power relations between male and female in matters of sex and marriage, distribution of household tasks, parenting styles, and assumptions of responsibility for the well-being of children. We know very little about these family formation and gender functioning patterns and how they affect reproductive and child health. Much, therefore, needs to be done to expand the knowledge base through research on these areas for Puerto Ricans. The information is critical for developing intervention efforts that seek to reduce the high incidence of teenage pregnancy, inadequate or no prenatal care, low birth weight, child and spouse abuse, and to make inroads on the increasing incidence of acquired immunodeficiency syndrome (AIDS) among young Puerto Rican women.

Questions that need addressing through routine data collection and research efforts are:

- What are the risk factors associated with undesirable perinatal outcomes in Puerto Ricans residing on the mainland? Are the risk factors different from those operating in other mainland racial and ethnic groups? Are the risk factors interrelated in a unique pattern or structure? What is the etiological significance of the unique structure?
- How many Puerto Rican children residing on the mainland have special health care needs? How many of these children are under active medical management, enrolled in early intervention programs, etc.? What are the factors that determine whether a Puerto Rican child with special health care needs gets underactive medical management and/or participates in compensatory and early intervention programs?
- Overall, how healthy are Puerto Rican children residing on the mainland? Are there any specific acute and/or chronic conditions to which they are prone? What are the presumptive etiologies of these conditions and their degree of amenability to preventive efforts?
- What are the 10 leading causes of death for Puerto Rican infants, children, adolescents, and young adults? What have been the trends in the last three decades? Are the trends following national norms or do they deviate in some particular way? Within the 10 leading causes of deaths, what particular conditions are amenable to prevention?
- Exactly how does access and affordability affect the use of health services in Puerto Rican women and children? Are there cultural determinants of use? What are they and how do they operate? What cultural values, beliefs, and conceptions about disease etiology in the mainland Puerto Rican culture influence the recognition and interpretation of symptoms, and with what consequences for the personal decision to seek care?
- Patterns of between gender functioning are culturally anchored and because of that are slow to change and often become dysfunctional. What values and value orientations in the mainland Puerto Rican culture dictate power relations between male and

female in matters of sex and marriage, distribution of household tasks, parenting styles, and assumptions of responsibility for the well-being of children? What is the nature of these values and values orientation? Under what circumstances are they functional or dysfunctional? With what consequences?

NORMATIVE GROWTH AND DEVELOPMENT

It is doubtful that significant progress can be achieved in solving the problems faced by Puerto Ricans on the mainland without information on the normative health, growth, and development of their children, and the cultural, ecological, and structural forces that enhance and impede attainment of norms in these domains. These information sets are crucial for the early identification of at-risk children and for undertaking clinical remediation and prevention efforts on their behalf. In addition, the information is needed to understand the collective life span trajectories of Puerto Ricans as a function of time and changes in their collective life circumstances.

Longitudinal and normative information on health, growth, and development of Puerto Rican children residing on the mainland and in Puerto Rico is practically nonexistent. What little is available derives from studies seeking to document how Puerto Rican children differ from the dominant non-Hispanic Caucasian group or how better or worse they fare in relation to African-American and other Hispanic children. This comparative approach to the study of minority children characteristically ignores within-group variability, fosters the view that these children are inferior and incapable of improvement, and draws attention away from the societal forces responsible for undermining their health, growth, and development. In addition, race/ethnicity comparative studies for the most part ignore the confounding effects of social class, are outcome rather than process oriented, and use tests and measures normed and validated on the majority non-Hispanic Caucasian group. Studies on the impact of racism, migration, and acculturation on the development Puerto Rican children are nonexistent. The centrality of these processes/variables on development have in the past been empirically and clinically undervalued even though theoretically and clinically they stand out as potent influencers.

In a situation of extreme scarcity, basic needs are paramount. Thus, studies concerned with documenting variations and establishing norms on selected health, growth, and developmental parameters for Puerto Rican children would be the first priority. Such information, when obtained through purely cross-sectional designs, would be acceptable in the absence of none. Longitudinal and mixed-longitudinal designs would be more ideal to employ as these designs avoid significant shortcomings (i.e., the confoundings of age by the cohort effect in the cross-sectional design and the nongeneralizability of the age effects on the longitudinal design). In the more complex and expensive, cause and effect studies, the following areas of research need critical attention:

- Are there neonatal and infant characteristics in mainland Puerto Rican infants that affect the caregiving environment? Are there any long-term consequences of such early caregiving-infant interactions? Are there any particular cultural values or practices that exacerbate or ameliorate biological vulnerabilities in Puerto Rican children?
- How does the process of migration and acculturation affect parenting and the children's subsequent development? How do families negotiate the different rates of acculturation experienced by each individual member?
- What are the extrafamilial contexts that impact on the health, growth, and development of mainland Puerto Rican children? What are the linkages between children's experiences in the home and the school settings?
- What is the role of Puerto Rican fathers and other members of the extended family in their children's attainment of developmental competencies?

RESILIENCY AND EXCEPTIONAL ACHIEVEMENT

Each of us is said to be born with varying degrees of abilities or capacities, be that in the realm of health, physical growth, artistic talent, sociability, intelligence, etc. Such innate abilities are postulated not to be fixed but to provide a range of possibilities. Whether we achieve only a small part, most, or all of the potential we are born with, is said to depend largely on individual characteristics (e.g., persistence), the scope of opportunities we are given, and the experiences we are subjected to within our immediate and distant environmental contexts (e.g., the family and school environments).

As has been said repeatedly throughout this volume, Puerto Rican children on the mainland reside for the most part in racially and ethnically segregated urban communities characterized by physical deterioration, high concentration of poverty, extreme violence, illicit drug use, etc. In addition, they come from economically marginal households and their daily life from infancy on is subjected directly or indirectly to the demoralizing forces of racism, prejudice, and discrimination. Despite all of these destructive life forces, a large percentage of these children turn out to be well-adjusted adults who perform competently in many dimensions of life; a significant number go on to excel and reach levels of exceptionality in many life endeavors. The fact that most mainland Puerto Rican children ultimately turn out to be competent adults should not blind us to the fact that a large proportion of them have their innate potential significantly dwarfed by social and political forces beyond their control.

Knowing about the personal characteristics and the circumstances and processes that impinge favorably and unfavorably on the attainment of competencies in mainland Puerto Rican children is of crucial importance if we are to help these children realize their full potential. With the latter, if multigenerationally sustained, it would be possible bit by bit to raise the collective lot of this population group to the level of parity. To do so would require that research and routine information gathering efforts be focused on the circumstances and processes that make some mainland Puerto Rican children become competent and exceptional adults while others exposed to similar situations do not.

The ability to reach and surpass normative levels of competencies despite an overwhelming number of stressors and insults has been labeled as "resiliency." The study of resilience, "the plurality of abilities and capacities . . . an organism has . . . to bounce back or recover from a disappointment, obstacle, or setback . . .,"[1] offers not only a window to the processes that shape normativeness but also that of exceptionality and deviance. Most importantly, such an approach to the study of child development is more likely than others to lay bare those protective personal characteristics, social and cultural processes and circumstances that in complex interactions lead to competency rather than noncompetency in children and adults. With this information it would be possible to intervene early and prevent negative outcomes, or seek to maximize the potential that, without intervention, could lie dormant throughout a lifetime in these children.

Research questions that need elucidation through prospective longitudinal investigations are:

- What determines favorable outcomes in mainland Puerto Rican children who are defined to be vulnerable to specific negative outcomes on the basis of individual, family, racial, and social status?
- What are the unique patterns of the mainland Puerto Rican culture which either facilitate or hinder resiliency in these children? Are there values and patterns of caretaking in the native Puerto Rican culture that become obsolete or dysfunctional to the attainment of competencies on the mainland because of a lack of goodness of fit to the host culture? What are they, and how can they be modified to promote resiliency and achievement?
- Is resiliency in mainland Puerto Rican children, as the empirical literature suggests for non-Hispanic Caucasian children, to a large degree a function of the caretaker response to the child's unique characteristics? To what extent are caretaking practices based on empathic understanding of the child as a separate person supported by the culture of Puerto Rico and the adaptive one under which most Puerto Ricans operate on the mainland?
- What is the role of circular migration in hindering or promoting resiliency in mainland Puerto Rican children? Through what means is the role expressed? By fostering the development of cultural and social flexibility?
- What important agents and contexts outside of the home influence resiliency in mainland Puerto Rican children? Specifically, what is the role of the school environments and the quality of the schools?
- Racism and its derivatives, prejudice and discrimination, are ever-pervasive in the life of minority children in this country, Puerto Ricans included. How are these developmentally injurious forces dealt with by the Puerto Rican caretaker? What specific socialization practices of the mainland Puerto Rican culture prepare Puerto Rican children to deal in an open manner with racism and still maintain a healthy self-image?
- Do strong family ties and adherence, with pride, to cultural traditions constitute buffering or protective factors against the detrimental effects of poverty and racism? What aspects of health, growth, and development are more resilient to insult or environmental pressure to change?

POLICY

In a democracy, national policies are influenced by consent and prudence as well as by political expediency. Political expediency is often influenced by how powerful is the electorate that pushes a particular agenda; also, by how controversial the agenda is for the rest of the nation and how deeply embedded in the national conscience are the issues the agenda addresses. In such complex and highly fluid political environments, specific national and state policies wax and wane in importance and many vanish into oblivion.

Policies guiding what to do about social disparities in socioeconomic status, health, and development follow this vacillating off and on course. Today, concern for social disparities is at a very critical crossroad and prospects for significant progress are at the highest since the mid-1960s and the 1970s. This is so with respect to a universal health insurance program that assures access to quality medical care for all. Similarly high prospects are present for other areas such as universal child care and early childhood intervention.

Puerto Ricans residing on the mainland and in Puerto Rico gain when the political pendulum swings toward the high side of the social concern scale. Even then they do not do as well as they need to because in terms of numbers and influence (e.g., island residents do not vote in presidential elections) they are not a potent political force to be reckoned with. Moreover, as a group, Puerto Ricans do not participate in the national political process as much as the other groups which are competing for attention and scarce national resources do. This politically disadvantaged position requires the presence of federal and private enabling mechanisms that can act as pushers and steerers for the social, economic, health, and development agendas of Puerto Ricans.

Two federal mechanisms for seeking social equity are (1) a national planning process that produces reasonably precise assessments of situations and develops realistic options on how to proceed and (2) an assertive federal overseer with the needed resources and sufficient political muscle inside the federal bureaucracy to oversee and execute the planning process. Both of these enabling mechanisms are currently in place nationally in the realm of health, although at a very nascent stage, understaffed, and located too far from the top levels of federal decision making.

The public health component of the U.S. Department of Health and Human Services (DHHS) has a planning process in place and has developed a national plan for improving the nation's health. The document, entitled *The Year 2000 National Health Objectives*,[2] is available and the procedures for annually evaluating progress and making corrections are more or less in place. Puerto Ricans on the mainland should rejoice at *The Year 2000* document. The document argues in chapter 3 for making social equity in health and access to health care services the cornerstone of the nation's health agenda for the twenty-first century. That was, and still is, a daring political act. In many ways, *The Year 2000* is a blueprint for action whose follow-through requires that we adopt a proactive approach to the nation's health by instituting a rational planning process that assesses needs, coordinates resources, plans, executes, and monitors courses of action, and evaluates at set intervals the effectiveness of those courses of action.

Important issues not addressed by the document are (1) realistically, how much social equity can be achieved, (2) how long will it take to achieve it, (3) how many drastic changes in our political and social institutions need to be done to accomplish these objectives, and (4) what amounts and types of resources will be required to decisively impact on the existing social disparities. In addition, the document has an overemphasis on individual life-style changes and personal responsibility. Of crucial importance is that for many of the minority health concerns the target values or end points are sure-to-be-met milestones, as in most cases they merely represent the values derived by extending forward in time long-established trend lines. Thus, barring a national catastrophe, the declared objectives will be met even though nothing substantially different or additional has taken place. Within minority groups, African-Americans get a disproportionate share of attention from the document, while Puerto Ricans and Native Americans, who also occupy bottom rungs, are minimally and selectively referred to. Puerto Ricans could argue that the end point values targeted to be met for racial and ethnic minorities in the document should be closer to that of the majority group. These stated weaknesses, however, should not distract from the many possibilities the document, and the processes producing and updating the document, have.

Although slow to materialize and yet to reach its full potential, the Office of Minority Health of DHHS is a milestone. The Office has assumed responsibility within the federal health bureaucracy for data acquisition and centralization of minority health concerns, has a modest but numerically growing group of excellent professionals, and has the authorization and some funds to issue grants and enter into contracts. It is not located at the highest level of decision making. Partly because of that, it does not have the prestige, influence, or the power to be assertive. Moreover, from its very beginning the Office had, and still has, a pronounced African-American emphasis which affects credibility and trust and detracts from its mandate to seek equity in health and health services access for all minorities. The Office, however, is an excellent idea. With some changes and fine-tuning, the unit should realize some of its potential as the nation's watchdog of the health of minorities.

Given the availability of these nascent mechanisms, what then would be realistic and possible to do? The national planning process that produced *The Year 2000* objectives should be continued and strengthened. The definition of health should be expanded to include developmental concerns and socioemotional considerations. This should be done not in a token fashion but commensurate with the degree of importance these dimensions have with respect to health.

Most of what is wanted of states and the federal government regarding health rests heavily on their ability to capture, process, and analyze information from different sources. Federal and state data collectors and repository units can sometimes be self-serving and slow to act. Much more needs to be done to curb these structural tendencies and to establish mechanisms that promote cooperative ventures and centralization of activities. Above all else, decisions on data acquisition and analyses impacting on the federal and state governments' ability to define and monitor problems for a specific minority group should not be allowed to be made without prior multiagency consultation, particularly with the Office of Minority Health.

Federal data collecting units such as the Bureau of the Census and the National Center for Health Statistics have played and will continue to play very important roles in the routine data collection enterprise. The prospective value of the census information for health planning in general and for minority health in particular is enormous. It is important that it be used to project future needs under more than one assumption as to growth, composition, disease incidence, and prevalence rates, and progress in scientific knowledge. Given the high levels of fertility and migration currently evident for minority groups in this country, collectively these groups will constitute a sizable proportion of our total population in the not too distant future. Knowing the current and future numbers, coupled with the documented morbidity and mortality experience and health services use, will make it possible to plan for the health needs of minority groups and to estimate what national resources are needed.

Of the new information collected by the decennial census, only a fraction results in published analyses a year or two after processing and tabulation. The published information is mostly demographic, descriptive, and, at most, includes cross-tabulation of two variables. What information remains, particularly that amplifying the changes that have occurred between decades and the data collected under special studies, takes many years to appear in publications. Clearly, there is an imperative need to conduct hypothesis and theory driven multivariate analysis of census data about minorities. This could be done either through contractual arrangements between federal agencies (i.e., National Institutes of Health [NIH], U.S. Bureau of the Census, etc.) and universities, or through the auspices of private organizations. What is impeding this undertaking is a lack of initiative and commitment from the parties most directly affected by the problem.

It was not until 1979 that state vital statistics units begin to use the national origin identifiers recommended by the National Center for Health Statistics (NCHS). All of the states now collect and report to the NCHS information on Hispanic origin; and according to specific subcategories. Only a small number, however, tabulate and analyze vital statistics for their own use in the detail needed to define and monitor problems for specific subgroups (i.e., Puerto Ricans). The states use the Hispanic identifier even less for data on utilization of services. So under present conditions in most states it is not possible to determine how many Dominicans, Mexican-Americans, or Puerto Ricans need specific services. It is not also possible to know how many use the services of programs supported by federal and state funds. This is contrary to what federal legislation and policies of recent vintage seek to promote.

The 1989 amendments of Title V of the Social Security Act require that states develop a needs assessment and plan of action. The states have to report to Congress every year how they plan to use federal and state funds, how they used them in the prior year, and with what results. The Maternal and Child Health Bureau, in collaboration with the states, is now responsible for developing reporting requirements for the states. It is also responsible for developing a comprehensive program of technical assistance to help the states develop and carry out the mandated planning process.

There are several implications in the amended Title V legislation for the health and development of minority populations. The states, as part of the required needs assessment and plan of action, must address forcefully the problems of their minority constituencies, Puerto Rican included. The legislation also calls for the needs assessments and plans of action of states to reach down to the city and/or county levels. This requirement will assure addressing the problems of minorities at the locus where they are occurring. Moreover, if minorities represent significant numbers at the city or county levels but not in the state, this will assure satisfaction of their needs. Time will tell whether the promise inherent in Title V, as amended, will come true for minorities, particularly Puerto Ricans. Monitoring the situation to assure that it does happen is important. Federal, private sector, and Commonwealth of Puerto Rico advocacy efforts should constructively push for the monitoring. This assures that the initiated monitoring will be permanent and that problems detected through this process get addressed. Unfortunately, advocacy for mainland and island Puerto Ricans in the domains of health and growth and development is missing at most levels.

Ideally, the current and future version of the Office of Minority Health should be organized and run in a way that attention is paid to the health problems of all racial and ethnic minorities and solutions are attempted with the least possible amount of apparent favoritism. To do otherwise will undermine the trust and confidence that is needed from all the minorities to do what has to be done. The possibility of creating subunits or branches within the Office to handle the different minority groups should be considered. This mode of organization creates in-depth expertise, a prerequisite for seeking solutions to the complex and unique needs of specific minority groups.

Routinely collected statistics such as those derived from vital, medical, and health insurance records have many inherent weaknesses. These data are collected to define and monitor existing problems and because of that they are outcome oriented. This type of information only allows description and, at most, after-the-fact contentions about the causal processes driving the outcomes. Univariate and bivariate analyses, and even multivariate ones, of routinely collected outcome statistics needs to be followed with process oriented, hypotheses driven research. If we do not understand, for example, how children learn, experience, and internalize racism, we will never bring about the necessary changes.

The scarcity of research on the health and normative development of Puerto Rican children alluded to throughout this volume derives from multiple causes. First in importance among these is the past failure of the federal research funding agencies to encourage research on minorities. Some small progress has occurred. The National Institutes of Health, the National Institute of Mental Health, and the Centers for Disease Control recently issued requests for research applications on minority health including longitudinal studies on development. However, the amount of funds earmarked for these activities has been very small. The initiatives can only satisfy a small proportion of current and future information and scientific knowledge needs. What these underfunded initiatives suggest is a less than full commitment to support research on minority children. Less than full commitment to support research on the effects of racism is also present. Again, some progress was recently made on this but a significant push forward awaits wider support from private foundations, federal agencies, and the developmental psychology and pediatric communities.

Past experiences with respect to nursing research and women's health at NIH suggest rigidities in undertaking new program directions. For example, it was not until considerable congressional pressure was exerted, and the arrival of a new Institutes Director fully committed to supporting research on the major diseases of women, that a major initiative on women's health research became a reality. Similar rigidities appear to be present at NIH and at NIMH with respect to minority health research, even though in at least one instance it has been recognized that a special focus was needed. Thus today there is within NIMH a unit specifically charged with doing research on how individuals from ethnic and racial groups react differently to psychotropic agents. The fact that similar organism-specific biological nuances are now being demonstrated with respect to gender emphasizes the need to undertake research specific to race and ethnicity in the biological, social, and psychological realms.

The practical utility of routinely collected information and research on mainland Puerto Ricans is not optimal if similar data were not to be available for residents of Puerto Rico. The information and research findings on the island population would help to better understand the adaptation of Puerto Ricans to life on the mainland. The data would also aid administrators in defining maternal and child health problems in the island and help develop the solutions to these problems.

To solve the medical care problems of Puerto Ricans on the mainland would require a variety of efforts applied along different pathways. Central among these efforts would be improvements in the economic status of Puerto Rican families either through a special program initiative and/or general improvements in the national economy. It would also require the elimination of discrimination in employment and housing. Additionally, it would also call for some universal payment mechanism that would assure access to quality medical care as a right of citizenship. In the past, national efforts seeking improvements in these areas for all racial and ethnic groups have not been as successful as many have wished them to be. The current political climate suggest optimism.

One approach to the health and development problems of U.S. mainland Puerto Rican children worth considering is to launch an advocacy movement. So far as the mainland is concerned, the advocacy movement would require coordinated efforts at the federal, state, and city levels. In Puerto Rico advocacy would call for efforts principally directed by the Commonwealth government and legislature. Traditionally, the Commonwealth government has maintained considerable distance from the problems besetting Puerto Ricans residing on the mainland. This has been so unless the problems happen to threaten civil liberties or the lifelines of the island economy—tourism, commerce, and industry. The need for the Commonwealth government to do more than it has done in the past is critical to the success of any advocacy movement.

The advocacy movement should have at least the following three goals: (1) to raise the consciousness of the mainland and Puerto Rican public about the health and development needs of Puerto Rican children; (2) to maximize obtaining federal, state, and local funds for the support of services that should be forthcoming to Puerto Rican communities based on entitlement; and (3) to foster a mind-set in Puerto Ricans and non-Puerto Ricans that the solution to the needs of Puerto Ricans residing on the mainland and Puerto Rico are inescapably interwoven. A strong national association of Puerto Rican professionals in health and child development is essential to carry out the advocacy initiative. Such an association currently does not exist, and it needs development and active offices in Washington and San Juan.

SUMMARY AND CONCLUSION

This chapter offered and discussed a series of recommendation on what areas of information and research should be expanded for mainland Puerto Rican mothers and children. The recommended areas of expansion were: (1) migration; (2) community studies; (3) health services use and health status; (4) normative growth and development; and (5) resiliency and exceptional achievement. The content of these areas were acknowledged not to be mutually exclusive nor to be entirely specific to reproductive health or child development. The broad scope of the coverage collectively represented by these areas was felt to be required in order to develop empirically well-informed interventions in a number of interrelated problematic areas for mainland Puerto Rican women and children. On the section having to do with policy, a generic "minority group" approach was taken with occasional references to Puerto Ricans. This approach was deemed necessary as what is needed for Puerto Ricans more or less apply to other minority groups. Moreover, the mechanisms needed to attain what is being recommended by pragmatic, political and cost-effective reasons need to be inclusive of all race and ethnic minorities. The idea of an advocacy initiative is one that needs greater specificity and refinement and constitutes a future area of collaboration for both authors. In conclusion it must be reiterated that up to now what information and research findings have been available for mainland Puerto Ricans in the areas of health and development is meager and that only a very modest beginning, as represented by this volume, was possible. We hope that with the apparent resurgence of interest and federal support for minority health and development research, more and of greater quality will be forthcoming in the not too distant future.

REFERENCES

1. Demos EV: Resiliency in infancy, in Dungan TF & Coles R (eds.), *The Child in Our Times: Studies in the Development of Resiliency*, New York, Brunner/Mazel, 1989, pp. 3–23
2. *Healthy People 2000: National Health Promotion and Disease Prevention Objectives*, DHHS Publication No. (PHS)91-50212, 1993

No official support or endorsement of the views in this book by DHHS or the Public Health Service is intended or should be inferred.

Index

MIX
Papier aus verantwortungsvollen Quellen
Paper from responsible sources
FSC® C105338

If you have any concerns about our products,
you can contact us on
ProductSafety@springernature.com

In case Publisher is established outside the EU,
the EU authorized representative is:
Springer Nature Customer Service Center GmbH
Europaplatz 3, 69115 Heidelberg, Germany

Printed by Libri Plureos GmbH
in Hamburg, Germany